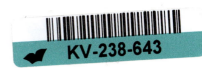

# Transplantation Surgery

*Other titles in the series:*

**Emergency Surgery and Critical Care**
*Simon Paterson-Brown*

**Upper Gastrointestinal Surgery**
*S. Michael Griffin and Simon A. Raimes*

**Hepatobiliary and Pancreatic Surgery**
*O. James Garden*

**Colorectal Surgery**
*Robin K. S. Phillips*

**Breast and Endocrine Surgery**
*John R. Farndon*

**Vascular and Endovascular Surgery**
*Jonathan D. Beard and Peter A. Gaines*

# A COMPANION TO SPECIALIST SURGICAL PRACTICE

*Series editors*

Sir David C. Carter
O. James Garden
Simon Paterson-Brown

# Transplantation Surgery

*Edited by*

## John L. R. Forsythe

Consultant Surgeon
University Department of Surgery
Royal Infirmary
Edinburgh

**W B Saunders Company Ltd**
London · Philadelphia · Toronto · Sydney · Tokyo

W B Saunders Company Ltd 24–28 Oval Road
London NW1 7DX

The Curtis Center
Independence Square West
Philadelphia, PA 19106-3399, USA

Harcourt Brace & Company
55 Horner Avenue
Toronto, Ontario, M8Z 4X6, Canada

Harcourt Brace & Company, Australia
30–52 Smidmore Street
Marrickville, NSW 2204, Australia

Harcourt Brace & Company, Japan
Ichibancho Central Building, 22-1 Ichibancho
Chiyoda-ku, Tokyo 102, Japan

A catalogue record for this book is available from the British Library

ISBN 0-7020-2146-6

Typeset by Paston Press Ltd, Loddon, Norfolk
Printed and bound in Great Britain by The Bath Press, Bath

# Contents

Contributors     vii

Foreword     ix

Preface     xi

Editor's note     xii

Acknowledgements     xiii

**1 Organ donation: ethical aspects**     1
*Christopher J. Rudge*

**2 Organ donation: logistics and technical aspects**     19
*Nigel D. Heaton*

**3 Matching the graft to the recipient**     45
*David Talbot and Derek Manas*

**4 Transplant immunology – for surgeons**     63
*Paul Gibbs*

**5 Immunosuppression: the old and the new**     89
*Neil R. Parrott*

**6 Kidney transplantation**     123
*John L. R. Forsythe*

**7 Liver transplantation**     147
*John A. C. Buckels*

**8 Pancreas transplantation**     167
*Richard D. M. Allen*

**9 Pancreatic transplantation (islet cell)**     203
*Reinhard G. Bretzel*

**10 Small bowel transplantation**     229
*Stephen G. Pollard*

**11 Heart, lung and heart–lung transplantation**     251
*Jonathan Forty*

**12 The depressed immune system in the transplant patient (infection risk and increased malignancy)**       **283**
*Gareth Morris-Stiff and Rozanne H. H. Lord*

**13 The economics of transplantation**       **307**
*Keith M. Rigg*

**Index**       **327**

# Contributors

**Richard D. M. Allen** *FRACS*
Director, National Pancreas Transplant Unit, Department of Transplant Surgery, Westmead Hospital, Sydney, Australia

**Reinhard G. Bretzel** *MD PhD*
Professor of Medicine, Acting Head, Third Medical Department, Fustus-Liebig-University, Giessen, Germany

**John A. C. Buckels** *MD FRCS*
Consultant Surgeon, Liver and Hepatobiliary Unit, Queen Elizabeth Hospital, Birmingham, UK

**John L. R. Forsythe** *MD FRCS*
Consultant Surgeon, University Department of Surgery, Royal Infirmary, Edinburgh, UK

**Jonathan Forty** *MA FRCS*
Consultant Cardiothoracic Surgeon, Department of Cardiothoracic Surgery, Freeman Hospital, Newcastle upon Tyne, UK

**Paul Gibbs** *FRCS*
Senior Lecturer and Honorary Consultant Surgeon, Liver Transplant Surgical Service, King's College Hospital, London, UK

**Nigel D. Heaton** *MBBS FRCS*
Consultant Surgeon, Liver Transplant Surgical Service, King's College Hospital, London, UK

**Rozanne H. H. Lord** *FRCS*
Consultant Transplant Surgeon, Department of Renal Transplant Surgery, Cardiff Royal Infirmary, Cardiff, UK

**Derek Manas** *BSc MBBCH FCS(SA)*
Consultant Surgeon, Renal and Liver Transplant Unit, Freeman Hospital, Newcastle upon Tyne, UK

**Gareth Morris-Stiff** *MB BCh FRCS*
Transplant Research Fellow, Department of Renal Transplant Surgery, Cardiff Royal Infirmary, Cardiff, UK

**Neil R. Parrott** *MD FRCS*
Consultant Surgeon and Senior Lecturer in Surgery, Department of Surgery, Manchester Royal Infirmary, Manchester, UK

**Stephen G. Pollard** *MA MS BSc FRCS*
Consultant Surgeon and Director of Liver and Intestinal Transplantation, St James's University Hospital, Leeds, UK

**Keith M. Rigg** *MD FRCS*
Consultant General and Transplant Surgeon, Renal Unit, Nottingham City Hospital NHS Trust, Nottingham, UK

**Christopher J. Rudge** *BSc FRCS*
Consultant Transplant Surgeon, Department of Renal Medicine and Transplantation, The Royal London Hospital, London, UK

**David Talbot** *MD FRCS(Ed)*
Consultant Surgeon, Renal and Liver Transplant Unit, Freeman Hospital, Newcastle upon Tyne, UK

# Foreword

General surgery defies easy definition. Indeed, there are those who claim that it is dying, if not yet dead – a corpse being picked clean by the vulturine proclivities of the other specialties of surgery. Unfortunately for those who subscribe to this view, general surgery is not lying down, indeed it is rejoicing in a new enhanced vigour, as this new series demonstrates.

The general surgeon is the specialist who, along with his other colleagues, provides a 24-hour, 7-day, emergency surgical cover for his, or her, hospital. Also it is to general surgical clinics that patients are referred, unless their condition is manifestly related to one of the other surgical specialties, e.g. urology, cardiothoracic services, etc. Moreover trainees in these specialities must, during their training, receive experience in general surgery, whose techniques underpin the whole of surgery. General surgery occupies a pivotal position in surgical training. The number of general surgeons required to serve a community, outstrips that required by any other surgical specialty.

General surgery is a specialty in its own right. Inevitably, there are those who wish to practise exclusively one of the sub-specialties of general surgery, e.g. vascular or colorectal surgery. This arrangement may be possible in a few large tertiary referral centres. Although the contribution of these surgeons to patient care and to advances in their discipline will be significant, their numbers are necessarily low. The bulk of surgical practice will be undertaken by the general surgeon who has developed a sub-specialty interest, so that, with his other colleagues in the hospital, comprehensive surgery services can be provided.

There is therefore a great need for a text which will provide comprehensively the theoretical knowledge of the entire specialty and act as a guide for the acquisition of the diagnostic and therapeutic skills required by the general surgeon. The unique contribution of this companion is that it comes as a series, each chapter fresh from the pen of a practising clinician and active surgeon. Each volume is right up to date and this is evidenced by the fact that the first volumes of the series are being published within 12 months from the start of the project. This is a series which has been tightly edited by a team from one of the foremost teaching hospitals in the United Kingdom.

Quite properly the series begins with a volume on emergency surgery and critical care – two of the greatest challenges confronting the practising surgeon. These are the areas that the examination candidate finds the greatest difficulty in acquiring theoretical knowledge and practical experience. Moreover, these are the areas in which advances are at present so rapid that they constantly test the experienced consultant surgeon.

This series not only provides both types of reader with the necessary up-to-date detail but also demonstrates that general surgery remains as challenging and vigorous as it ever has been.

**Sir Robert Shields** *DL, MD, DSc, FRCS(Ed, Eng, Glas, Ire),*
*FRCPEd, FACS*
President, Royal College of Surgeons of Edinburgh

# Preface

*A Companion to Specialist Surgical Practice* was designed to meet the needs of the higher surgeon in training and busy practising surgeon who need access to up-to-date information on recent developments, research and data in the context of accepted surgical practice.

Many of the major surgery text books either cover the whole of what is termed 'general surgery' and therefore contain much which is not of interest to the specialist surgeon, or are very high level specialist texts which are outwith the reach of the trainee's finances, and though comprehensive are often out of date due to the lengthy writing and production times of such major works.

Each volume in this series therefore provides succinct summaries of all key topics within a specialty and concentrates on the most recent developments and current data. They are carefully constructed to be easily readable and provide key references.

A specialist surgeon, whether in training or in practice, need only purchase the volume relevant to his or her chosen specialist field plus the emergency surgery and critical care volume, if involved in emergency care.

The volumes have been written in a very short time frame, and produced equally quickly so that information is as up to date as possible. Each volume will be updated and published as a new edition at frequent intervals, to ensure that current information is always available.

We hope that our aim – of providing affordable up-to-date specialist texts – has been met and that all surgeons, in training or in practice will find the volumes to be a valuable resource.

**Sir David C. Carter** *MD, FRCS(Ed), FRCS(Glas), FRCS(Eng), Hon FRCS(Ire), Hon FACS, FRCP(Ed), FRS(Ed)*
Chief Medical Officer in Scotland, Formerly Regius Professor of Clinical Surgery, University Department of Surgery, Royal Infirmary, Edinburgh

**O. James Garden** *BSc, MB, ChB, MD, FRCS(Glas), FRCS(Ed)*
Professor of Hepatobiliary Surgery at the Royal Infirmary, Director of Organ Transplantation, University Department of Surgery, Royal Infirmary, Edinburgh

**Simon Paterson-Brown** *MS, MPhil, FRCS(Ed), FRCS(Eng), FCSHK*
Consultant General and Upper Gastrointestinal Surgeon, University Department of Surgery, Royal Infirmary, Edinburgh

# Editor's note

Although part of a surgical series, this volume is not just for surgeons. It is for all those who play an important role in the transplant procedure. Thus it has been designed to interest nursing staff who care for organ failure patients, transplant co-ordinators, theatre staff, immunology laboratory staff, paramedical personnel, physicians and surgeons. Modern techniques in transplantation and new forms of immunosuppression, emphasised throughout this volume, have increased the complexity of clinical and ethical dilemmas which face the whole team caring for the transplant patient. Appropriate response to such dilemmas is required to ensure the continued success of transplantation medicine.

# Acknowledgements

I am indebted to all the authors who have contributed to this volume for their perseverence and expertise. I am grateful to my fellow editors for assistance and advice in the initial planning of this book. Thanks are also due to Rachael Stock and Linda Clark from WB Saunders for their enthusiasm and support. Invaluable secretarial skill provided by Susan Keggie and Bridget Kerr made this volume possible. Last but not least, thank you to my wife, Jo, without whom nothing would ever happen.

# 1 Organ donation: ethical aspects

*Christopher J. Rudge*

**Introduction**

It is perhaps overstating the case to suggest that the clinical problems of organ transplantation have been overcome, but as the other chapters in this volume will show, the success rates for virtually all solid-organ transplants are now in excess of 80% (1 year graft survival) and in certain situations may exceed 90%. Long-term graft loss and the morbidity associated with life-long immunosuppression remain of great concern but one of the most pressing problems is the availability of adequate numbers of transplantable organs. Estimates of the organ shortage vary somewhat from organ to organ but a general conclusion would be that the donor supply would need to be doubled in order to provide the necessary numbers of organs. In the face of a falling death rate from road traffic accidents and intracerebral haemorrhage in many countries[1] and a critical shortage of intensive care beds (from where most cadaver organs are retrieved) the shortage of suitable donors seems likely to continue, or indeed to worsen.

Various options have been discussed in attempts to increase the number of organs available. Because every transplant procedure involves a donor as well as recipient there are inevitable ethical concerns raised by organ donation. This chapter discusses, in simple terms, basic ethical principles that are commonly used in medicine before attempting to apply the principles to various aspects of organ donation.

**Principles in medical ethics**

In Western philosophy there are two general ethical theories that are widely used when discussing medical ethics.[2] The first may be called duty-based ethics or deontology and is the principle that underlies the traditional concept of the doctor–patient relationship. The theory stresses the essential 'uniqueness' of each individual and the responsibility that this places on the doctor to do everything in his power to treat the individual patient in the best possible way. Each doctor–patient relationship exists in its own right and treatment is dictated by the needs of the individual alone. This principle has been used since the Hippocratic Oath as the basis for many National and International Commitments to good medical practice.

An alternative theory, utilitarianism, takes a broader view and looks towards the ambition of achieving the greatest good for the greatest number. In many countries the difficulties now experienced in the provision of adequate funding for the provision of all available health-care to all patients that may benefit has led to discussions – implicit or explicit – on the rationing of health care and utilitarianism is at the heart of much of this debate. It can lead, for example, to the decision that a highly expensive form of treatment for an individual with a poor prognosis should be withheld in favour of a cheaper treatment (of perhaps less dramatic benefit) to a larger number of patients.

Within the doctor–patient relationship four general principles have been described that make up an ethical framework for medical practice.

1. Primum non nocere: first of all, do no harm. To the well intentioned this may appear self-evident but it is, of course, almost impossible to achieve. Every drug has possible side effects, minor or major, and every surgical procedure does harm to the patient in addition to good. The principle is usually taken in practice to imply that any harmful effects of a given treatment should be kept to a minimum and are justified only when the potential benefits of the treatment are balanced against the risks.

2. Beneficence: do good. Once again, an apparently self-evident premise for good medical practice. Taken together these two principles are the basis for much decision-making in medicine. The likely benefits of any treatment are balanced against the possible risks before any treatment decision is made. This allows us quite ethically to recommend a course of treatment with significant potential risks if we are satisfied that the potential benefits, and the likelihood that the benefits will occur, more than balance the risks.

3. Autonomy. Autonomy, and the respect for autonomy, are areas of major philosophical interest. However, in medicine the essential component of autonomy is respect for the individual, with treatment of the individual being given purely in his or her own interests – the patient should not be used as a means to an end. A significant component of autonomy is 'informed consent, freely given' – the patient should understand the problem and any options for treatment, should understand the risks and benefits of the treatments and should give informed consent to the treatment that is to be given. Moreover, the whole process should be carried out without any form of coercion or pressure – the decision should be freely made.

4. Justice. Treatment should be given without regard to factors such as race, age, gender or any other irrelevant aspect of the patient's persona. Moreover, it should have the rather general virtues of fairness, honesty, balance and lack of prejudice.

To summarise, the general principles of medical ethics stress the need to do as much good as possible to the patient whilst doing the minimum amount of harm. Considerable attention must be given to the rights of the patient to be given full, or at the very least adequate, information in a manner that allows the patient to make up his or her mind about a proposed line of treatment. Their decision should be made, as far as possible, free from undue external pressures. Finally, treatment should be available, and be given, in a fair and just manner.

It is not always easy to apply these principles to clinical practice and to determine that a particular proposal is clearly ethical or unethical. The principles may conflict with one another or be mutually incompatible, information may not be available that is required to allow a principle to be applied and it may well be possible to justify an 'unethical' practice because the only possible alternative is *more* unethical.

## Specific issues in organ transplantation

### Cadaver donors

#### *Definition of death*
It is now widely accepted that brain stem death is a valid medical definition of death and whilst the law is not explicit, there is also acceptance of brain stem death as a legally acceptable definition of death. Mason and McCall Smith[3] have argued that a death certificate should be issued whilst the brain-dead potential donor is still maintained on a ventilator. Virtually all the major world religions have accepted brain death and the opportunity this gives for cadaveric organ donation for transplantation.[4] In this situation it is usual for the wishes of the potential donor to be respected, if these are known, together with those of the relatives.

#### *Consent for organ donation*
The legal framework that regulates organ donation falls into one of two main types. In the United Kingdom and many other European countries there is a requirement to confirm from the next of kin that they have no objection to organ removal and have no reason to believe that the donor would have objected. Some countries, most noticeably Belgium and Austria, have introduced opting-out legislation that places the responsibility firmly on the individual who does *not* wish to donate organs after death to register that objection – if no objection is registered organ removal may proceed after the donor's death with no requirement for explicit consent from the donor's next of kin. Many practising transplant surgeons take the view that whatever the legal position they as individuals would be unwilling to remove organs from a cadaver without the certain knowledge that it was the donor's wish and, if that knowledge were not available, that the next of kin had shown no objection to organ removal. An example, perhaps, of the conflict between duty-based ethics (which would encourage the doctor

to treat the donor only in the light of the individual's wishes) and the utilitarian approach which would certainly justify (on the grounds of the greatest good) organ removal from a donor who had not registered an objection.

Organ removal from the brain-stem dead, heart-beating cadaver is now uncontroversial – the donor has died, the law or at least a Code of Practice[5] sets out clearly the situation regarding consent for donation and few awkward ethical issues are raised. However, the shortage of organs for transplantation has pushed transplant surgeons into attempts to find other ways of enabling donation to occur. The two policies that have been introduced are elective, or interventional, ventilation and the use of kidneys from non-heart beating donors. Both have generated extensive legal and ethical discussions.

### *Interventional ventilation*

Interventional ventilation was first reported from Exeter, UK[6] where a joint initiative between general physicians, intensivists and transplant surgeons had developed a protocol of ventilatory support for patients who stopped breathing after major intracranial haemorrhage, solely and exclusively in order to allow the patient to be declared brain dead and thus to be an organ donor. Without ventilation such patients would die in a hypoxic, hypotensive, state that for practical reasons excludes solid organ donation. The Exeter protocol emphasised that interventional ventilation for such patients should only be instituted with the consent of the patient's next of kin, and was given support by the British Medical Association. However, both legal and ethical problems have been raised by those unhappy with the procedure.

The legal objection relates to consent. If the donor had expressly desired, during his lifetime, that artificial ventilation for organ donation be instituted then adequate consent would have been given. However, it is not felt that the general expression 'I would like my organs used after my death' can apply to this specific, non-therapeutic intervention. Legal opinion further holds that no-one, during the patient's lifetime, can give consent for treatment that is not directly in the patient's interest. Permission is required to intervene – to ventilate the patient at a stage when the donor is on the verge of respiratory arrest but still has a cardiac output – i.e. is neither brain dead nor dead in the cardiorespiratory sense. Doctors may only treat such a patient without consent if it is in the patient's own interests and the next of kin are not able to give legally valid consent. The relatives may give consent to organ donation after death has occurred but at that stage it is too late to institute ventilation for organ donation. This (untested) legal opinion – that interventional ventilation could constitute a common law assault and is therefore illegal – has led the British Department of Health to suspend the procedure for the time being.

The donor may of course still act as a non-heart beating donor (see below) although this is a far less successful form of organ donation.

It is possible that the law may be clarified or modified so as to allow interventional ventilation to be carried out legally. There remain several ethical aspects of the procedure that are of great concern, primarily to intensive care staff who would be called on to manage such patients.[7] One of their main concerns centres around the possibility that ventilation of a patient at the time of respiratory arrest may be followed not by brain stem death but by enough recovery of respiratory activity as to allow the patient to survive for a significant time in the persistent vegetative state (PVS). This could only be seen as a tragedy for the patient, his relatives and his friends. This is an unquantifiable risk at present – there were no cases in the reports from Exeter – and if the clinical selection criteria for interventional ventilation are followed rigidly the risk may be extremely small. However, the risks and implications of the development of PVS significantly alter the ethical aspects of the procedure. It is an interesting exercise to apply the basic principles outlined at the start of the chapter to the subject of interventional ventilation – not least as a demonstration of the ways in which the principles may conflict.

Let us examine interventional ventilation in terms of the two main ethical theories. Duty-based ethics requires the doctor to do the best for the individual patient regardless of outside factors. Unless the patient was known to have a strong desire to donate organs after his death it is difficult to argue that such a radical change to the nature and timing of the patient's death is in his best interests. Of the four ethical principles discussed above the first two – do no harm, do good – would also imply that interventional ventilation carries risks (PVS) without benefit. The third, autonomy, cannot be respected, as the donor is not in a position to give consent and, finally, justice: it has certainly been argued that to manipulate a patient's death in this way is distasteful, that it threatens the rights, dignity and respect that should be accorded to the dying, and is therefore unacceptable.[7]

Thus the balance of this analysis would suggest that interventional ventilation is, at best, ethically dubious and possibly unethical.

The alternative ethical theory of utilitarianism can be simplified (over-simplified?) into the concept that 'morality is all about maximising happiness and minimising misery: that one's actions are right insofar as they tend to that end, wrong insofar as they tend to decrease happiness or increase misery'.[8] Interventional ventilation has no effect on the patient's happiness or misery but may confer significant happiness on the relatives (who commonly feel that organ donation offers some good out of an otherwise hopeless and tragic event), and will give not only happiness but perhaps life to the recipients of the donor organs. The risk of PVS barely alters the argument – the patient will not suffer (although he may 'live' longer) and the relatives can accept that they made every effort to allow organ donation to take place. Put at its most basic, can it be wrong to do something that the patient may have wanted, the relatives certainly want, the doctors agree to and which can benefit several organ recipients. Interventional ventilation can therefore be argued to be morally and ethically acceptable.[9]

So – two ethical theories lead to conflicting conclusions. Where does this leave us? Most transplant surgeons would wish to see legal clarification that allowed interventional ventilation to be instituted lawfully. They would accept, however, that the procedure would only be introduced if all concerned (admitting clinician, intensivist, ITU nurses and, most importantly, the potential donor's relatives) were fully informed and gave free and full consent. For some clinicians the case presented above may lead to a conviction that the practice is unethical and that they would not wish to be involved. Others may conclude that it is acceptable. There are precedents for such a compromise – for example the freedom of doctors to choose whether or not to participate in the termination of pregnancy.

One final, more practical issue complicates the matter further. Intensive care facilities in the United Kingdom are woefully inadequate and many intensivists feel that scarce resources should not be used to treat a patient assumed to have no chance of recovery. To do so may go against the ethos of the unit – that every patient is treated there on the assumption that survival and recovery are possible – or, more seriously, may limit the ability of the unit to admit such patients. This is clearly of major concern and thus even if the legal and ethical issues were clarified this lack of facilities may determine the adoption of interventional ventilation in many hospitals.

### Non-heart beating donors [10]

Following respiratory and cardiac arrest all solid organs suffer anoxic damage while at body temperature. Only the kidneys can be removed from such patients and transplanted successfully, and they must be cooled within, at most, about 60 min of cardiac arrest. There are two circumstances in which non-heart-beating kidney removal may be undertaken. The first of these can be called semi-elective: the patient may be on a ventilator, not brain dead, but so irreversibly brain damaged that the decision to discontinue ventilation is made, or brain dead but the relatives wish to be with the patient at the time the ventilator is switched off. Alternatively the patient may be comatose and dying, not on a ventilator – for example the same group of patients for whom interventional ventilation would be considered. When death occurs these patients can be certified dead and then moved immediately to an operating theatre for organ removal. Permission for this is obtained from the relatives in the usual manner and the practice raises few ethical issues; although the hurried transfer to the operating theatre may be distasteful it is not unethical.[11]

The second situation is more controversial, as it involves organ removal from patients dying unexpectedly and suddenly, usually in hospital accident and emergency units. Such patients may be suitable kidney donors if the kidneys can be cooled within minutes of death. This is best achieved by the insertion, usually through the femoral artery, of a double balloon aortic catheter for *in situ* kidney cooling. It is not always possible to obtain permission from the next-of-kin at this stage (although of course their permission would be required before the kidneys were removed) and the issues raised are therefore the legality and morality of the procedure carried out on a dead body without permission.[12,13] A number of units around the world, notably in the Netherlands and the United States, have attempted to increase donation rates by use of this technique. The Leicester group have the most active non-heart-beating donor programme in the UK which was introduced only after detailed discussions with the local coroner. In addition they attempted, through the local media, to obtain widespread publicity (and public approval) for their proposal in advance. Their experience to date suggests that no major objections have been raised[14] but there are those who instinctively feel uncomfortable with such a programme.

## The allocation of cadaveric organs

Although the law in most countries has defined the ways in which consent for cadaveric organ removal may be given, and by whom, the law does not clarify the 'ownership' of those organs once removed. It is generally accepted that ownership of the organs rests with the State, which is assumed to have delegated its authority to the hospital and transplant team.[15] The transplant team therefore have a responsibility to the State to ensure that the best possible use is made of donated organs and it also follows that the relatives of a donor are not in a position to dictate how the organs should be used. Andrews[16] has argued for a clearer legal definition of the ownership and value of donated organs. The principle of justice is particularly relevant to the processes by which cadaver organs are allocated to particular patients.[17,18] Any system that attempts to provide guidelines for organ distribution must, if it is to merit respect and authority, be based on some theory of justice. Gillon's admirable book *Philosophical Medical Ethics* contains a lucid description of the theory of distributive justice on which the following discussion is (in part) based.* However, two general options that have also been put forward should be mentioned, if only to dismiss them. Neither appears acceptable to practising clinicians. Cahn[19] has suggested that if not all who need scarce resources can have them then none should, and Ramsey[20] and Childress[21] mention, among other methods, that allocations could be made by randomisation – a proposal strongly supported by Doyal.[22] A third alternative, equally unacceptable, is of organ allocation by social 'worth': as Dossetor[15] so pertinently asks 'is a Bishop worth more than a prostitute?' This is a much more understandable temptation and one to which most clinicians involved in organ allocation are likely to have been exposed (and even to have succumbed). However, morally and ethically it is indefensible and breaches all the aspects of justice, fairness, equality and impartiality. Closely related to social worth is merit – the patient's ability to return to work, or to look after children, for example. Do these patients somehow 'deserve' the transplant more than the single, the unemployed, the retired? Once again these are aspects of selection which may influence clinicians forced

*The Author gratefully acknowledges permission from Professor R Gillon and the *British Medical Journal* for permission to base part of this text on *Philosophical Medical Ethics* (John Wylie and Sons, Chichester 1985).

to make almost impossible decisions on the spot, but they imply personal value judgements and prejudices which really are not acceptable.

Two systems are available that satisfy the requirements of justice. The first of these has been called welfare maximisation. If identifiable factors are known to produce better results then allocation according to those factors would maximise the benefit gained from each available organ. The most obvious example of such a scheme is the distribution of cadaver kidneys by HLA matching. The United Kingdom kidney allocation scheme puts 'beneficially matched' recipients as a priority and such a scheme is clearly in line with the principle of justice. If no factors were known to influence graft survival it could be argued that organs should preferentially be transplanted into younger recipients on the grounds that they have a longer life ahead of them and therefore would 'make use of' the transplant for longer than the older recipient.[23] If graft survival were indefinite it is self-evident that a 20-year old recipient is likely to 'use' a transplant for many more years than a 60-year old.

But systems such as these are not perfect. If HLA matching is used as the sole criterion for kidney allocation there is a minority of patients who are likely to be prejudiced against. For example a patient with an unusual tissue type – perhaps because different ethnic groups have different antigen frequencies – may have to wait very much longer to receive a transplant than a patient with a common tissue type. The system therefore has a form of justice but can hardly be said to be fair. Moreover, many clinicians – most markedly those involved in liver and thoracic organ transplantation – would argue strongly that whatever system is used must take note of clinical need – the allocation system with which doctors tend to feel most comfortable as it fits in most closely with the traditional doctor–patient relationship. At the extremes few would disagree with this, for example that an available liver should go to a patient with terminal liver failure likely to die within days rather than a second patient with compensated, stable chronic liver failure likely to survive for some months without a transplant. Not all situations are as clear cut as this, however, and indeed clinical need may mean different things to different people. Prolongation of life, reduction in suffering and an improved quality of life are all desirable objectives but may be mutually incompatible. An example would be the distribution of the thoracic organs from a single donor – two lungs and the heart. Three patients could receive one organ each (single lung transplantation may dramatically improve the quality of life of a patient with emphysema) or one patient terminally ill with cystic fibrosis may receive a heart and double lung transplant. For patients with chronic renal failure maintained on dialysis, clinical need and clinical desire may easily be confused. Most dialysis patients desire a transplant, which undoubtedly can lead to an improved quality of life, but need implies significant clinical, as opposed to social, benefit. Not only is the term clinical need therefore not precise, but it is very likely to rely on subjective criteria that cannot be standardised. Doctors may feel comfortable with it but in many ways it creates more problems than it solves if it is to be used in a demonstrably just manner.

There are two groups of patients that cause particular difficulties when discussing organ allocation: those with self-induced disease and those who are non-compliant with their treatment. The most clear-cut example of self-induced disease is probably alcohol-related cirrhosis of the liver leading to liver failure, with cigarette smoking associated with coronary artery disease another example. Transplant surgeons have debated the morality of liver transplantation of alcoholics for many years without always reaching a consensus. If the patient has truly given up alcohol then there seems to be every reason to consider the patient equally with all others with liver failure. However, the unreformed alcoholic offers a more difficult problem, one which is analogous to that faced by renal transplant surgeons when a patient loses a first, potentially successful, transplant through non-compliance with medication.[24] It is often argued that such patients have 'had their chance' and should not be considered for a second transplant unless there is good evidence that they have 'reformed'. A time on dialysis may be used, not in a punitive sense, to assess whether the patient complies with the fluid and dietary restrictions, medication and routine, the carrot of a second chance of a transplant being dangled before them. Given the shortage of suitable organs it is easy to argue that available kidneys should be given to those who are going to look after them and although this may be criticised as being judgemental it is entirely understandable. In the real world, as opposed to the abstract world of ethical theory, such patients are found in every unit and difficult decisions as to their management have to be made.

Everybody – recipients, donor families, clinicians, managers – is entitled to expect organ allocation to be carried out in a fair, equitable and non-discriminatory manner. Moreover, not only must justice be done it must be seen to be done. To quote Gillon:

> Thus if in the context of allocating scarce medical resources, practical systems were set up for resolving conflicts about which value, in a particular case, should have priority, and if those systems took account of the fundamental moral values of respect of autonomy, beneficence and non-maleficence, and if their deliberative structures incorporated Aristotle's formal principle of justice with its demands of formal equity, impartiality and fairness then they would be just systems and their deliberations could be expected to yield just results despite (perhaps because of) the conflict within them. I doubt if better than that is achievable. Is less acceptable?[8]

## Live donor transplantation

Ethical concerns in live donor transplantation centre almost exclusively around the donor. In order to donate an organ the donor must be healthy and normal (the definition of a normal person has been said to be 'someone who hasn't had enough tests') but the procedure to remove the organ inevitably involves a degree of harm and of risk. In the UK all live donor transplants are governed by the Human Organ Transplant Act (1989) which sets out those genetic relatives of the recipient that may act as donors, and establishes a mechanism that allows non-relatives to act as donors in certain circumstances. There is a common law principle that no person may give consent to his being killed or seriously injured but, given the relative safety of the donor operations (see below) this principle has not been invoked as a serious obstacle to live donation. It is useful to look again at some of the basic principles of medical ethics to see how they apply to discussion of the ethics of live donor transplantation.

First, there is the utilitarian approach. If one accepts the principle that transplantation is better than the alternatives (dialysis in the case of end-stage renal failure, death in the case of terminal liver, heart or lung failure) and further that the supply of human cadaveric organs does not match the need, then clearly live donor transplantation is doing good. A more detailed analysis comes from application of some of the principles of the duty-based approach.

(1) 'Do no harm' and (2) 'Do good' is the heart of the problem because, looked at exclusively from the donor's point of view, live donation does physical harm to the patient while doing no physical good.[25,26] Certainly physical benefits accrue to the recipient, and in almost every case it can be argued that the benefits to the recipient outweigh the harm and the risks to the donor, but that is not quite the point. It can also be argued that the donor receives psychological and social benefits from donation (increased self-esteem, benefits from the improved quality of life of the recipient) although whether these rather speculative and ill-defined benefits outweigh the risks of major surgical complications or even death is debatable. It is interesting to speculate on the outcome of an approach to an ethics committee requesting approval for a programme of live donor transplants if that approach were made today, without the benefit of over 40 years' experience of live donor kidney transplantation. The case presented above would certainly justify such a committee in concluding that the proposal was unethical. Fortunately (from the transplant community's point of view), that 40 years' experience has produced considerable evidence to show that live donor nephrectomy carries an extremely small mortality risk to the donor, acceptable short-term morbidity, and probably no significant long-term morbidity despite theoretical fears.[27–29] It is now widely, although not uniformly, agreed that in principle kidney donation by living donors is acceptable. Donation of liver segments, distal pancreas, lung lobes or small bowel by living donors are more controversial as the risks to the donor are perceived (although not established) to be greater than is the case with kidney donation.[30–33]

Pursuing that line of argument, of course, leads immediately to the question: 'what level of risk to the donor is acceptable?' Live donor nephrectomy carries a risk of death of approximately 1:1600, i.e. 0.06%[27] and is perhaps acceptable. A live donor heart transplant is an absurd example of an unacceptable risk (i.e. 100%!). But is a procedure deemed acceptable if the mortality can be shown to be not 0.06% but 0.6%, or 1.6% – what is the cut-off? This is not a speculative question. Removal of a lung lobe from donors is already occurring as is live donor small bowel resection. It is not, however, a question to which any immediate answer is available, nor is there an obvious methodology for deriving an acceptable risk unless comparison is made with other activities that are known to carry risk but which society accepts – for example mountain-eering, hang-gliding or round-the-world sailing.

(3) 'Informed consent, freely given'; if the discussion about do no harm, do good relates to the general acceptability of live donor trans-plantation in ethical terms the principle of 'informed consent, freely given' is central to the suitability/acceptability as a donor of a given individual. The complexities surrounding this apparently simple proviso have generated considerable debate in medico-ethical circles and are of very real concern to surgeons involved in clinical transplantation.

How can there be problems with 'informed consent'? First, and most simply, because information may not be available that allows a truly informed decision to be made. As mentioned above, there are plenty of data concerning the risks and benefits of live donor nephrectomy but virtually none concerning lobectomy for lung transplantation. However, this lack of information does not nullify consent that is given, provided the donor is aware that his 'informed' consent is based on little or no information. Second, there is a well-documented tendency for prospec-tive or possible donors to make their decision – particularly the decision to donate – at a very early stage and then not to 'hear' any of the further information that is given to them.[34] They have made up their minds and they do not want the facts to get in the way. That this possibility is well recognised does not make it any easier to be certain that the donor's consent is truly informed.

Is the consent 'freely given'? The external pressures that may be put on a potential live donor are not difficult to imagine. Family pressure to help the recipient, bribery, coercion and manipulation may occur and may indeed be almost unavoidable. It has been suggested that these pressures can (to some extent) be alleviated by the use of a donor advocate – a counsellor independent of the recipient's clinicians, who is able to guide the donor to their own decision.[34] It has even been proposed that clinicians should invent medical contraindications if they are aware that the donor's consent is less than genuine. Less easy to detect are the 'internal' pressures that may influence a prospective donor. Although live-donor theory emphasises that altruism must be the guiding motive for donors it is almost impossible to separate the donor's desire to help the recipient from the donor's desire to 'do the right thing', or the unwillingness of the donor to be seen to be letting down the recipient, from the proposal that once donation is mentioned there is only one right answer. Once again a donor advocate may be able to talk more openly and honestly with the donor than can the recipient's clinicians, thus protecting the donor from the pressures, internal and external, that may distort the principle of 'informed consent, freely given'.

Despite these problems and anxieties it is widely accepted that for a relative to donate a kidney is, in principle, acceptable. Live-related renal transplantation is seen in some countries, e.g. Norway, as the best, and perhaps the only, way to ensure an adequate supply of kidneys. Other live-related transplants – of liver, lung, pancreas and small bowel – remain more controversial. Whether it is ever appropriate for those under the age of medical consent or those mentally incompetent to give informed consent to act as living related donors (of non-regenerative organs) is a complex issue[35] which fortunately is rarely of clinical relevance.

The use of non-related live donors has become increasingly common as better immunosuppressive regimens have resulted in acceptable results despite the lack of HLA matching. Emotionally related donors (for example spouses) have been shown to give results at least as good as those obtained with well-matched cadaver kidneys.[36] The ethical issues raised by the use of non-related donors are intrinsically the same as those for relatives, with one exception. Altruism is widely held to be the only acceptable motive for a live donor and altruism between relatives is assumed (perhaps naively!) to be the norm. It is equally possible to accept that a spouse may wish to donate a kidney for the most honorable of motives. However, once the principle is accepted that donor and recipient need not be related there is a slippery slope that can lead eventually to outright commercialisation of live donors. Daar[4] discusses the stages on this slippery slope in detail – this chapter will limit itself to the issue of payment for kidneys.

### Commercialisation and live donor transplants

It has already been mentioned that altruism is widely held to be the only acceptable motive for a live donor. In particular the Western dominated transplant community has made clear its outright rejection of payment to live donors for their organs, a practice which has been repudiated by the International Transplant Society. A British Minister has said that 'the concept of kidneys for sale is entirely unacceptable in a civilised society'.[37] The sale of organs offends against the ethical principles of justice in that inevitably it becomes an alternative available to the rich but denied to the poor, and of course it is the poor who would be exploited by acting as paid organ donors. In recent years there have been regular media stories describing the activities, particularly in Asia, of kidney brokers – middlemen who arrange for the poor to donate a kidney for payment and who profit themselves from the arrangement. Many of the stories are harrowing: the donors rarely seem to benefit as much as expected from the transaction and, moreover, the medical supervision and assessment of both donor and recipient has been reported to fall below acceptable standards.[38] Thus there is widespread agreement that this form of exploitative, profit-led commercialisation of live donor transplantation is unacceptable.

On the other hand a number of authors have questioned whether this instinctive rejection of paid organ donation is necessarily an appropriate response.[39] It has been emphasised that it is a specifically Western view,[3,15,40] coloured by our experience of a National Health Service under which the state provides (in theory) all necessary medical care. In a truly free market health system the situation could be described as one in which an anxious buyer meets a willing seller.[3] From the donor's point of view the balance of risk against benefit (discussed above) is, if anything, more in favour of live donation if the donor received payment than if the donation is purely altruistic, i.e. there is some benefit to balance against the known risks. Also discussed above is the question of the donor's autonomy and the acceptance that in practice both external and internal pressures may be at work as the potential donor comes to a decision. Financial rewards for the donor certainly influence his or her decision but that does not of itself render the consent less informed or less freely made. Indeed there have been reports of donors wishing to sell a kidney in order to raise money for medical treatment of another family member – surely an altruistic motive.

The final point raised to justify paid organ donation is that the alternative, i.e. the consequences of prohibiting paid donation, may equally be ethically dubious. In many countries dialysis is not freely available. To receive a transplant may save the life of the recipient and allow a second patient to receive dialysis, who would otherwise die. It can certainly be argued that paid organ donation may be not only ethical but desirable in such countries.[41]

It can be seen from this discussion that there are strong arguments leading to condemnation of paid organ donation and alternative arguments to support it. Much of the condemnation centres around unacceptable exploitation of poor, often poorly educated and certainly poorly informed donors by middle-men and organ brokers who themselves profit from the exploitation. Distaste for such a system must not be allowed to condemn the principle of paid organ donation out of hand. It is certainly possible to argue that a well-run, well controlled system of payment for live donors may on balance do more good than harm. 'As long as there are adequate safeguards, any ethical or legal fastidiousness demanding that donation be only gratuitous could condemn the sick'.[42] Put another way: 'the ethical distinction between allowing one poor and needy citizen to run the risk of brain damage in the boxing ring and denying another the right to sell a kidney may prove hard to define'.[43]

## Xenotransplantation

A number of isolated attempts have been made over the past 30 years to use animal organs for transplantation. Most, but not all, of these transplants have been performed in extreme circumstances and have used primate organs, and most of the organs have failed (or the patients died) within days or weeks. The 9 month survival of a chimpanzee kidney transplanted into a woman in 1964[44] is the best result so far achieved. More recently interest and research into the immunobiology of the xenograft response has intensified, driven largely by the increasing gulf between the need for transplantable organs and the number of human organs available.

It is outside the scope of this chapter to review the progress in xenotransplantation research[45] that has led at least one group to announce that they anticipate starting a carefully planned and controlled series of xenotransplants within one to two years. For a variety of reasons the pig has been studied most closely and the Cambridge group have succeeded in producing, and breeding, transgenic pigs carrying a human gene whose products are involved in the regulation of complement activation. Results to date suggest that this genetic modification circumvents the classical xenograft response although whether this is enough to give the potential for long-term graft survival is not yet clear. However, let us consider for the moment that the problems have been overcome and that within the foreseeable future it will be possible to breed, on a large scale, genetically modified pigs whose hearts, lungs, kidneys and perhaps even livers could be successfully transplanted into humans. Society in general may quite reasonably ask some very searching questions as to the acceptability of this development. The case for the prosecution asks three questions – and answers 'no' to all of them. The defence, of course, answers 'yes'.

Firstly, is it acceptable for humans to manipulate the genetic constitution of another species? Is this not a science-fiction scenario that has gone horribly wrong with the creation of half-pig–half-man creatures. Where will it end – this is surely the thin end of the wedge leading to who knows what, and humans have no right to meddle with another species in this way. A religious element may be brought into this – humans are interfering with the wonder of God's creation. The counterargument runs something like this: humans, by way of reason and intellect, have been given the opportunity to do things for the benefit of humankind. We are 'superior' to the rest of the animal kingdom (whether we like it or not) and we must use our abilities to improve the lot of our species. We manipulate the genetics of other species already – by selectively breeding race-horses for speed or stamina, for example, or breeding cattle to produce larger milk yields or more tender meat. There is nothing wrong with this (exceedingly small) alteration of a pig's DNA given the potential benefits that may follow from it.

Second, is it acceptable to breed animals – pigs – purely to act as organ donors. Is this exploitation of another species that should be accorded the same rights as humans. But we eat animals (and breed them selectively for that purpose), we use their skins or hides (and have done since time immemorial) and in recent years we have used porcine insulin and heart valves in medicine. If breeding animals to keep ourselves warm and well fed is acceptable then it must be doubly so to breed them to save our lives.

Third, can we be certain that it is safe to 'mix' animal and human tissues. In particular, are there infective agents (mainly viruses) that are not pathogenic to pigs but which would become virulent and pathogenic when introduced into humans. And does this risk extend far beyond the organ recipient into the wider world. This is more a scientific objection than a moral one and it is the hardest for the proponents of xenotransplantation to consider. Although every possible step may be taken to avoid transmission of all known pathogens the transmission of unknown, unrecognised pathogens is, by definition, a possibility. Expert opinion may be that this risk is slight, or very slight, or extremely slight but a risk it remains.[46]

A number of other criticisms have been made of the use of pig organs but they are all really variants of those discussed above. Ultimately the discussion can be reduced to one fundamental issue: do animals have rights, and are they the same rights that we accord to humans? For those who believe that the answer to this question is 'yes' we should apply all the ethical principles to the problem and would demonstrate immediately that xenotransplantation is unethical. However, if it is accepted that humans are in someway superior to animals, that a human life is intrinsically worth more than that of an animal, than given due regard for the details (the conditions in which the pigs are reared, kept and slaughtered and so forth) xenotransplantation will be seen as a development that offers life to patients who otherwise would die – and is therefore acceptable.

A recent report[47] has considered this subject in great detail and concluded that in principle the development and breeding of transgenic pigs for the purposes of xenotransplantation is ethically acceptable. The report emphasises the concerns about possible transmission of animal infections to humans and for this, and other, reasons expresses considerable reservations about the use of primates. Finally, the report recommends a strong regulatory system to oversee the introduction and conduct of a programme of clinical xenotransplants.

**Summary**

The introduction to this chapter is, of necessity, a very simplistic attempt to provide a theoretical ethical basis for the discussion of the issues raised by transplantation. However, without such a basis the discussion proceeds along the lines that conscience, good character and integrity are sufficient to allow very difficult subjects to be discussed, and even more difficult decisions reached, in a satisfactory manner. Gillon[8] shows clearly that although these attributes are an integral part of the character of a good doctor they are not of themselves enough. As has been emphasised, ethical theories do not necessarily produce clear answers to all the questions but they allow a structured discussion of difficult alternatives. Ultimately decisions have to be made and some system has to be adopted that assesses the weight that must be given to various possible solutions. For example, would live donor transplantation still be acceptable if there were a surfeit of human organs? If animal organs can be transplanted successfully is that more desirable than using human organs – particularly if human donation involves interventional ventilation or non-heart-beating donors? Is interventional ventilation more 'ethical' than live donor liver or lung transplantation?

No doubt future developments in transplantation, opening more opportunities for the successful treatment of more patients, are likely to produce increasingly difficult choices for clinicians. Discussion of these issues must be firmly based on principles of medical ethics although accepting that although absolute principles may be available, absolute answers are more difficult to come by.

## References

1. New B, Solomon M, Dingwall R, McHale J. A question of give and take. Research Report 18, Kings Fund Institute, 1994.
2. Beauchamp TL, Childress JF. Principles of biomedical ethics. Oxford: Oxford University Press, 1989.
3. Mason JK, McCall Smith RA. Law and medical ethics, Chapter 14, 4th edn. London: Butterworth, 1994.
4. Daar AS. Transplantation in developing countries. In: Morris JP (ed) Kidney transplantation, 4th edn. Philadelphia: Saunders, 1994, pp. 478–503.
5. Cadaveric Organs for Transplantation: A Code of Practice. Health Department of Great Britain and Northern Ireland. London: HMSO, 1983.
6. Feest TG, Riad HN, Collins CH et al. Protocol for increasing organ donation after cerebrovascular death in a district general hospital. Lancet 1990; 335: 1133.
7. Willetts SH. Transplantation and interventional ventilation on the intensive therapy unit. BMJ 1995; 310: 714–8.
8. Gillon R. Philosophical medical ethics. Chichester: John Wiley, 1985.
9. Collins CH. Elective ventilation for organ donation – the case in favour. Care Crit Ill 1992; 8: 60.
10. Anaise D, Smith R, Ishimuru M et al. An approach to organ salvage from non-heart beating cadaver donors under existing legal and ethical requirements for transplantation. Transplantation 1990; 49: 290.
11. Younger SJ. Respect for the dead body. Transplant Proc 1990; 22: 1014.
12. Anaise D, Rapaport FT. Use of non heart beating cadaver donors in clinical organ transplantation – logistics, ethics and legal considerations. Transplant Proc 1993; 25: 2153–5.
13. Kootstra G. Statement on non-heart beating donor programmes. Transplant Proc 1995; 27: 2965.
14. Veitch P. Personal Communication.
15. Dossetor JB. Ethics in transplantation. In: Morris PJ (ed.) Kidney Transplantation, 4th edn. Philadelphia: Saunders, 1994; pp. 524–531.
16. Andrews LB. My body, my property. Hastings Centre Report 1986; 16: 28.
17. Rhodes R. A review of ethical issues in transplantation. Mt Sinai J Med 1994; 61: 77–82.
18. Anon. General principles for allocating human organs and tissues. Transplant Proc 1992; 24: 2227–35.
19. Cahn E. Cited by Calabresi G, Bobbitt P. Tragic choices. New York: Norton, 1978.
20. Ramsey P. The Patient as Person, 10 edn. New Haven: Yale University Press, 1979, pp. 239–75.
21. Childress J. Who shall live when not all can live? Soundings: An Interdisciplinary Journal 1970; 53: 339–55.

22. Doyal L. The role of the public in health care rationing. Critical Public Health 1993; 4: 49–53.

23. Lockwood M. Quality of Life and Resource Allocation. Philosophy and Medical Welfare.

24. Schweitzer RT, Rovelli M, Palmeri D, Vossier E, Hull D, Bartus S. Non compliance in organ transplant recipients. Transplantation 1990; 49: 375.

25. Michielsen P. Medical risk and benefit in renal donors: the use of living donation reconsidered. In: Land W and Dossetor JB (eds) Organ Replacement Therapy. Berlin: Springer-Verlag, 1991, p. 32.

26. Schreiber H-L. Legal implications of the principle nihul nocere as it applies to live donors. In: Land W and Dossetor JB (eds) Organ Replacement Therapy. Berlin: Springer-Verlag, 1991, p. 13.

27. Bay WH, Lee AH. The living donor in kidney transplantation. Ann Int Med 1987; 106: 719–27.

28. Williams SL, Oler J, Jorkasky DK. Long term renal function in kidney donors: a comparison of donors and their siblings. Ann Int Med 1986; 105: 1–8.

29. Najarian JS, Chavers BM, McHugh LE, Matas AJ. 20 Years or more of follow up of living donors. Lancet 1992; 340: 807–10.

30. Singer PA, Siegler M, Whittington PF et al. Ethics of liver transplantation using living donors. N Eng Med 1989; 321: 620.

31. Whittington PF, Singer PA, Broelsch CE. Living donor non renal transplantation: a focus on living related orthotopic liver transplantation. In: Land W and Dossetor JB (eds). Organ Replacement Therapy. Berlin: Springer-Verlag, 1991; p. 116.

32. Shaw LR, Miller JD, Slutsky AS et al. Ethics of lung transplantation with live donors. Lancet 1991; 338: 678.

33. Caplan A. Must I be my brother's keeper? Ethical issues in the use of living donors as sources of liver and other solid organs. Transplant Proc 1993; 25: 1997–2000.

34. Russell S, Jacob RG. Living related organ donation: the donor's dilemma. Patient Education and Counselling 1993; 21: 89–99.

35. Doyal L, Henning. Ethics of transplantation in children. Ballières Clinical Paediatricians 1993; i: 1061–85.

36. Terasaki P, Cecka JM, Gjertson DW, Takemoto S. High survival rates of kidney transplants from spousal and living unrelated donors. N Engl J Med 1995; 333: 333–6.

37. Warden J. Kidneys not for sale. BMJ 1989; 298: 1670.

38. Salahuddin AK, Woods HF, Pingle A et al. High mortality among recipients of bought living unrelated donor kidneys. Lancet 1990; 336: 725.

39. Dossetor JB. Rewarded gifting: ever ethically acceptable? Transplant Proc 1992; 24: 2092.

40. Dossetor JB, Manickavel V. Ethics in organ donation: contrasts in two cultures. Transplant Proc; 23: 2508.

41. Reddy KC. Organ donation for consideration: an Indian viewpoint. In: Land W and Dossetor JB (eds) Organ Replacement Therapy. Berlin: Springer-Verlag, 1991; p. 173.

42. Davies I. Live donation of human body parts: a case for negotiability? Med-Legal Journal 1991; 59: 100.

43. Bignall J. Kidneys: buy or die. Lancet 1993; 342: 45.

44. Reemtsma K, McCracken BH, Schlegel JU et al. Renal heterotransplantation in man. Ann Surg 1964; 160: 384.

45. Cozzi E, White DJG. The generation of transgenic pigs as potential organ donors for humans. Nature Medicine 1995; 1: 964–6.

46. Chapman LE et al. Xenotransplantation and xenogeneic infections. N Engl J Med 1995; 333: 1498–1501.

47. Nuffield Council on Bioethics. Animal to human transplants. London, 1996.

# 2 Organ donation: logistics and technical aspects

*Nigel D. Heaton*

**Introduction**

Solid organ transplantation has transformed the outlook for patients with end-stage organ failure. Since the introduction of cyclosporin the number and type of organ transplants performed world-wide has increased remarkably, leading to the development of techniques for multiorgan retrieval and specialised teams to perform these operations. The success of organ transplantation has meant that the demand for suitable organs for transplantation has continued to increase rapidly, leading to a shortage of suitable donors and unfortunately to potential recipients dying while awaiting engraftment. If this scenario is to be improved it is important for doctors to be familiar with the donation process, to be able to identify potential donors in the critically ill and to manage them appropriately. Three types of organ donation will be considered in this chapter, including living donation, heart beating and non-heart beating cadaveric donation.

**Brain stem death**

Cadaveric organ donation remains the most important source of grafts for all forms of transplantation. The concept of brain stem death is essential to the process of cadaveric heart beating organ donation.[1] Potential donors include any patient deeply unconscious on a ventilator as a result of severe irreversible brain injury of known aetiology and include patients who have suffered spontaneous intracranial haemorrhage, acute neurological or neurosurgical trauma and cerebral anoxia from diverse causes. The initial step following identification of a potential organ donor is the assessment of clinical signs of brain death.[2] Two sets of brain stem function tests should be performed by two independent physicians before brain stem death is confirmed. In a deeply comatose person, maintained on a ventilator, the criteria to be satisfied that brain stem death has occurred are listed in Table 2.1.[3]

**Table 2.1** *The clinical criteria for diagnosing brain death*

1. Fixed and dilated pupils not responding to bright light
2. Absent corneal reflexes
3. No motor response to painful stimuli
4. No reflex activity unless of spinal cord origin
5. No oculocephalic reflex (dolls eyes)
6. Absent vestibulo-ocular reflexes (tested by flushing ice cold water into the ear and observing eye movement)
7. No gag or cough reflex to bronchial stimulation by the passage of a suction catheter
8. No respiratory movements if mechanical ventilation is stopped for long enough to ensure the arterial $Pco_2$ rises above the threshold for stimulation of ventilation (greater than 60 mm Hg)

Ingestion of alcohol, neurodepressant drugs, such as barbiturates, neuromuscular blocking agents and the presence of metabolic abnorm-alities such as hypernatraemia, can reversibly impair brain function and mimic the clinical picture of brain death. It is an absolute requirement that sufficient time should elapse for the effect of any such drug intoxication to wear off before performing brain stem testing. Permanent functional death of the brain stem equates to brain death and once this has occurred further artificial support is of no benefit and should be withdrawn. It is considered good medical practice to recognise when brain stem death has occurred and to act accordingly, sparing relatives from the further emotional trauma of sterile hope.[1] Doctors who have been involved in determining the brain stem death of a donor should not be involved in organ retrieval or the subsequent transplantation of any organ from that donor.

## Organ donation

Over the past 5 years a ceiling has been reached in organ donation. There has been a fall in the overall number of donors by approximately 30%, but a compensatory increase in the number of organs retrieved from each donor. The suitability of the majority of brain stem dead donors to become multiorgan donors is borne out by a study of intensive care units in the United Kingdom which identified 497 potential donors out of 5803 patients dying on intensive care with no general contraindications to organ donation. The suitability of the various organs for transplantation was recorded as a percentage of the overall number of potential donors: kidneys, 95%; eyes, 91%; liver, 90%; heart, 63%; lungs, 29%.[4]

The fall in the number of donors is in part due to a reduction in the number of deaths from road traffic accidents and from intracranial haemorrhage which has continued over the past 20 years. There is also a trend towards an older donor population, for example in the United Kingdom there are approximately 850 donors each year with 10% being aged 60 years or older.[5] There is also considerable variation in donor rate between different countries. The current UK organ donation is 16 per million population (pmp) which compares unfavourably with most other European countries, particularly Spain which has a donation rate of 28 pmp and the Channel Islands of 42 pmp. In Spain there was a doubling of the number of donors at a time when deaths from road traffic accidents were falling dramatically and this was felt to result from changes in the organisation of the donor co-ordinator network.[6]

Spain established 17 regional donor co-ordinators who link with local co-ordinators to organise daily visits to all hospitals and ITUs. The number of co-ordinators grew from 56 in 1990 to 118 in 1992. The majority of the co-ordinators are doctors (accounting for 55% of the overall number) or nurses, all of whom are part-time and they are responsible to the hospital and its medical director not to the transplant teams. They are based on ITUs and remain in post for between two and four years. In addition to organ procurement, they provide educational support, administration, identify resources aned provide a link to the media. The starting point for this reorganisation was an audit which identified a major shortfall in the number of organ donations as compared to the potential number from records of brain stem death. The success of the Spanish programme can be judged by the increase from 14 donors pmp in 1989 to 25 per million in 1994 with an overall increase in the number of organ donors from 550 to 960 per year. Smaller hospitals have been identified as being very important in increasing donor numbers and although Spain accounts for only 0.6% of the world's population, it performs 12% of worldwide liver transplants.[6]

Other factors influencing the donor number include the density and age of the population. It has been suggested that failure to request donation after brain stem death could account for a significant number of donors, however, this number appears to be relatively small.[7] The incidence of intensive treatment unit (ITU) beds does have a major impact on the incidence of brain stem death. Because of the insufficient number of ITU beds in the United Kingdom there is great pressure not to admit patients to ITU if they are considered to have a poor outcome despite ventilation, and such patients instead are managed on the ward.[8] Increased provision of facilities for ventilation and ITU beds would allow more patients to be managed in this way and would increase the number of potential organ donors. This formed the basis of the Exeter protocol of 'elective ventilation'. All patients with cerebrovascular accidents were admitted to ITU and this resulted in an increase in the number of potential kidney donors from 19.8 to 37.5 donors per million population.[9,10] There have been ethical objections to elective ventilation which have halted this practice (see Chapter 1).

Organ donation is voluntary and has been encouraged by schemes such as 'donor cards' which indicate that the carrier is willing to act as a donor in the event of untimely death. However, rates of card ownership vary – 25% in America, 30% in UK, 9% in Holland and only 2% in Germany. In addition, donor cards can be overruled by next of kin, although this is not a common occurrence. This has led to the use of a mechanism where an individual 'opts in', for example consent to the inclusion of their name on a computerised national registry (as in the UK). The effectiveness of such an 'opt in' scheme is unproven and seems unlikely to increase the number of donors over the long term. Some European states including Belgium and France have legislation for presumed consent or 'an opt out' scheme in which there is presumed consent to organ donation at death unless the person has previously registered an objection to organ donation with the State. These countries have a 'soft' opt-out scheme in that relatives are allowed to object and will be heeded. In Austria, the views of the close relatives may not be taken into account. This scheme does appear in the short term to improve organ donation. Whether this is sustained in the long term is less certain. The potential for poor publicity for organ donation in cases where dispute arises by refusal of the family may counteract the benefits of such legislation.

The most important aspect in this difficult subject, is to improve the way in which families are asked about organ donation and although time consuming and emotionally demanding the need for professionally trained coordinators to approach relatives of brain-dead patients cannot be overstated.[6] This would seem to return us to the Spanish system with investment in coordination. The cost of the 'Spanish solution' of central and regional offices with a relatively large number of coordinators was identified at approximately $6 million per year. The estimated potential savings due to the increased number of donors allowing increased kidney transplantation rather than dialysis was estimated at $53 million. However, Spain has two and half times the number of intensive care beds compared with the United Kingdom and unless this problem of ITU shortage is addressed the benefits of such a scheme would be limited. The importance of audit in monitoring performance of hospitals, intensive care units, coordinators and retrieval teams can be seen from the Spanish experience. Problems of 'burn out' for donor coordinators are well recognised and career alternatives are kept for Spanish practitioners in contrast to current practice in many countries.

## Donor transplant coordinator

Transplant coordinators initially developed in the late 1960s and 1970s from staff attached to renal units helping to arrange donor retrieval and kidney transplantation. Arrangements became more formalised and they are now employed by transplant units or procurement agencies.

The donor transplant coordinator is responsible for the multiorgan donor retrieval within a large geographical area and is usually based within a regional kidney transplant centre. Responsibilities include assisting in donor management, gathering all relevant information regarding the potential donor, and relaying the details to a transplant support service (Eurotransplant, United Kingdom Transplant Support Service) or a procurement agency, as well as the appropriate recipient transplant centres. The donor coordinator supports the donor family in making an informed decision about organ donation and continues to maintain contact with the donor families. The donor coordinator is responsible for arranging the organ donation process, coordinating multiorgan retrieval and possible assistance to the surgical teams in retrieving the organs. The organisation of the retrieval teams is vital to ensure the least possible disruption to donor hospitals. The promotion of tissue and organ transplantation within all referring hospitals and within the community is an important part of the job. This may involve significant interaction with the broadcast media and the press. Good news stories about transplantation and feedback information to referring hospitals ensure continued support to the transplant unit.

### *Offers of organ donation*

A telephoned offer of a potential donor is made by the Transplant Support Service or Procurement Agency to the recipient transplant co-ordinator. This individual is responsible for collecting relevant donor details to allow the surgeon to make a preliminary assessment. Based on the suitability of the donor, a retrieval team travels to the donor hospital. In the case of heart and lung transplants the recipient is prepared and the transplant surgical team organised to ensure the cold ischaemia time for the grafts are as short as possible.

**Non-heart beating donation**

The increasing shortage of donor organs has led to attempts to increase the pool of donor organs in several different ways. The concept of non-heart beating donors is not new as prior to the introduction of brain stem death legislation it was the only method of cadaveric organ donation.[12] The introduction of heart beating donation resulted in a loss of interest in this potential source of organs, but interest has been rekindled particularly for kidney retrieval. The circumstances under which non-heart beating donors may present vary from patients who are dead on arrival at hospital when there is clear evidence that resuscitation is not possible, those dying after unsuccessful resuscitation, patients with a hopeless prognosis who will die on withdrawal of ventilatory or inotrope support and lastly brain dead patients who unexpectedly arrest and cannot be resuscitated.[13] At present there is no legislation which would allow organ retrieval from patients who are dead on arrival in hospital without consent being given by relatives and this source of donors will remain limited without legislation for presumed consent. Patients who die after unsuccessful resuscitation may be considered as potential donors if they are under 65 years of age, have had a circulatory arrest for less than 30 min and a period of cardiac massage and ventilatory support of less than 2 hours. Consent must be given by relatives before organ retrieval is undertaken.[14]

Several different techniques have been described to remove organs from non-heart beating donors, but all share the aim of rapid cooling of the organs to be retrieved (Fig. 2.1). Perhaps the most common method is insertion of a double balloon catheter to the aorta via a femoral

**Figure 2.1** *Non-heart beating cadaveric retrieval: showing the placement of an intra-aortic balloon to perfuse the kidneys prior to retrieval.*

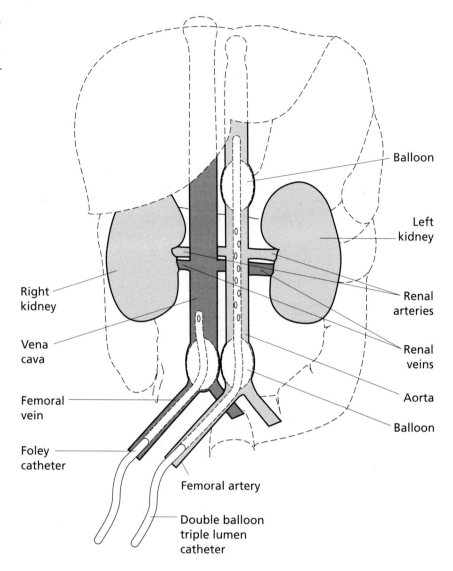

arteriotomy. This allows preferential perfusion of the organs destined for transplantation. Preservation fluid is flushed through the lumen of the catheter and blood is vented from a femoral venotomy. Once the perfusion has been performed, the relatives can be interviewed and consent obtained for laparotomy and organ retrieval.

Non-heart beating donation may supplement the supply of cadaveric kidneys by at least 20%, however, such grafts have a higher risk of delayed and primary nonfunction than for heart beating donor kidneys.[15] The number of centres performing non-heart beating donor retrieval is increasing and it is therefore likely to become an important source of grafts for kidney transplantation. Preliminary experience has been reported of the use of livers from non-heart beating donors, but the overall results are not sufficiently satisfactory at present and liver grafts from this source are likely to be few for the present.[16,17]

**Donor medical management**

Good management of the donor after diagnosis of brain stem death is increasingly being seen as a neglected area. Correct management is vital if use is to be made of all potential donors.[18–21] The aims of medical management of the brain dead organ donor should include the early recognition and treatment of haemodynamic instability, maintenance of an adequate systemic perfusion pressure to ensure the best possible post-transplant graft function and avoidance of complications related to brain death with continuing supportive care (Table 2.2).

The principles of good supportive care should include:

- Frequent turning of the patient to prevent pressure sores developing;
- Lubrication and protective closure of the eyes;
- Frequent suctioning of the airways and manual lung inflation to prevent atelectasis and pneumonia;
- Nasogastric aspiration and free drainage to keep the stomach empty and prevent aspiration of gastric contents;
- Central venous pressure catheter to guide the use of fluid replacement and vasopressors;
- Urinary catheter to monitor hourly urine output;
- Warming blankets to maintain a temperature above 35°C, to avoid hypothermia and consequent impairment of cardiac, renal and hepatic function.

The commonest haemodynamic abnormality seen in brain dead patients is hypotension due to the destruction of pontine and medullary vasomotor centres. A systolic pressure of less than 80 mm Hg is inadequate for optimal liver and kidney function. Maintaining a minimum systolic pressure of 90–100 mm Hg is necessary to ensure adequate perfusion to all vital organs. Hypotension should initially be treated by correcting hypovolaemia using central venous or pulmonary wedge pressure to ensure that the donor is not fluid overloaded as this may jeopardise the use of the lungs for transplantation. Catecholamines should be used in combination with fluid replacement and gradually reduced as blood pressure improves. Dopamine is the preferred vasopressor because of its potential for maintaining renal and

**Table 2.2**  *Likely medical problems in potential donors*

| |
| --- |
| Haemodynamic instability and the need for inotropes |
| Fluid management |
| Treatment of diabetes insipidus |
| Hormone levels |
| Management of ventilation |
| Hypothermia |

mesenteric blood flow provided the dose is kept at or below 10 $\mu$g kg$^{-1}$ min$^{-1}$.[22] Above this level, if additional inotropic support is needed, dobutamine is preferred to isoprenaline as it causes less of an increase in myocardial oxygen demand. Evidence of myocardial injury has been reported in brain stem dead patients unrelated to the cause of death. It is believed to result from intense sympathetic nervous system activity secondary to raised intracranial pressure resulting in the release of myocardial catecholamines.[23] Alterations in the levels of circulating hormones have been described after brain death. Low levels of free tri-iodothyronine (T3) in donors have been reported in association with elevated reverse T3 and unchanged TSH levels. Replacement with intravenous T3 appears to reduce the requirement for inotrope dosage in unstable brain dead donors.[24] Hyperglycaemia may occur and require insulin therapy and occasionally corticosteroid can help to improve cardiovascular stability.

A urine output of at least 100 ml h$^{-1}$ especially in the hour preceding retrieval, has been shown to be one of the most important factors determining renal allograft function in the recipient.[25] If the urine output is inadequate after volume expansion with a satisfactory blood pressure, mannitol or frusemide should be administered to establish diuresis. Maintenance fluids should be in the form of dextrose saline as hypernatraemia is a common problem in donors. Maintenance fluids should contain dextrose to ensure preservation of adequate stores of intrahepatic glucose, particularly if the donors have not received any nutrition in the preceding 24 h. Destruction of the hypothalamic–pituitary axis results in central diabetes insipidus. Desmopressin is the preferred vasopressin for the management of diabetes insipidus because of its long duration of action and low pressor activity. The intense splanchnic vasoconstrictor activity of other vasopressin preparations can cause reduced blood flow to the liver and kidneys causing post-transplant graft dysfunction.

Ventilation should be maintained at an inspired oxygen level sufficient to ensure arterial saturation of 95–100% with normal blood gases. Physiotherapy should be continued to minimise atelectasis. Positive expiratory pressure may be used to maintain lung expansion, but excessive ventilatory pressures must be avoided if possible. Sputum samples should be sent for Gram stain and cultures and antibiotics should be given if appropriate.

Maintenance of a core temperature of greater than 33°C is necessary to ensure an accurate diagnosis of brain stem death and also decreases the risk of cardiovascular instability. The use of radiant warmers, thermal mattresses and warmed inspired gases may all be required to maintain the core temperature within the normal range.

## Assessment of potential donors

The selection of donors is likely to vary from centre to centre depending on the organ to be transplanted, the overall supply of donor organs, the experience of the transplant centre and the size of the recipient transplant waiting list. A thorough history and physical examination are essential to the initial assessment of donor suitability. Initial details of the donor may be sparse but a provisional acceptance can be made from the donor age, weight, cause of death, time in hospital and renal/liver function tests. Before the donor retrieval team is dispatched, however, a more detailed assessment of the donor history should have been made.[26] This should include:

- The date of admission to the hospital.
- The cause of brain stem death, duration and history of the presenting illness. If the cause of death is trauma, whether there are other sites of significant injury.
- The timing of endotracheal intubation and ventilation of the donor.
- Details of the patient's medical condition since admission, particularly if there were any episodes of hypotension or resuscitation.
- Any significant medical history which should include details of previous surgery, alcohol and smoking habits, drug usage, and allergies.
- The current medical status of the donor (pulse rate, blood pressure, temperature, urine output and peripheral perfusion).

There are a number of conditions which exclude a donor from further consideration (Table 2.3).[27]

High risk groups such as prostitutes or intravenous drug abusers, who are HIV antibody negative should be considered on an individual basis along with the urgency of the potential recipient. A history of cardiac arrest and prolonged hypotension does not contraindicate organ donation and the suitability of individual organs would depend on their postresuscitation function. There has been a gradual rise in the maximum age of organ donation, but some units are reluctant to use organs from donors over 70 years of age for liver and kidney donation although this is changing.[27]

### Relative contraindications

There are no hard and fast rules regarding a good or poor potential donor, however, an assessment of the potential risk of graft dysfunction can be made. Cardiac or respiratory arrest, prolonged resuscitation or a systolic blood pressure of less than 70 mm Hg for more than 30 min

**Table 2.3**  *Exclusion criteria for organ donation*

| |
|---|
| Severe untreated systemic sepsis |
| Acquired immunodeficiency syndrome |
| Active viral hepatitis B and C |
| Viral encephalitis |
| Malignancy excluding primary brain tumours |
| Risk of rare viral disease such as Jakob–Creutzfeldt disease and recipients of human pituitary growth hormone |

without a period of at least 12 h cardiorespiratory stability are not encouraging factors.[28]

The presence of Type II diabetes mellitus would exclude pancreas transplantation and is often associated with fatty change in the liver which may be a contraindication to liver donation. Brain stem death in association with diabetic coma is associated with severe electrolyte disturbances which may preclude donation. The length of hospital stay of greater than 5 days has been associated with an increased incidence of liver dysfunction or primary non-function and this may be linked to the lack of either nasogastric feeding or intravenous nutrition prior to donation.[29] Infusion of dextrose prior to organ donation may help improve early graft function.

A history of chronic disease affecting an organ is a contraindication to donation. Alcohol abuse and potential liver disease is more difficult to assess from the history and liver function tests, unless the latter are wildly deranged. The commonest abnormality of the liver at retrieval is the presence of a fatty liver in about 30% of donors. There may be underlying metabolic disorders due to diabetes mellitus, steroid therapy or alcohol abuse, but the fatty change may be due to simple imbalance of diet. The liver can be assessed for fat content by inspection. Particularly worrying are the presence of a globular shape with the loss of the sharp edges of the liver and a firm or hard consistency. If there is doubt then a liver biopsy and frozen section will help in the further assessment of fat content. Greater than 30–40% fatty change is a contraindication to use. Liver-based inborn errors of metabolism are rare and may not be a contraindication to organ donation. Meningococcal meningitis may be a cause of brain stem death and provided effective treatment with high dose penicillin has been given, organ donation should be considered. If the treatment period has been short then the recipient should be given 5 days prophylaxis post-transplant.

## Assessment for individual organs

### Heart donor selection[30,31]

- Donors younger than 60 years of age
- No history of pre-existing coronary or valvular heart disease
- Normal chest radiograph
- Normal 12 lead ECG

Inotrope requirement of less than $10 \mu g \ kg^{-1} \ min^{-1}$ of dopamine to maintain systolic pressure greater than 90 mm Hg after correction of hypovolaemia.[30] An echocardiogram may be helpful to assess myocardial function in donors receiving more than $10 \mu g \ kg^{-1} \ min^{-1}$ of dopamine to maintain adequate blood pressure and those who have had cardiac arrest, prolonged hypotension or chest trauma (see also Chapter 11).

### Lung donor selection[32,33]

- Donors younger than 60 years of age
- No history of primary pulmonary disease
- Normal chest radiograph
- Adequate gas exchange ($Pa_{O_2} > 50$ kPa on 100% $O_2$ with 5 mm Hg positive end expiratory pressure)
  (see also Chapter 11)

A history of chronic lung disease, heavy smoking, pulmonary aspiration and parenchymal trauma should all be excluded in heart–lung donors. High alveolar–arterial oxygen gradients and tracheal colonisation with bacteria or fungi are contraindications because of the associated increase in recipient morbidity and mortality. Minor chest radiograph abnormalities are noted in 27% of donors and do not contraindicate the possibility of lung donation.[32]

### Pancreas donor selection[34]

- Donors younger than 50 years of age (majority of donors 20–40 years, mean age around 25 years)
- No history of significant cardiac disease
- No history of alcohol abuse
- No major obesity
- No Type II diabetes mellitus
  (see also Chapter 8)

### Liver and kidney donor selection[29,35]

Donors with a history of chronic liver disease and viral hepatitis are excluded. Alcohol abuse and potential liver disease is more difficult to assess from history and liver function tests unless the latter are wildly deranged. Marked elevations in serum transaminase levels can occur in donors subjected to short periods of hypotension or asystole. However, if the levels of transaminase are falling rather than rising then the liver can be used. Donors with a history of chronic renal insufficiency are excluded from kidney donation. Serum creatinine levels higher than 170 $\mu$mol l$^{-1}$ are associated with decreased graft survival, and should be carefully assessed before being used. There is no upper age limit for exclusion.

Investigations to be requested for the acceptance of a donor include:

- Blood tests
  ABO and Rhesus blood group match
  haemoglobin, platelets, white blood count
  urea, creatinine, sodium, potassium
  liver function tests (bilirubin, alkaline phosphatase)
  $\gamma$-glutamyltransferase, aspartate transaminase, albumin

arterial blood gases
blood for subsequent HLA studies
- Chest radiograph
- Electrocardiogram
- Any positive blood or sputum cultures
- Viral studies
  HIV
  Hepatitis B surface antigen and if possible core antibody
  Hepatitis C antibody
  Cytomegalovirus
  Epstein–Barr virus (consider in young children)

**Composition of the donor retrieval team**

The surgical team taking responsibility for the retrieval of the intra-abdominal organs should normally consist of two surgeons, a scrub nurse and a technician/perfusionist. The anaesthetist is usually provided by the donor hospital and assists in theatre in the intraoperative management of the donor. Each member of the team will have identified duties. The senior surgeon of the team must review the donor and the hospital notes to recheck the suitability of the donor, the laboratory results, blood pressure, pulse and temperature or ITU charts, drug charts and documentation of brain stem death with permission for organ donation. In addition, he or she is responsible for the collection of donor details which will include anatomy and appearance of the donor organ.

**Surgical equipment**

The surgical team travels with an instrument set prepared and sterilised ready for use. An ice box is taken containing 4 litres of University of Wisconsin solution, 2 litres of normal saline and 4 litres of Marshall's solution to ensure that they remain at 4°C. All sutures, antibiotics, heparin and other drugs and equipment are carried with the donor team. Large quantities of sterile ice are required.

**Organisation of organ retrieval**

Good communication between donor and recipient hospitals is essential if misunderstandings about the donor status, timing of donor retrieval and coordination of multiple retrieval teams are to be avoided. Organ retrieval is often performed in hospitals which are infrequently involved in multiorgan donor retrieval operations and the extra work entailed by the donor operation may place great strain on the staff and facilities and if performed in an unprofessional manner may deter hospitals from referring potential donors in the future. The donor team must at all times be aware of their responsibilities to ensure that the procedure is performed professionally.

The donor team uses either an adapted minibus for the road travel or fixed wing aircraft for longer distances. For journeys longer than 3 h by road, a fixed wing aircraft is used providing there is a convenient airport close to the donor hospital. Geography may dictate long travel times and require transplant units to have access to jet aircraft. This is vital in countries like America and regions such as that covered by Eurotransplant.

## Organ preservation

Continuing efforts are being made to extend the limits of preservation for all groups.[36,37] These have included the use of hypothermic storage which remains a key element. Current preservation times for the heart and lungs are 4–6 h, pancreas and liver 20 h and kidneys for over 40 h. Several solutions have been used for cold preservation and storage. University of Wisconsin (UW) solution was originally developed for pancreas preservation, but is now accepted as the best preservation fluid for liver, pancreas and kidney retrieval. UW solution contains hydroxy-ethyl starch to support the colloid pressure, lactobionate and raffinose which help to prevent cell swelling and interstitial oedema. Also present is allopurinol which inhibits xanthine oxidase and helps to prevent oxygen free radical generation during ischaemia and reperfusion. Glutathione restores cell reducing potential which also reduces oxygen free radical generation. Other constituents include adenosine to enhance adenosine triphosphate synthesis after reperfusion, dexamethasone, magnesium, phosphate buffer, insulin, potassium ($120\,\mathrm{mmol\,l^{-1}}$) and sodium ($30\,\mathrm{mmol\,l^{-1}}$). There are many alternative solutions. One of the most popular is Marshall's solution which has a composition similar to intracellular fluid. It is less viscose than UW solution and may be preferred for the initial wash-out phase of perfusion with the more expensive UW fluid employed after the effluent has become less bloody.

## Intraoperative management

- All documents must be reviewed in theatre before commencement of procedure (including those certifying brain death). The care of the donor in theatre follows the same basic physiological principles as for any other major surgical procedure.
- Optimal oxygenation and cardiac output should be maintained.
- Arterial blood gas and haemoglobin should be measured at regular intervals.
- Blood loss should be replaced with blood or colloids to maintain a haematocrit of around 30%.
- Urinary output should be maintained around $60$–$100\,\mathrm{ml\,h^{-1}}$.
- Hypotension should be managed with adequate fluid replacement and if appropriate inotropic support. Initially dopamine is recommended as at low infusion rates it causes vasodilatation of renal and mesenteric vessels, tending to minimise end-organ damage. If more than $10\,\mu\mathrm{g\,kg^{-1}\,min^{-1}}$ is given this effect is lost and its uses are limited due to the tachycardia and vasoconstriction produced. Although inotropes may be necessary they should be weaned if possible to allow maximal vasodilatation in the donor organs prior to preservation and removal. However, this must not be at the expense of a satisfactory perfusion pressure.

- Hypertensive episodes which may occur should be treated by vaso-active drugs or anaesthetic agents.
- Spinal reflexes are present in donors and muscle relaxants should be given.

## Surgical technique

### Liver and kidney retrieval[38,39]

At the start of the procedure antibiotics such as benzylpenicillin 1.2 g, gentamycin 160 mg and cefuroxime 1.5 g should be given intravenously. The chest and abdomen are opened through a full length midline incision through the sternum and abdomen even in the case of removal of abdominal organs alone (Fig. 2.2). The sternum is divided using a Gigli saw or if available a power saw. The liver is initially mobilised by dividing the falciform ligament down towards the inferior vena cava. A laparotomy is then performed to assess the suitability of the organs. A careful search is made for any abnormality such as tumour or an unrecognised focus of sepsis.

After this the liver is mobilised by dividing the left triangular ligament. A careful search is made for a left hepatic artery arising from the left gastric artery by observation and palpation of the lesser omentum. Any such vessel must be carefully preserved. The porta hepatis is then inspected and the anatomy of the hilar structures identified. The common bile duct is ligated and divided at the upper border of the duodenum. Again it is important to palpate behind the duct for a right hepatic artery from the superior mesenteric artery (SMA). The common hepatic artery can then be identified and followed back to the coeliac trunk. If there are no accessory or anomalous arteries and there is a single common hepatic artery then the splenic and left gastric arteries can be ligated in continuity so as to ensure the preservation fluid is delivered to the appropriate organs and not wasted. The portal vein can be skeletonised, but extensive dissection should be avoided.

The caecum and right colon are then mobilised together with the small bowel mesentery to reveal the distal inferior vena cava and abdominal aorta. The distal abdominal aorta is isolated and prepared for subsequent cannulation. The superior mesenteric vein is then identified at the junction of the transverse mesocolon and the root of the small bowel mesentery just to the right of the SMA. A section approximately 2 cm in length is prepared for subsequent cannulation. Then either the descending thoracic aorta or the infradiaphragmatic aorta is isolated and a tape passed around it in preparation for cross clamping. This initial dissection should take about 45 min. Dissection of the kidneys can be left until the end of the procedure although some surgeons prefer to perform mobilisation before perfusion. This enables ice to be placed around the kidney at the time of perfusion. The cardiac team is then allowed to proceed with their dissection. The superior and inferior vena cava are isolated. A cannula is inserted into the ascending aorta and connected to

**Figure 2.2**  *Heart-beating cadaveric retrieval: full length midline incision to reveal the contents of the chest and abdomen.*

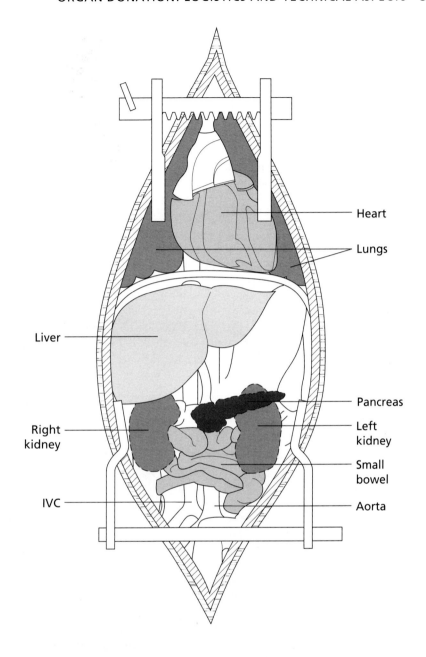

a system for infusion of cardioplegic solution later. Prior to cannulation of the descending aorta and superior mesenteric vein the donor is given 20 000 i.u. of heparin.

Cannulae are inserted into the aorta for perfusion of the abdominal organs and into the portal vein through an incision in the superior mesenteric vein for perfusion of the liver (Fig. 2.3). Once the cannulae are in, the heart team removes the heart and ventilation is stopped. The inferior vena cava is then incised just below the pericardium and the

**Figure 2.3** *Heart-beating cadaveric retrieval: showing placement of the cannulas in the intra-abdominal aorta and superior mesenteric vein for subsequent perfusion of the liver and kidneys.*

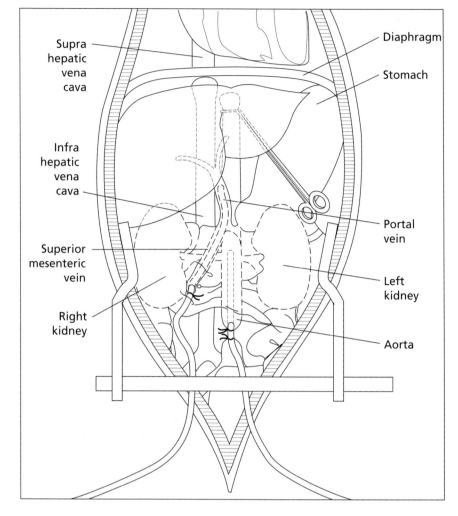

heart and liver are allowed to empty. After a few seconds the aorta is cross clamped at the arch and above the diaphragm and cold perfusion of the heart and abdominal organs is started simultaneously. The pericardial sac and the abdominal cavity are filled with cold saline solution at 4°C to achieve surface cooling. Cold UW solution is perfused through both cannulae (alternatively Marshall's kidney perfusion solution can be given through the aortic cannula). Each litre of UW solution contains 240 mg benzylpenicillin, 16 mg dexamethasone and 40 i.u. of insulin. Approximately 2 l of preservation solution should be perfused through each cannula. The fundus of the gallbladder is opened, bile is removed and the biliary tree is thoroughly flushed with cold normal saline solution.

The heart is removed first. If the lungs are to be removed as well they are excised en bloc with the heart and separated on the back table. The liver and pancreas are excised next. The kidneys are removed last. Spleen and lymph nodes are also removed for use in tissue typing. The common and external iliac arteries and veins should be retrieved intact by sharp dissection taking care to avoid intimal trauma by pulling on the vessels. They are preserved in their own containers containing UW solution and transported in ice together with the liver and pancreas.

Further dissection of the liver takes place towards the end of the perfusion. The common hepatic artery is dissected down to the origin of the coeliac trunk which is excised with a surrounding patch of aorta (Carrel patch). Accessory arteries should be identified and care taken in dissection of either a left hepatic artery back to the left gastric artery which can be retrieved with the coeliac trunk or a right hepatic artery arising from the superior mesenteric artery when the coeliac trunk should include both aortic origins on a common patch. Care must be taken not to injure the renal arteries during dissection of the superior mesenteric artery.

At completion of liver perfusion the portal vein is divided at the junction of the splenic and superior mesenteric veins. The infrahepatic inferior vena cava is divided above the renal veins and part of the right adrenal is left intact to ensure that there is a good length of right adrenal vein to ligate on the back table. The suprahepatic inferior vena cava is mobilised with a cuff of diaphragm and the retrohepatic cava is freed and the liver removed.

The liver is taken to a prepared table for further perfusion of the hepatic artery and portal vein with 250–500 ml of UW solution to each. The flush solution coming out of the liver should be relatively clear and not bloody. The bile duct should be flushed with some UW solution to ensure there is no residual bile in the biliary tree. The liver is then packed in three successive polyethylene bags, the first of which contains UW solution and then stored in an ice chest to be transferred to the recipient hospital.

The kidneys are then retrieved. The right colon is mobilised and the duodenum Kocherised. The aorta, IVC and right kidney are exposed. The aorta and IVC are exposed to the level of the renal vein. The superior mesenteric artery is identified. The kidneys are mobilised by sharp dissection through Gerota's fascia. The ureters are divided below the level of the pelvic brim. Care should be taken to include periureteric tissue in dissection of the ureters to avoid devascularisation. Both the aorta and IVC are encircled above the renal vessels. During the procedure cold saline can be poured over the kidneys to keep them cool. The IVC and aorta are divided anteriorly in a vertical plane and a good cuff of IVC and aorta containing the renal vessels are taken for the right and left kidneys. Care must be taken to identify and preserve any accessory renal vessels and to include them if possible in the vascular patch. The kidneys are then excised and placed in a sterile bag containing ice-cold Marshall's solution and packed in two sterile bags each tied individually having expelled all the air and then the bag is placed in a box containing ice for transport.

## Pancreas retrieval

Pancreas removal would always take place as part of a multiorgan retrieval operation. Following mobilisation of the liver, the right colon is mobilised and the C loop of the duodenum is exposed. The duodenum is then Kocherised to mobilise the head of the pancreas. The common hepatic artery is traced proximally to identify the origin of the splenic artery and a sling is passed around it. The superior mesenteric artery is mobilised below the body of the pancreas and traced up to its origin. Both the portal vein and aorta are perfused with one litre of UW solution through each. Overperfusion of the pancreas leads to graft swelling and this can be avoided by clamping the origins of the splenic and superior mesenteric arteries which had previously been isolated. Further details are given in Chapter 8.

The pancreas is transported in UW solution at 4°C. The back table preparation usually takes about 2 h. The splenic artery and vein are ligated at its hilum and the spleen removed. The splenic and superior mesenteric arteries are cleared of surrounding fibrofatty tissue in preparation for subsequent anastomosis. The distal end of the SMA and vein are ligated. A Y graft of donor common iliac artery bifurcation is prepared and anastomosed to the proximal end of the SMA and splenic arteries, respectively. The first and fourth parts of the duodenum are separated from the head of the pancreas by carefully ligating and dividing the feeding vessels. The length of the duodenum attached to the pancreas should be kept as short as possible to preserve an adequate blood supply.

## Heart and lungs

Just prior to stopping ventilation the superior vena cava is ligated and the inferior vena cava is divided to empty the right heart and the left atrial appendage is opened to empty the left side of the heart. After emptying the heart the aorta is cross-clamped and cardioplagic solution, which contains a high concentration of potassium, is given to arrest the heart and cools the myocardium. If the lungs are being retrieved ventilation is continued and the lungs are perfused via the pulmonary arteries with preservation solution such as EuroCollins solution which will allow 6 h of cold ischaemia. The heart and lungs can then be excised en bloc by dividing the superior vena cava and transecting and stapling the trachea with the lungs fully inflated.

## Small bowel retrieval

Donor retrieval of the liver and small bowel en bloc follows the same basic principles as for the liver alone. A nasogastric tube should be inserted to instil antibiotics to include colistin, tobramycin or neomycin and amphotericin. Following a midline incision the donor aorta is mobilised and the inferior mesenteric artery is ligated. The duodenum and head of pancreas and the right colon are fully mobilised. The portal vein is cannulated via the inferior mesenteric or splenic vein. Once the cannulas are in the aorta and portal vein, heparin is given, the supra-coeliac aorta is cross-clamped and UW solution infused giving 1 l into the aorta and 2 l into the portal vein. Blood is vented via the suprahepatic cava above the diaphragm and/or via the infrahepatic inferior vena cava below the renal veins. Larger volumes of preservation solution may cause bowel oedema and subsequent graft dysfunction.

The liver is then resected en bloc with the pancreas and small bowel. Included in this are the common hepatic artery and coeliac trunk on a Carrel patch of aorta together with the superior mesenteric artery. The portal vein, duodenum and head of pancreas are removed in continuity with the superior mesenteric artery and vein and the whole small bowel. The small bowel is divided at the level of the second part of the duodenum and the distal ileum using an intestinal stapler. Subsequent dissection either to separate an isolated small bowel graft or as a combined liver–small bowel graft is undertaken as a back table procedure. It is essential to retrieve a length of common and external iliac artery and vein for vascular reconstruction during the recipient operation. The graft should be transported in UW solution at 4°C and transplanted within 6 h of preservation. (Further details are given in Chapter 10.)

## New techniques and surgical variations

Over the last ten years the number of donors considered for multiorgan donation has continued to increase and on occasion there may be multiple retrieval teams present to perform sequential dissections which may prolong the procedure. Several 'rapid' techniques have been described to retrieve the intra-abdominal organs, particularly the liver and pancreas, in an attempt to minimise dissection and retrieval injury.[40,41]

The majority of centres have employed a technique of careful dissection in the donor as previously described. Rapid retrieval of a block of tissue to include the liver and pancreas has been advocated. Following the standard midline incision, the right colon is mobilised and reflected to the left and the duodenum Kocherised to reveal the distal abdominal aorta and inferior vena cava which are then prepared for subsequent cannulation. The left renal vein marks the proximal extent of the mobilisation to avoid injury to renal arteries or an unrecognised right hepatic artery from the superior mesenteric artery. A search is then made for an accessory left hepatic artery from the left gastric artery and triangular ligament and gastrohepatic ligament are divided. The aorta is isolated just below the diaphragm. The fundus of the gall bladder is opened and the bile is aspirated and then flushed with saline. After the other retrieval teams have completed their dissection 20 000 units of heparin are given intravenously and a cannula inserted in the distal aorta. The infradiaphragmatic aorta is clamped and the aorta flushed with 3–4 l of UW solution depending on the size of the donor.

The aorta is divided just below the clamp and the SMA is then exposed. The aorta is then incised anteriorly just below the SMA origin and a patch of aorta is taken which includes the SMA and coeliac axis, leaving the origins of the renal arteries well alone. The retroperitoneal tissue is dissected to free the whole bloc posteriorly.

## Allocation of organs

Since the demand for organs has outstripped the supply, the transplant clinician is often faced with many possible recipients for each organ. In most cases the organ is given to a patient with a compatible blood group although liver transplantation is sometimes carried out across this barrier where the risks of poorer graft outcome are outweighed by greater risk of death before a blood group compatible organ becomes available. In renal transplantation the HLA match remains one of the most important factors in determining who should receive the kidney graft. However, there is variation even in this aspect of organ allocation given that the geography of large countries such as United States of America will sometimes encourage the use of a slightly less good match, but much shorter cold ischaemic times. Since there are many potential renal failure patients for each possible graft, many details of the patient may be used to aid organ allocation over and above the tissue match. These include age of the patient, age of the donor, time on dialysis, level of antibodies and number of previous transplants. Many clinicians prefer to make the final decision about organ allocation based on the above details, but without any strict protocol to guide them. They feel that such flexibility enables the best recipient/donor combination. However, the complexity of these decisions has encouraged point scoring systems with each of the above details awarded points which are then totalled for each potential recipient. The patient with the most points is the likely recipient of the kidney graft. Proponents of such a system argue that it is demonstrably objective and this provides a defence against charges of bias towards one patient or towards one section of patients.

Most centres include all renal transplant or all potential renal transplant recipients on the same level of urgency for transplantation. This is because renal failure patients can fall back onto dialysis except in unusual circumstances where there is a crisis in achieving access for that dialysis. This is not the case for patients in acute fulminant liver failure. Many countries have put in place special schemes whereby such patients are offered an organ preferentially. In the United Kingdom, this scheme is coordinated by the United Kingdom Transplant Support Service Authority (UKTSSA). When a patient fulfils strict criteria for inclusion on a 'super urgent' list for liver transplantation, UKTSSA ensure that this patient takes precedence over others waiting on the list for a liver transplant.[42] This degree of urgency is necessary as it is assumed that such urgent patients have a prognosis of less than three days.

**Living-related organ donations**

Despite theoretical and practical advantages, living donation of organs has not found widespread ethical acceptance given that the only benefit to the donor is psychological. The use of living related donors in kidney transplantation is widely practised in North America and Scandinavia, but not in the United Kingdom. Reservations remain about the ethics of subjecting a healthy donor to surgery for the benefit of a relative.[43] The risks of a significant complication after living-related kidney donation are about 2% with a reported mortality of 1:1600.[44] Reported complications include operative problems such as haemorrhage, pneumothorax, wound infection and hernia. Longer-term problems include depression and mild proteinuria, but progressive deterioration of renal function 20 years after donation does not appear to occur.

Living-related liver donation of the left lateral segment is likely to have a higher complication rate. To date there has been one donor death, from pulmonary embolus 3 days after liver donation, reported after approximately 500 living-related liver transplants. Other complications occurring in about 5% of cases have included bile leak, bleeding, small bowel obstruction, wound infection and incisional hernia.[45] The long-term risks of hepatectomy are unknown. However, in countries lacking legislation to diagnose brain stem death, living-related liver transplantation is a significant development in the management of children with end-stage liver disease.[46,47] There is a small, but definite need for this operation in selected cases. The current increase in the number of liver transplants being performed inevitably increases the competition between adult and paediatric transplant programmes for liver grafts, particularly younger donors. Split liver transplantation is helping to offset these problems but children who face a potentially long wait for transplantation should, if their families are considered suitable, be offered living-related liver transplantation.

### Donor selection and assessment

In the initial approach to the family, it is most important to put forward the options available for transplantation. The paediatric hepatologist or nephrologist and nurse specialists provide the initial approach regarding liver or kidney transplantation and may if requested provide information about living-related donation. In considering family suitability, such factors as parental health and employment and the number and health of children become important. Common sense has to be applied to the screening of potential donors, excluding families from living donation, for example, if there are several dependent children, a single parent, or if there are serious financial implications for the family.

Simple screening tests should be performed to ensure the potential donors have no health risks with normal cardiac, respiratory, renal and liver function and that there is an ABO blood group match. These tests will exclude approximately 50% of parents as potential donors. Medical and psychiatric assessments of potential donors are performed by medical staff (not involved in the transplant programme) to verify the voluntary nature of the donation and establish that there are no additional donor risk factors. An important part of the independent assessment is ensuring that the family understands the nature of the operation, the alternatives and the risks involved.[44] Consent in our institution has to be given on two occasions separated by a two week interval to allow adequate time to reconsider the decision to go forward as a potential donor. An important part of the consent is to assure the parents/donors that alternatives to living-related transplantation are available. The relationship of the donor to the recipient must be confirmed by genetic HLA typing by a recognised testing centre.

### Living-related kidney donation

It is important to exclude renal disease by performing urine analysis, 24 h urinary protein excretion, intravenous urography and measurements of the creatinine clearance. If the donor is suitable medically then renal angiography should be performed to exclude any arterial or venous abnormality.

### Living-related liver donation

To ensure that the size of the liver graft is a suitable size match for the recipient, estimations can be made from a comparison of body weight. More precise estimations of the left lateral segment size can be made by CT scan or nuclear magnetic resonance scan and potential grafts with a volume of less than 350 ml accepted (for children under 5 years of age). We have used selective hepatic angiography to assess the arterial supply to the donor liver and at present would consider that a bilateral arterial duplication is a contraindication to living-related liver donation. In countries without cadaveric transplant programmes such vascular anomalies are not considered an absolute contraindication and back table reconstruction of the arterial supply has been successfully performed by microvascular surgeons using operating microscopes. In these units angiography is not considered an essential part of the donor investigation as they are prepared to reconstruct any arterial variant found at donor surgery.

### Donor surgery

#### *Kidney*

Most centres prefer to use the left kidney because of the greater length of the left renal vein. The patient is positioned lying on the right side with a break in the table underlying the 12th rib. The incision is made from the tip of the 12th rib towards the umbilicus as far as the lateral border of the rectus sheath. The underlying muscle layers are divided taking care not to enter the peritoneal cavity or the pleural space. The peritoneum is displaced and Gerota's fascia incised. The kidney is mobilised by gentle dissection. The hilum is identified and the left renal vein is mobilised anteriorly. The left adrenal and gonadal veins are ligated and divided and the renal vain is mobilised to the junction with the inferior vena cava. The posterior aspect of the kidney is freed and the artery mobilised up to the aorta. After complete mobilisation of the kidney the ureter is mobilised taking care not to devascularise it. Both renal vessels are clamped with vascular clamps and the kidney removed and flushed on the back table with cold preservation solution (containing heparin and antibiotics as for cadaveric preservation). The wound is then closed.

### Liver

The patient is explored through a bilateral subcostal incision which can be extended in the midline to the xiphisternum (Mercedes incision). The falciform ligament is divided and the triangular flaps comprising the skin and abdominal muscles are sutured to the chest wall and a retractor positioned to expose the liver. The falciform and left triangular ligaments are divided and the left lobe is mobilised. The right lobe can be mobilised to isolate the supra- and infrahepatic inferior vena cava.

The porta hepatis is then dissected to identify the common hepatic artery and its bifurcation. Having identified the left branch of the hepatic artery, the left branch of the portal vein is isolated and caudate lobe branches are transfixed and divided. The left hepatic duct should be isolated, but not divided until after the parenchymal dissection has been completed. The left hepatic vein is then isolated. The liver capsule is incised using point diathermy to mark the plane of dissection to the right of the falciform ligament. The liver parenchyma is divided using an ultrasonic dissector taking care to ligate or transfix all vessels and biliary radicles that are encountered to minimise blood loss. After completion of the parenchymal dissection the left branch of the portal vein, left hepatic artery and left hepatic vein are clamped and the left lateral segment excised. Haemostasis is achieved and fibrin glue applied to the cut surface. The graft is taken to the back-table and immediately perfused with cold UW solution (containing heparin and antibiotics as for cadaveric preservation). Reconstruction of the donor portal vein and artery may be necessary, but depends on the recipient anatomy and vessel size.

## Conclusion

The success of solid organ transplantation has led to a universal shortage of donor organs and an increasing number of potentially suitable patients dying without treatment. There has been a gradual reduction in the overall number of donors because of the fall in deaths from road traffic and cerebrovascular accidents. Increased awareness and good publicity concerning the benefits of organ donation and transplantation increase the number of donors, but the effect is short lived. Debate continues over the potential advantages of 'opt out' versus 'opt in' organ donation policies at a national level but even successful 'opt out' legislation is unlikely to provide sufficient donors for a comprehensive clinical service. Exclusion of patients on the basis of age, disease or social circumstance is not ethically right. Improved patient selection, better use of marginal grafts, fewer organs lost to logistical problems and improved graft survival are all important. Living-related donation is an option to be considered for selected patients and families. Xenotransplantation may provide a solution for heart and kidney transplantation, but is unlikely to be satisfactory for liver replacement in the near future.

### Acknowledgement
I am grateful to Dr Vilca-Melendez for the diagrams.

# References

1. Department of Health and Social Security. Cadaveric organs for transplantation. A code of practice including the diagnosis of brain death. London, Health Departments of Great Britain and Northern Ireland, 1983.
2. Kaufmann HH, Lynne J. Brain death. Neurosurgery 1986; 19: 850–6.
3. Criteria for the diagnosis of brain stem death. Working party review 1995. J R Coll Phys 1995; 29: 381–2.
4. Gore SM, Ross Taylor RM, Wallwork J. Availability of transplantable organs from brain stem dead donors in intensive care units. Br Med J 1991; 302: 149–53.
5. New W, Solomon M, Dingwall R, McHale J. A question of give and take: improving the supply of donor organs for transplantation. London. King's Fund Institute. 1994; Research Report 18.
6. Matesanz R, Miranda B, Felipe C. Organ procurement in Spain: impact of transplant coordination. Clin Transplant 1994; 8: 281–6.
7. Bodenham A, Berridge JC, Park GR. Brain stem death and organ donation. Br Med J 1989; 299: 1009–10.
8. Gore SM, Hinds CJ, Rutherford AJ. Organ donation from intensive care units in England. Br Med J 1989; 299: 1193–7.
9. Feest TG, Riad HN, Collins CH et al. Protocol for increasing organ donation after cerebrovascular deaths in a district general hospital. Lancet 1990; 335: 1133–5.
10. Collins CH. Elective ventilation for organ donation – the case in favour. Care Crit Ill 1992; 8: 57–9.
11. Michielson P. The introduction of an opting-out law in Belgium doubled organ retrieval. In: Sirchia G et al. (eds). Proceedings of the Second

International Meeting on Organisational Aspects of Transplantation, Ospedale Maggiore Policlinico di Milano, Milan, 1992.
12. Arnold RM, Youngner SJ. Back to the future: obtaining organs from non heart beating cadaver donors. Kennedy Inst Ethics J 1993; 3: 103–11.
13. Oomen A, Daemen JHC, Cumberland BG, Koostra G. Non-heart beating donors: a useful way to decrease the organ shortage. Challenges in immunosuppression No 2. High Wycombe, Holmes and Marchant Counseller, 1996.
14. Koostra G, Ruers IJM, Vroemen JPAM. Non-heart-beating donor: contribution to the organ shortage. Transplant Proc 1986; 18: 1410–12.
15. Koostra G, Wijnen R, van Hooff JP, van der Linden CJ. Twenty per cent more kidneys through a non-heart beating program. Transplant Proc 1991; 23: 910–11.
16. Casavilla A, Ramirez C, Shapiro R et al. Experience with kidney and liver allografts from non-heart-beating donors. Transplantation 1995; 59: 197–203.
17. D'Alessandro DM, Hoffman RM, Knechtle SJ et al. Successful extrarenal transplantation from non-heart-beating donors. Transplantation 1995; 59: 977–82.
18. Bodenham A, Park GR. Care of the multiple organ donor. Intensive Care Med 1989; 15: 340–8.
19. Jordan CA, Snyder JV. Intensive care and intraoperative management of the brain-dead organ donor. Transplant Proc 1987; 19: 21–5.
20. Brink LW, Ballew A. Care of the paediatric organ donor. Am J Dis Child 1992; 146: 1045.
21. Wijnen RMH, van der Linden CJ. Donor pretreatment after pronouncement of brain death:

a neglected intensive care problem. Transplant Int 1991; 4: 186–90.

22. Whelchel JD, Diethelm AG, Phillips MG, Rhyder WR, Schein LG. The effect of high-dose dopamine in cadaver donor management on delayed graft function and graft survival following renal transplantation. Transplant Proc 1986; 18: 523–7.

23. Novitzky D, Rhodin J, Cooper DKC, Ye Y, Min KW, DeBault L. Ultrastructural changes associated with brain death in the human donor heart. Transplant Int 1997; 10: 24–32.

24. Novitzky D, Cooper DKC, Morrell D, Isaacs S. Change from aerobic to anaerobic metabolism after brain death and reversal following tri-iodothyronine therapy. Transplantation 1988; 45: 32–6.

25. Lucas BA, Baughn WK, Spees EK, Sanfillipo F. Identification of donor factors predisposing to high discard rates of cadaver kidneys and increased graft loss within one year post transplantation. Transplantation 1987; 43: 253–8.

26. Odom NJ. Organ donation. Br Med J 1990; 300: 1571–3.

27. Gore SM, Armitage WJ, Briggs JD et al. Consensus on general medical contraindications to organ donation? Br Med J 1992; 305: 406–9.

28. Odom NJ. II – Logistical disincentives to organ donation. Br Med J 1990; 300: 1573–5.

29. Pruim J, Klompmaker IJ, Haagsma EB, Bijleveld MA, Slooff MJH. Selection criteria for liver donation: a review. Transplant Int 1993; 6: 226–35.

30. Copeland JG, Emery RW, Levinson MM et al. Selection of patients for cardiac transplantation. Circulation 1987; 75: 2–9.

31. Emery RW, Cork RC, Levinson MM et al. The cardiac donor: a six year experience. Ann Thorac Surg 1986; 41: 356–62.

32. Harjula A, Starnes VA, Oyer PE, Jamieson SW, Shumway NE. Proper donor selection for heart-lung transplantation. J Thorac Cardiovasc Surg 1987; 94: 874–80.

33. Winton TL, Miller JD, Scavuzzo M, Maurer JR, Patterson GA. Donor selection for pulmonary transplantation. Transplant Proc 1991; 23: 2472–4.

34. Sutherland DER, Gruessner RWG, Gores PF et al. Pancreas and islet transplantation: an update. Transplant Rev 1994; 8: 185–206.

35. Makowka L, Gordon RD, Todo GS et al. Analysis of donor criteria for the prediction of outcome in clinical liver transplantation. Transplant Proc 1987; 19: 2378–82.

36. Belzer FO, Southard JH. Principles of solid organ preservation by cold storage. Transplantation 1988; 45: 673–6.

37. Collins GM, Bravo-Shugarman M, Terasaki PI. Kidney preservation for transportation: initial perfusion and 30 hours ice storage. Lancet 1969; ii: 1219–22.

38. Starzl TE, Hakala TR, Shaw BW et al. A flexible procedure for multiple cadaveric organ procurement. Surg Gynecol Obstet 1984; 58: 223–30.

39. Starzl TE, Miller C, Broznick B, Makowka L. An improved technique for multiple organ harvesting. Surg Gynecol Obstet 1987; 165: 343–8.

40. Margreiter R, Konigsrainer A, Schmid Th, Takahashi N, Pernthaler H, Ofner D. Multiple organ procurement – a safe and simple procedure. Transplant Proc 1991; 23: 2307–8.

41. Goyet J de Ville, Reding R, Hausleithner V, Lerut J, Otte J-B. Standardized quick en bloc technique for procurement of cadaveric liver grafts for pediatric liver transplantation. Transplant Int 1995; 8: 280–5.

42. Halliday NP. Provision of transplant services. Balliere's clinical gastroenterology 1994; 8: 399–410.

43. Busuttil RW. Living-related liver donation. Transplant Proc 1991; 23: 4–45.

44. Singer PA, Siegler M, Whittington PF et al. Ethics of liver transplantation with living donors. N Engl J Med 1989; 321: 620–2.

45. Broelsch CE, Whitington PF, Emond JC et al. Liver transplantation in children from living related donors. Ann Surg 1991; 214: 428–38.

46. Ozawa K, Uemoto S, Tanaka K et al. An appraisal of pediatric liver transplantation from living relatives. Initial clinical experiences in 20 pediatric liver transplantations from living relatives as donors. Ann Surg 1992; 216: 547–53.

47. Morimoto T, Ichimiya M, Tanaka A et al. Guidelines for donor selection and an overview of the donor operation in living related liver transplantation. Transplant Int 1996; 9: 208–13.

# 3 Matching the graft to the recipient

*David Talbot*
*Derek Manas*

**Introduction**

The surgical techniques of renal transplantation were described long before the realisation of the need to match graft and recipient. Operative success was therefore turned into immunological failure by hyperacute rejection.[1] The ideal match between identical twins allowed successful renal transplantation and encouraged further development in this field. As immunosuppressive therapy has become more sophisticated and powerful, clinicians may believe that similarities between donor and recipient are not vital. However, the results of solid organ transplantation continue to demonstrate an improved graft survival after matching the donor and the recipient in a number of different ways.

Blood group and tissue typing remain important factors to match between donor and recipient. Developments in the technique of tissue typing have contributed to improve graft survival. In contrast, a number of groups have argued that enhanced graft survival is seen in the face of poor tissue match provided the ischaemic times are kept as short as possible. Such debate fuels argument between those who say that the organ should travel to the best match and those who say that a reasonable match nearer to the donor is preferable. In addition, avoiding reaction between preformed antibody in the recipient and donor tissue may be vital. Increased sensitivity of assays for detection of antibody have refined this form of testing between donor and recipient. Age has also become a factor with the increasing use of elderly donors: most clinicians involved in solid organ transplantation will avoid a large mismatch in age between the donor and the recipient. Finally, there are alternative strategies in matching different organs such that each of the factors mentioned above may need to be considered for each type of organ transplant.

**Age matching**

In the past, recipient age in excess of 55 years was considered an absolute contraindication to all forms of solid organ transplantation. However, advances in anaesthesia, improved preoperative assessment and better intensive care have resulted in an increasing number of elderly recipients undergoing successful transplantation. The selection process becomes more vital with advancing age of potential recipient. If this process is run well, results can be very satisfactory.[2]

## Kidneys

### The recipient

Patients in their eighth decade can be safely transplanted if carefully selected.[3] It is now quite evident that age alone is not the major factor which defines risk for anaesthesia; the physiological age is far more important than the chronological age. Further, it has been demonstrated[4] that the incidence of myocardial infarction, cerebrovascular accident and complicated peripheral vascular disease remain constant whether or not the elderly renal failure patient remains on dialysis or receives a kidney transplant.

The older diabetic patient with end-stage renal failure remains problematic. Liberal use of invasive and non-invasive imaging allows detection of elderly atherosclerotic diabetics who have non-correctable lesions or limited potential for rehabilitation. These patients may be best advised to remain on dialysis and not undergo transplantation.[5]

At the opposite end of the spectrum, experience suggests that recipients below the age of 5 years fare less well than older children. In contrast, the results of live-related donation in the 1–5 age group have been more rewarding.

### The donor

Results of renal transplantation demonstrate that donor age has an important influence on long-term graft survival.[6] Figures for donors older than 55 years are significantly worse when compared with donors younger than 55 years (half-life of the graft is 6 years and 10 years, respectively). In addition, kidneys from older donors transplanted into patients with high immunological risk demonstrated a 1 year graft survival below 50%.

Similarly, kidneys from donors under 10 years old have a graft survival significantly less than those over 10 years.[7] Other groups have confirmed these results and recommend conservative use of young donor kidneys into young adult recipients.[8]

### Matching

Donor and recipient age match has little or no known relevance between the ages of 5 and 60 years. In contrast, an attempt should be made to match for age if the donor or recipient fall outside this range.

Although certain groups have had acceptable results,[9] surgical practicalities of a high risk anastomosis and relative adult kidney 'bulk' in small recipients make a good argument for age matching in the young recipient. In addition, if recipients over the age of 65 years are dying from cardiovascular disease, with functioning grafts from young donors, the dialysis community is not gaining maximum benefit from the scarce donor pool. As a result, many centres adopt a selective policy in the elderly recipient 'old kidneys for old recipients'.

## Hearts

### The recipient

Before 1985, no patient aged over 50 years who received a heart transplant survived for more than 2 years.[10] Due to better monitoring of the graft, improved immunosuppression and advanced intensive care techniques, improved survival has been experienced in several centres.[11] Recipients up to the age of 60 years are assessed by most centres. However, the potential complications which increase with age due to comorbidity, coupled with the limited resources of any transplant centre mean that older candidates need to be reviewed in a very critical manner. Again, a policy of 'older donors for older recipients' may be followed. However, the number of suitable older donors is very limited due to the presence of other disease processes in the donor which preclude retrieval. Therefore, older potential recipients may not have the same opportunities of a cardiac transplant.[12]

### The donor

During the last decade, the criteria for donors has gradually been extended in an effort to meet the increased demand. As a result the donor age limit has risen from 35 years to 55 years. However, data from the International Society for Heart and Lung Transplantation Registry has revealed an increased mortality for recipients if the heart has come from a donor aged over 40 years.[13] There is a fear of unrecognised coronary artery disease or previous myocardial infarction with increasing age of the donor. Current recommended practice is to consider all donors up to the age of 40 years and appropriate screening and consideration of donation is arranged for potential donors up to 55 years old. Older donor hearts with significant coronary artery disease have been used as 'human bridges'[14] but only in exceptional circumstances.

## Livers

### The recipient

Results of orthotopic liver transplantation have improved considerably over the past decade. In the period before 1980 a 1-year survival rate of 32% was reported. Most centres are now reporting survival rates in excess of 80%.[15] This improvement is in part due to better immunosuppression with cyclosporin, but also due to better postoperative management, refinements in surgical technique and improved patient selection. But such success has meant that the age limit for transplantation is being liberalised. Ten years ago a recipient age range of 1 to 55 years was a standard recommendation.[16] Most centres would now consider extremes of age as a relative contraindication and any potential recipient over the age of 65 years or under the age of 1 month would be evaluated on an individual basis. The potential for complete recovery and rehabilitation after liver transplantation requires to be fully assessed.

### The donor

Failure of the donor liver to function adequately following transplantation (primary non-function) is devastating to the patient and requires retransplantation. As yet no practical method is available to assess viability of the graft prior to implantation. For a long time, older donors with long-standing medical conditions were excluded as a way of avoiding such complications. Unfortunately this was no guarantee of adequate allograft function even with the availability of on-site frozen section histology to identify the unacceptable donor livers.[17]

Faced with the death of potential recipients on the waiting list, most centres have attempted to expand the donor pool by relaxing donation criteria. This involves use of so-called 'marginal livers'. Included in this group are older donors and those with associated medical conditions such as diabetes, hypertension and ischaemic heart disease. Gruenberger et al.[18] considered the influence of donor criteria on postoperative graft function and found donor age not to be a significant risk factor in determining early function provided liver function tests were normal. Recent unpublished data from Mount Sinai Medical Centre (New York), (personal communication) have confirmed this fact in a group of donors with a mean age of 73 years.

### Matching

Matching of the donor and recipient pair for age is not a pre-requisite for successful liver transplantation. In the adult population, 'old donors for old recipients' is certainly not a practical option in view of the limited donor pool and size restraints which need to be taken into account. In the paediatric age group, lack of paediatric donors has, over the last decade, led to the expanded use of reduced size adult grafts, split-liver grafts[19] and living related lateral segment grafts[20] from adults or large children. Although early results demonstrated a steep learning curve, segments of adult livers into children have reduced paediatric waiting list mortality to below 10% and overall survival reported by most units is very acceptable.[21]

## Size matching

### Kidneys

Matching kidneys for size appears to be important under certain circumstances. According to Brenner's hyperfiltration hypothesis, kidneys with reduced renal mass will progress towards failure due to hypertrophy of the remaining nephrons to meet the excess load, eventually leading to nephron exhaustion. Hyperfiltration may be related to size and this could be relevant in conditions of major size mismatch, for example when small kidneys from donors aged 4 months to 6 years are transplanted into large recipients weighing more than 100 kg.[22] Experimental work in rats has shown that reducing renal mass to one-fifth normal results in hyperfiltration and from a clinical point of view, lower graft survival rates have been reported when the donor's graft was too small for the recipient.[23] Vincenti *et al.*[24] showed that in kidneys from donors aged 6 months to 4 years, solitary kidneys had a 12% lower 1-year graft survival rate when compared with a similar group of 302 en bloc paired kidneys in recipients more than 15 years old.

## Heart

An attempt should be made to match the muscle mass of the donor heart to the expected cardiac output requirement of the recipient. The difference between donor and recipient body size and weight should be no greater than 20%. This should prevent the 'too small' heart from a large filling pressure and fast heart rate in order to achieve the appropriate increase in cardiac output. Most centres accept hearts from donors with a donor/recipient weight ratio of 0.8 or greater. However, donor body weight does not always predict heart size and muscle mass; often added weight simply reflects obesity. The body height should also be considered, as this often reflects cardiac output. Therefore, in obese inactive recipients height may be more appropriate in terms of matching heart size to young non-obese donors. Finally, pulmonary hypertension in the recipient requires a donor heart equal to or greater than the estimated heart size for the recipient's ideal body weight.[12]

## Liver

Donated livers are matched with recipients on the basis of weight combined with ABO compatibility. Donor size should be as closely matched to the recipient as possible.[25] In most adult programmes this does not present a problem because donor weight usually predicts the graft size. Potential recipients with significant ascites or very small 'shrunken' livers (e.g. primary biliary cirrhosis), very often have enough space in their abdominal cavities for a much larger donor liver. Occasionally, recipient or donor weight simply reflects obesity and in these instances donor height may need to be considered.

In recent years reduced volume allograft techniques have been developed to overcome the shortage of cadaveric organs for infants and young children, as well as adults with fulminant hepatic failure or early graft failure, when a donor of appropriate size cannot be found. Broadly speaking three techniques exist: 'cut-down', 'split liver' and live-related donation.

The technical details are beyond the scope of this chapter but, unlike whole liver transplantation, unexpected size mismatch between the reduced size donor liver and the recipient's liver has become one of the most common graft-related complications. Although Bismuth and

Houssin[26] reported their first success in 1984, optimal size of the reduced-size donor liver for safe grafting remains largely undefined. Recent animal work suggests that recipient survival rates decrease when the ratio of the donor to recipient liver weight is less than 0.35:1, i.e. when the donor liver mass is reduced to 35% or less of the recipient. On the other hand, reduced recipient survival rates were also found when the ratio was increased to 1.56:1 or more and the range of ratios for successful rat liver transplantation was therefore noted to be from 0.53:1 to 1.26:1.[25] From a practical point of view, a size reduction for a left lateral segment transplantation should conform to a donor:recipient weight ratio of less than 10:1 and preferably of the order of 7:1. Optimal size matching remains unknown, but it is clear that donor liver size should be as close to recipient size as possible for best survival, especially in reduced volume allografts or marginal donors.

**Tissue typing**   From the early days of transplantation the need for some similarity in tissue antigens was appreciated. At its simplest this was by ABO blood grouping. In general, blood group O donors were universal donors and could be used for A or B recipients as well as blood group O. In practice, there are more people of blood group O waiting for any organ than patients of other blood groups. Therefore group O donors donate to group O recipients in the vast majority of cases. In a similar manner, other rules of blood transfusion are followed except lesser blood groups such as Rhesus or Duffy do not have a significant effect on organ transplantation. The liver transplant is a relatively immuno-privileged site. Therefore, one can consider placing a blood group-incompatible liver into a recipient, if the circumstances of that recipient indicate that delay to obtain a matched graft would be dangerous, e.g. fulminant hepatic failure or primary graft non-function. However, this action also carries increased risk of rejection and poorer long-term graft survival. In this difficult situation, the relative risks must be balanced for each individual.

With the identification of the major histocompatibility complexes in the mouse, steps were taken to identify and classify these in humans. The class I major histocompatibility antigens which are carried by all cells, are identified as A, B and C of the human leucocyte antigen (HLA) and are encrypted on chromosome 6. Similarly the class II antigens which are carried by antigen presenting cells and certain other activated cells are denoted as DR of the human leucocyte antigens.

The C antigen of HLA relates to complement components, does not have much variation between individuals and so has no clinical relevance to transplantation. The A and B antigens are identified as significant to the course of transplantation because they are present on all peripheral circulating lymphocytes, and prone to large variation. The relevance of the DR antigen was determined later because lymphocytes from peripheral blood consist of approximately 85% T lymphocytes which in their inactivated state are free of DR antigen. Therefore, to type

**Table 3.1**  *Complete list of HLA-A, HLA-B and HLA-DR antigen specificities (World Health Organization Report from 11th Workshop on HLA Nomenclature, 1991). As technology has advanced, subsets or 'splits' have been defined within more broad specificity number, e.g. A9 → A23, A24. This is expressed as A9, A23(9), A24(9). Provisional or 'working' classifications are shown as Bw4, Bw6.*

| A | | B | | | | DR | |
|---|---|---|---|---|---|---|---|
| A1 | A32(19) | B5 | B3901 | B54(22) | B76(15) | DR1 | DR16(2) |
| A2 | A33(19) | B7 | B3902 | B55(22) | B77(15) | DR103 | DR17(3) |
| A203 | A34(10) | B703 | B40 | B56(22) | B7801 | DR2 | DR18(3) |
| A210 | A35 | B8 | B4005 | B57(17) | Bw4 | DR3 | DR51 |
| A3 | A36 | B12 | B41 | B58(17) | Bw5 | DR4 | DR52 |
| A9 | A43 | B13 | B42 | B59 B | | DR5 | DR53 |
| A10 | A66(10) | B14 | B44(12) | B60(40) | | DR6 | |
| A11 | A68(28) | B15 | B45(12) | B61(40) | | DR7 | |
| A19 | A69(28) | B16 | B46 | B62(15) | | DR8 | |
| A23(9) | A74(19) | B17 | B47 | B63(15) | | DR9 | |
| A24(9) | | B18 | B48 | B64(14) | | DR10 | |
| A2403 | | B21 | B49(21) | B65(14) | | DR11(5) | |
| A25(10) | | B22 | B50(21) | B67 | | DR12(5) | |
| A26(10) | | B27 | B51(5) | B70 | | DR13(6) | |
| A28 | | B35 | B5102 | B71(70) | | DR14 | |
| A29(19) | | B37 | B5103 | B72(70) | | DR1403 | |
| A30(19) | | B38(16) | B52(5) | B73 | | DR1404 | |
| A31(19) | | B39(16) | B53 | B75(15) | | DR15(2) | |

for DR antigen the minority B lymphocytes have first to be separated and then typed. The presence of haplotype pairing means that for each gene locus of the major histocompatibility complex there are two antigens produced, according to genetic inheritance. Each individual carries two specificities for each of A, B and DR, unless identical antigens are inherited from both parents (such people are said to be 'homozygous') (Table 3.1).

The process of recipient tissue typing is performed on peripheral blood lymphocytes. The donor is typed also by peripheral blood lymphocytes prior to organ harvesting. The lymphocytes are separated by centrifugation over ficol.[27] This generates a mixture of B and T lymphocytes which formerly were separated using sheep red cells made more adherent by pretreatment with 2-aminoethisothiouronium bromide. The sheep red cells form rosettes around T lymphocytes which have receptors for the erythrocytes whereas B cells do not. These rosettes can be separated by centrifugation over ficol and then the enriched T cells treated with ammonium chloride which lyses the more sensitive sheep erythrocytes.[28] The separated B lymphocytes can then be typed for class II. This somewhat quaint technique has been superseded by the use of monoclonal antibodies to T or B cells which are conjugated to iron particles. The relevant coated cells can then be drawn to the side of the test tube by the application of a magnet. The remaining cells are removed by pouring off the liquid cell suspension and the magnetic cells suspended in new liquid after the magnet is removed.

After isolation of the lymphocytes the cell suspension is aliquoted into a tissue typing plate which contains known antisera in different wells. Because the volumes used are very small (1$\mu$l of serum to 1$\mu$l of cell suspension) the plates are covered in a thin film of oil, the cell suspension being added below it. After incubation, either at room temperature or 37°C a small volume of complement is added. This is usually a freeze dried compound derived from animal sera and reconstituted prior to use. The most effective animal source of complement for use with human antisera has been found to be the rabbit. After a further period of incubation the cells are then tested for viability. This is done using a viability stain which at the most simplest is eosin or methylene blue. Greater sensitivity is found with fluorescent stains such as propidium iodide, acridine orange or carboxyfluorescein diacetate. In this way it is even possible to automate the assay for reading by measuring the intensity of fluorescence with a photomultiplier tube. However, varying numbers of cells in the well produce different intensities of fluorescence and are, therefore, prone to error.[29]

In this way the tissue typing plate will provide a number of positive and negative wells and knowing the distribution of the antisera the tissue type can be identified. A class I plate is used for separated T lymphocytes and a class II plate for B cells. In this way an A, B and DR type can be determined.

### DNA typing

One of the problems in conventional serological tissue typing as described above is that it depends on living cells retrieved from the donor. As the sample of blood, spleen or lymph node is obtained from a living being the sample starts to deteriorate from the moment it is removed. This has little relevance for the first few hours but after this time period the background cell death increases. Consequently serological typing with time becomes complex as more background staining causes the reading of results to become more difficult. This means that the initial type is the most important. However, it is known that a fair degree of variation in sensitivity and reproducibility exists between laboratories with up to 47.9% discrepancy rates.[30] This is particularly applicable to the more difficult class II antigens and of these split determinants are particularly troublesome. Consequently the description of graft function according to tissue match between donor and recipient must be entirely dependent on the reliability of the tissue typing laboratories. This fact must account for some of the variation in conclusions seen with DR matching in the early days.[31] Secondly, the donor is often tissue typed on peripheral blood before retrieval. If the number of B cells is low, as is often the case, then the class II result can be difficult to obtain. Such difficulties have been overcome with the use of DNA typing.

The methods developed are restriction fragment length polymorphism (RFLP) analysis and the more rapid polymerase chain reaction–sequence specific oligonucleotides (CPR-SSO). In the former genomic DNA from lymphocytes is digested by specific restriction endonuclease enzymes. The resulting liquid is aliquoted into gels and separated by electrophoresis. The gels with single-stranded DNA are then treated with radiolabelled probes which are specific DNA probes or class II DNA from homologous donors with known identity. They are then exposed to photographic paper which is developed and the hard copy identifies the tissue type according to the distribution of the probes.[32] The PCR-SSO relies on the isolation of a specific length of DNA which is selected by the relevant oligonucleotide probe and cleaved by enzymes with the resulting length of DNA amplified by PCR. This system, though rapid, can be difficult because of the PCR which also amplifies inappropriate contaminating DNA.[30] Improvements have come with the use of PCR-sequence specific primers.[33]

By using these DNA methods of determining class II antigens, tissue typing laboratories could improve the standard of typing and produce much more uniformity of results between centres. This meant that conclusions on the benefit of matching could be made with more certainty. Consequently reports on large numbers of renal transplants emerged from multicentre studies. Large discrepancies were detected between DNA typing and serological typing: 9.7% to 86.7%.[30] Correcting of the DR type by DNA typing, allowed examination of the true effect of DR mismatch on graft survival. A significant advantage was detected for a DR match.[34] Less change was made on class I matching by the new DNA methods as this had been more accurately evaluated by the older serological typing techniques.

## The benefit of HLA matching

With the success of living related transplantation, cadaveric programmes attempted to reproduce good results by HLA matching between donor and recipient. Part of the success of the living-related programmes was due to the short ischaemic times but the endurance of national organ sharing schemes is testimony to the widely held views that matching is important. The first loci which were considered important were class I (A and B) principally because they were the first to be typed. Of the two, the most important was held to be the B locus. Since the description of class II antigen it has been thought to be more important still, because antigen presentation was strongest when supported by class II antigen. Now most organ sharing schemes are positively biased in favour of DR matching. The former traditional approach was to describe the number of matched loci between donor and recipient.

For example a recipient of A1;B2,16;Dr2,4 and donor A1,2;B12,16;DR2 would be described as 1,1,1 match. However, this has since been changed because the importance was the difference between donor and recipient seen from the recipient's view point. Therefore, this combination would be described as a 1,1,0 mismatch.

Large multicentre series including the international registries have consistently shown that the worst results were found with six antigen mismatches and the best with 0. The strongest locus was found to be DR.

### Heart/liver

Organs other than renal grafts were not as clear initially but that situation is also now changing. Heart transplantation obeys the rules of matching with best results seen in a six antigen match.[35] Corneal transplants also appear to follow the trend with improved outcome with A and B HLA matching in some series[36] though this opinion is not universal. Liver transplantation revealed an opposite effect principally in one condition, namely primary biliary cirrhosis. This is essentially an autoimmune condition such that a maximally mismatched liver had a better outcome than did a well-matched combination. Other non-auto-immune liver conditions such as alcoholic cirrhosis had an improved outcome with matching.[34]

With the emergence of new immunosuppressive agents it has always been tempting to conclude that there is 'now' no role for donor/recipient matching. This was the situation with the emergence of cyclosporin when improved survival figures suggested that tissue matching need only be of minor importance. The important data to refute this came much later; even though the survival curves showed little benefit from matching in the early post-transplant period, between 5- and 10-year post-transplantation, the strongest positive indicator of outcome was a zero DR and B locus mismatch. Therefore, care should always be shown in claiming that a new drug has improved the survival until 10 years post-transplant. Though the area under the survival curve has changed, there has been no improvement beyond tissue matching since the advent of azathioprine and prednisolone in the 1960s.

### Lymphocytotoxic crossmatching

In the mid 1960s when only steroids and radiotherapy were available with the emergence of a new agent called azathioprine, human organ allotransplantation was a therapy with few successes. At that time it was noted that grafts were lost either very early, within minutes or after a week to 10 days. There was a keen interest in exploring the mechanisms of hyperacute rejection to give a chance to the immunosuppressive agents that were available. From this came the discovery that if donor cells were incubated with sera from the recipient, preformed antibodies could be identified in some cases. This finding was associated with hyperacute rejection. The more simplified cytotoxicity assay was developed by Paul Terasaki which used small volumes of sera and a low number of cells with an external source of complement.[29] This assay tested for complement binding antibody (IgG and IgM). By varying the temperature of incubation different conclusions could be extrapolated regarding the nature of the antibody; room temperature for IgM and 37°C for IgG.

The overwhelming conclusion from these early series was that it was mandatory to test for antibodies before transplantation. The situation was further clarified by identifying the importance of IgG, IgM accounting for a positive reaction but having limited relevance to organ rejection. This was done by deactivation of IgM with dithiothreitol. A cytotoxic crossmatch test remaining positive despite this indicated an IgG antibody. The separation of B from T cells led to the generally accepted principle in renal transplant units that a positive cross-match due to IgG to donor T cells was a contraindication to transplantation. This was due to immunological sensitisation of the recipient to donor class I antigen. Although some units suggested that transplanting in the face of a positive cytotoxic crossmatch in sera held from time past (historic sera) was acceptable, all units agreed that a positive current result in sera was not.

The evolving liver and cardiac transplant units dabbled in cytotoxic cross-matching but by and large concluded that the detection of donor directed antibodies carried no relevance to the outcome of transplantation.

## Panel reactivity

After transfusions, pregnancy and particularly after previous transplants the potential recipient often has anti HLA antibodies. These present a problem in so far as finding a suitable donor is more difficult. The incidence of these antibodies can be kept to a minimum by reducing the mismatch between donor and recipients as much as possible. The problem in a potential recipient can be described in terms of panel reactivity. This is done by taking about 20 different cell sources for lymphocytes and placing these in different wells and allowing incubation with test sera. The number of positive wells are then described as a percentage of the total. This describes adequately the degree of the problem though does not differentiate between IgG or IgM which has to be determined separately. In addition the target of the antibody is not known. This can be examined by varying the cell sources so that an approximate idea of the antibody specificity can be obtained by serology.

A better technique has now been developed which is an enzyme linked immunoabsorbent assay (ELISA) method. Here the wells are preloaded with soluble HLA antigens. The test serum is added and after washing anti-human IgG is added conjugated with peroxidase. This agent converts the inactive dye (such as phenylenediamine) which is added to each well after washing. The plates are then analysed by a plate reader which with the correct code will give the precise target of the recipient IgG. Using the same technique antibodies to other targets can be detected.[38] Excellent reproducibility has been produced between laboratories (99%) in comparison with that seen in the lymphocytotoxic crossmatch (78%).[39]

Potential renal recipients with high panel reactivity are difficult to transplant. However, those with additional access problems for dialysis require transplantation as a matter of urgency. Therefore, active measures are required to remove the cytotoxic antibodies and reduce the risk of hyperacute rejection. The subsequent survival of the graft is then dependent on the effectiveness of the immunosuppressive used. The removal of the antibodies is performed by either regular plasmaphoresis or immunoadsorption. The latter process consists of the passage of the patient's own blood through columns containing staphylococcal protein A which absorbs the majority of the patient's immunoglobulin. After treating in this way the recipient is either maintained in a deficient state by administration of cyclophosphamide or by non-HLA specific immunoglobulin (which is effective by negative feedback) until a suitable graft is obtained. Alternatively the next available graft is implanted no matter what the mismatch. The problem with the first approach is the risk of sepsis in the immunosuppressed state and the second approach has the risks of rejection in the mismatched, sensitised recipient. Both approaches are used by different groups in an attempt to treat this problematic group of patients.

### Flow cytometric cross-matching

Since the advent of conventional cytotoxic cross-matching in the 1960s research workers have frequently questioned whether this assay was enough. The conventional assay demanded donor directed antibody at sufficient concentrations to activate complement and produce cell death. In the case of IgM, the cytotoxic cross-match assay was probably sufficient as one molecule of IgM, being a pentamer, could activate complement and so penetrate the membrane. However, IgG had to be at sufficient concentrations to have two molecules close enough to bind complement. In addition the definition of a positive assay by the tissue typist inspecting the well for increased uptake of stain could also be open to error. Improvements were made at a simple level by changing the viability stain. Fluorescent viability stains such as propidium iodide, for dead, and carboxy fluorescein diacetate for living cells conferred an advantage in reading the wells and thereby the sensitivity of the assay was improved.

At about this time flow cytometry became available which allowed individual cell analysis rather than an automated system detecting the fluorescence of a whole population of cells. The latter system was therefore largely surpassed.

Garavoy[29] was the first to use flow cytometry for cross-matching. The donor cells after incubation with the test serum were incubated with an

**Figure 3.1**
*Diagrammatic
representation of the
flow cytometer.*

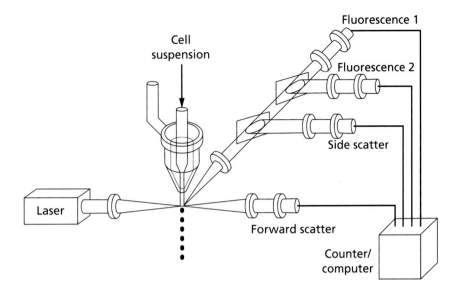

anti-immunoglobulin conjugated with a fluorescence label, usually fluorescein. The cells were then passed in a stream of liquid through a fine nozzle and at the point where the jet broke into droplets a laser beam was aligned to pass through the liquid. The light emerging was measured by photomultiplier tubes (Fig. 3.1). Forward scatter of the laser from the stream was measured and was proportional to the size of the cell. Other photomultiplier tubes were arranged at right angles to the laser beam and these were used to assess the fluorescence of the cells. This obviously depended on the fluorescent label attached to the cells before passing the cells through the flow cytometer and the band pass filter used. The early flow cytometric cross-match used a simple single stain which was an anti-immunoglobulin conjugated with fluorescein. The flow cytometer was set to select the lymphocytes by their forward (size) and side scatter (granularity) characteristics. A third photomultiplier tube was used to assess the degree of fluorescence of these selected cells. In this way mixtures of B and T lymphocytes were obtained which produced a double peak histogram. This was because B lymphocytes had a degree of naturally occurring surface immunoglobulin in addition to immunoglobulin which was taken up passively. These two peaks of fluorescence then varied independently of each other when alloreactive sera was added. Consequently interpreting these different peaks was sometimes difficult.

The original flow cytometric cross-match was improved first by separating the T and B lymphocytes manually by sheep red cell rosetting and centrifugation. Consequently the fluorescent histograms only had one peak for each cell/sera combination. The manual separation was replaced when flow cytometers were developed with four photomultiplier tubes. This allowed an additional stain to be used (usually phycoerythrin) which was conjugated to a monoclonal antibody against either T or B lymphocytes. This meant that the T or B cells could be identified electronically so that the computer software connected to the flow cytometer would only evaluate these positively stained cells. These selected cells would be evaluated for their fluorescein fluorescence which related to the surface concentration of immunoglobulin derived from the test sera.

Since the introduction of this assay system there has been great debate as to its relevance. In the case of renal transplantation some groups felt that the method was oversensitive and that it precluded potentially successful recipients from transplantation. Others felt that it only had relevance in sensitised recipients. A fair degree of variation occurred with the precise method of performing the assay and this probably accounted for some of the different conclusions. If a centre with an established reliable method followed its recipients for all complications after transplantation, it was found that some grafts with donor T lymphocyte directed IgG as detected by flow cytometry (anti class I) had an uncomplicated course. However, the majority had delayed graft function or frequent or refractory rejection leading to graft loss in some cases.[29] These findings have been reinforced by Ogura and Terasaki[29] who found an increased incidence of graft failure in first and regraft recipients with donor-directed IgG by flow cytometry.

The relevance for the flow cytometric crossmatch for other organs is not as well evaluated as it is for renal transplants. A limited number of reports have suggested that FACS cross-matching may be relevant in cardiac transplantation which follows on from a similar finding with the conventional cytotoxicity test. For livers it is a little more controversial because for many years cytotoxicity was considered of no relevance due to high levels of autoantibodies occurring in liver patients. The demonstration of donor T cell directed IgG specifically has been accepted as more relevant than pan immunoglobulin. The flow cytometric cross-match at face value offered nothing if no effect could be seen even at high levels of immunoglobulin. However, it did offer a way of detecting IgG only. To this end some workers demonstrated an effect with treatable rejection; however, no impact was found with the more important graft failure.[40] This either illustrated the special nature of the liver or the size and ability to absorb immunological rejection. Other workers have found no relevance to liver grafts.[41]

## Local versus imported organ usage

The success of transplantation has been accompanied by an increasing demand for fair and appropriate allocation of organs. Availability remains a major problem. Data suggest that the number of patients awaiting transplantation greatly exceeds the number of available donor organs and this will continue to grow. Many centres have modified their donor and recipient criteria, as previously discussed, in an attempt to prevent an increasing number of potential recipients dying while awaiting transplantation. If no suitable candidate is available locally then the organ is 'offered-out' nationally through national or international organ sharing bodies. Sharing of suitably matched organs addresses to some extent the worldwide donor organ shortage.

In kidney transplantation, the use of shipped organs has become a routine procedure. As early as 1988, Wagner *et al.*[42] showed it to be a safe practice and in their centre, the early function and short-term outcome of the shipped kidneys was certainly no worse than the locally retrieved organs. We also know that optimal matching of cadaveric kidneys for the HLA-A, -B and DR antigens is associated with less acute rejection episodes and improved long-term survival. Exchanging kidneys between centres offers a mechanism for sharing kidneys shown to have only a single HLA-A or -B antigen mismatch and thereby optimising results. However, organ sharing usually leads to prolonged cold ischaemic times (CIT). CIT over 24 h has been shown to be associated with significantly increased rate of delayed graft function (DGF). This in turn may be associated with at least one biopsy proven rejection episode,[43] with a potentially negative effect on early function, hospital stay and long-term outcome. All these factors escalate costs. Fortunately it has been shown that by exchanging HLA-matched kidneys, which experience less rejection (5% vs 42%), there is a cost saving at 1 year. This is due to the fact that less post-transplant dialysis is required in comparison to HLA mis-matched recipients.[44]

With respect to liver transplants, there was no significant difference in early function, between shipped and locally harvested livers provided the procurement was done by an experienced team.[45] Interestingly, mean cold ischaemic times were not significantly different and this may be related to the general tendency to transplant during daylight hours. In addition, the formation of retrieval zones served by specific transplant teams is far more cost effective and allows a 'super-urgent' exchange scheme (i.e. donor liver for patients who it is thought would not survive more than 3 days), to work very efficiently.

Unlike abdominal organs, the thoracic organs have a relatively short preservation time of 4–6 h and so allocation and sharing of these organs is more complex and often quite emotive because of the sense of urgency felt by recipients and their families. Consideration needs to be given to urgency status of the recipient (e.g. patients who are on ventricular assist systems) as well as distance and travel time needed. This is particularly true in countries like the USA where the donor centre may be more than 1000 miles from a potential recipient. Consequently sharing of these scarce organs with short preservation times is not as well developed as kidneys or livers.

This chapter has attempted to describe the different approaches taken to improve the chances of a particular donor/recipient combination being as successful as possible. The steps described are used to a greater or lesser extent whenever an organ becomes available in every transplant centre in the world.

# References

1. Ullman E. Tissue and organ transplantation. Ann Surg 1914; 60: 195–219.
2. Cantarovich D, Baranger T, Tirouvanzian R et al. One hundred and five kidney transplants with cyclosporin A in recipients over sixty years of age. Transplant Proc 1993; 25: 1323–4.
3. Vivas CA, Hichet DP, Jordan MP et al. Renal transplantation in patients sixty five or older. J Urol 1992; 147: 990–3.
4. Horina JH, Holzer H, Reisinger EC et al. Elderly patients and chronic haemodialysis. Lancet 1992; 339: 183–4.
5. Derfler K, Kletler K, Balche P et al. Predictive value of thallium-201 dipyridamole stress scintigraphy in chronic haemodialysis and transplant recipients. Clin Nephrol 1991; 36: 192–202.
6. Gjertson DW. Multifactorial analysis of renal transplantation. In: Terasaki P, Cecka J (eds) Clinical transplant 1992. Los Angeles, California; UCLA Tissue Typing Laboratory.
7. Ploeg RJ, Visser TH, Stijnen G et al. Importance of donor age and quality of donor kidneys on graft survival. Transplant Proc 1987; XIX: 1523.
8. Neumayer HH, Huls S, Schreiber M, Riess R, Luft F. Kidneys from paediatric donors – risk vs benefits. Clin Nephrol 1994; 41: 94–100.
9. Creagh TA, McLean PA, Donovan MG, Walshe J, Murphy DM. Older donors and kidney transplantation. Transplant Int 1993; 6: 39–41.
10. Cooper DKC, Lanza R, Boyd ST et al. Factors influencing survival following heart transplantation. Heart Transplant 1983; 3: 86.
11. Frazier OH, Macris PM. Progress in cardiac transplantation. Surg Clin North Am 1994; 74: 1169–82.
12. Olivari MT. Selection of candidates for heart transplantation and their pretreatment management. In: Shumway SJ, Shumway NE (eds) Thoracic transplantation. Oxford: Blackwell Science, 1995.
13. Hosenpud JD, Novick RJ, Breen TJ et al. The registry of the international society for heart and lung transplantation: 11th official report. J Heart Lung Transplant 1994; 13: 561–70.
14. Thomson DJ, Kostuk W, Pfugfelder P et al. De novo CABG in a heart transplant recipient. J Heart Transplant 1988; 7: 460–70.
15. Starzl TE, Demetris AJ, Van Thiel DH. Liver transplantation. N Engl J Med 1989; 321: 1092–9.
16. Calne RY, Williams R, Rolles K. Liver transplantation in the adult. World J Surg 1986; 10: 422–31.
17. D'Alessandro AM, Kalayoglu M, Sollinger H et al. The predictive value of donor liver biopsies on the development of primary non function after liver transplantation. Transplantation 1991; 51: 157.
18. Gruenberger TH, Steininger R, Sentur TH et al. Influence of donor criteria on post-op graft function after orthotopic liver transplantation. Transplant Int 1994; 7(suppl): S672–S674.
19. Otte JB, de Ville de Goyet J, Sokal E et al. Size reduction of a donor liver is a safe way to alleviate the shortage of size matched organs in paediatric liver transplantation. Ann Surg 1990; 211: 146.
20. Broelsch CE, Whitington PF, Emond JC. Orthotopic liver transplantation in children from living related donors: surgical technique and results. Ann Surg 1992; 214: 428.
21. Emond JC, Heffron TG, Kartz EO et al. Improved results of living related liver transplantation with routine application in a paediatric programme. Transplantation 1993; 55: 835.
22. Terasaki PI, Koyama H, Cecka JM, Gjertson D. The hyperfiltration hypothesis in human renal transplantation. Transplantation 1994; 57: 1450–4.
23. Cecka JM, Terasaki PI. Matching kidneys for size in renal transplantation. Clin Transplant 1990; 4: 82.
24. Vincenti F, Amend WJC, Kaysan G et al. Long-term renal function in kidneys demonstrating compensatory hyperfiltration with no adverse effects. Transplantation 1983; 36: 620.
25. Hua-Sheng XU, Pruett TL, Scott Jones R. Study of donor-recipient liver size match for transplantation. Ann Surg 1994; 219: 46–50.
26. Bismuth H, Houssin D. Reduced size liver grafts in hepatic transplantation in children. Surgery 1984; 95: 367–70.
27. Boyum A. Separation of leucocytes from blood and bone marrow. Scand J Clin Lab Invest 1968; 21 suppl. 97.

28. Hokland P, Hokland M, Heron I. An improved technique for obtaining E rosettes with human lymphocytes and its use for B cell purification. J Immunol Methods 1976; 13: 175–82.

29. Talbot D. The flow cytometric crossmatch in perspective. Transplant Immunol 1993; 1: 155–62.

30. Mytilineos J, Scherer S, Dunckley H et al. DNA HLA-DR typing results of 4000 kidney transplants. Transplantation 1993; 55: 778–81.

31. Opelz G. HLA matching analysis of cyclosporin-treated cadaver kidneys transplanted in 1986. Transplant Proc 1987; 19: 3557.

32. Bidwell J. DNA-RFLP analysis and genotyping of HLA-DR and DQ antigens. Immunol Today 1988; 9: 18–23.

33. Olerup O, Zetterquist H. HLA-DRB1*01 subtyping by allele specific PCR amplification: a sensitive, specific and rapid technique. Tissue Antigens 1991; 37: 197.

34. Opelz G, Mytilineos J, Scherer S et al. Analysis of HLA-DR matching in DNA-typed cadaver kidney transplants. Transplantation 1993; 55: 782–5.

35. Opelz G, Wujciak T. The influence of HLA compatibility on graft survival after heart transplantation. The Collaborative Transplant Study. N Engl J Med 1994; 330: 816–19.

36. Bradley BA, Vail A, Gore SM et al. Penetrating keratoplasty in the United Kingdom: an interim analysis of the corneal transplant follow up study. Clin Transplant 1993; 293–315.

37. Thiel G, Bock A, Spondlin M et al. Long term benefits and risk of cyclosporin A (Sandim-mun) – An analysis at 10 yrs. Transplant Proc 1994; 26: 2493–8.

38. Kao KJ, Scornik JC, Small SJ. Enzyme-linked immunoassay for anti-HLA antibodies – an alternative to panel studies by lymphocytocity. Transplantation 1993; 55: 192.

39. Buelow R, Chiang TR, Monteiro F et al. Soluble HLA antigens and ELISA – a new technology for crossmatch testing. Transplantation 1995; 60: 1594–9.

40. Talbot D, Bell A, Shenton BK et al. The flow cytometric crossmatch in liver transplantation. Transplantation 1995; 59: 737–40.

41. Donaldson PT, Thomson LJ, Heads A et al. IgG donor specific crossmatches are not associated with graft rejection or poor graft survival after liver transplantation. Transplantation 1995; 66: 1016–23.

42. Wagner K, Henkel M, Neumayer H. Shipped kidneys: are they worse? A single center study. Transplant Proc 1988; 20: 869–71.

43. Troppmann C, Gillingham KJ, Benedetti E et al. Delayed graft function; acute rejection and outcome after cadaver renal transplantation: a multivariate analysis. Transplantation 1995; 59: 962–8.

44. Christiaans MHL, Van den Berg-Loonen PM, Nieman FHM et al. Cadaveric kidney exchange on the basis of HLA-matching is already cost effective in the first year of grafting. Transplant Proc 1993; 25: 1685–6.

45. Jonas S, Bechstein WO, Kech H et al. Transplantation of shipped donor livers. Transplant Int 1993; 6: 206–8.

# 4 Transplant immunology – for surgeons

*Paul Gibbs*

**Introduction**  The rapid development of clinical solid organ transplantation over the past 40 years has often outstripped knowledge of the immunological mechanisms involved in the rejection and subsequent failure of the engrafted organ. Gradually, however, understanding of these processes has increased so that transplant immunology is now recognised as a distinct subspecialty within immunology and a fairly detailed description of the response of the recipient's immune system to a graft is possible. This chapter gives only a brief outline of the current understanding of the immunological events which occur following solid organ transplantation.

**Definitions**  Clinical and experimental transplantation is performed in three distinct contexts: syngeneic where the organ is transplanted within the same or identical pure bred animal; allogeneic where the recipient is a non-identical member of the same species; and xenogeneic when the recipient is a member of a different species. Xenotransplants can be divided into concordant, where the species are relatively closely related (e.g. mouse to rat) or discordant where there is greater evolutionary divergence (e.g. pig to primate). In addition the organ can be placed in its normal anatomical position (orthotopic) or into an abnormal site (heterotopic). Heterotopic transplantation is used in human renal transplantation and in many experimental animal models, human liver and heart transplantation is usually orthotopic. This chapter will be largely confined to a description of allograft immunology as this is currently the most clinically important, although there will be some discussion of recent developments in xenotransplantation.

**Early experimental work: the role of Sir Peter Medawar**

The basis of transplant immunology was established by Sir Peter Medawar in a series of experiments from 1944 onwards. Using mainly skin transplant techniques he demonstrated that skin transferred between genetically unrelated mice failed to gain a blood supply and became necrotic within a few days. This 'rejection' took place at a faster rate if a further piece of skin from the same donor was transplanted onto the same recipient whereas skin from a third unrelated animal became necrotic in the same time as the first graft.

Medawar termed these events first and second set responses and went on to demonstrate that rejection was a systemic event and that the second set phenomenon was also donor specific. He was also able to postulate the existence of at least seven proteins (termed antigens) capable of provoking an immune response in rabbits.[1] These experimental findings established the basic tenets of transplant immunology which can be expressed as follows.

1. Graft rejection is donor specific.
2. Rejection possesses memory and responds to a second graft in an accelerated manner.
3. First set rejection is cell mediated.
4. Second set rejection is largely antibody mediated.

This pioneering work opened the way for a series of advances which were made over the following 20 years. These included the concept of lymphocytes having a regular circulation around the body and their importance in both antigen–antibody and cell-mediated responses;[2] the revelation of a fundamental functional division between thymus-processed (T) and bursa-processed (B) lymphocytes[3] and the development of a theory of self-tolerance together with a demonstration of the ability to induce tolerance during the neonatal period.[4]

Subsequent experience in humans (who are clearly much more genetically diverse than inbred laboratory animals) has demonstrated three patterns of rejection based on clinical presentation and histological criteria.

### Hyperacute rejection

This is caused by preformed circulating cytotoxic antibodies which are present in the recipient's serum. It occurs within the first few hours after grafting, often before the operation has been completed, when cells in the donor organ express antigens previously 'seen' by the recipient's immune system so that the recipient's serum contains antibodies against these same antigens. Immediate loss of the graft with endothelial cell disruption, platelet margination, complement activation and thrombosis occurs.[5]

### Acute rejection

This most commonly occurs between days 5 and 14 after transplantation but can occur at any time within the first three months, or even longer after transplantation if the immunosuppression is reduced or the immune system is activated by an unrelated event such as a viral infection. It is cell mediated and is the equivalent to the first set rejection response seen in the original Medawar experiments. In renal transplantation the timing of the first rejection episode can be accelerated if a second graft shares antigens with a previous transplant, the clinical equivalent of the second set response caused by memory T cells present as a result of previous exposure to these same antigens.

### Chronic rejection

This is the least characterised form of rejection and has probably several aetiologies which are manifest by a common end pathway of ischaemic graft damage. Where immunological causes are suspected it has been postulated to be due to ongoing microvascular endothelial damage by either antibody or cell-mediated processes. Graft deterioration is often slow and insidious and the histological findings are characteristic for a particular organ. They include accelerated coronary atheroma in cardiac transplantation which has been associated with the presence of anti-endothelial antibodies,[6] ischaemic injury to renal glomerulae and the disappearance of small bile ducts in liver grafts (vanishing bile duct syndrome, VBDS). Much debate remains over the relative importance of immunological processes in the progressive deterioration seen in chronic rejection. There is usually no significant inflammatory cell infiltrate and although antibody-mediated damage has been suggested to be the source of some of the damage, the only well established association found to date has been with the heart.[6] One characteristic of chronic rejection is that once a certain stage is reached no currently available therapeutic manipulation has been effective in altering the final outcome which is invariably graft failure.

## Origin of the rejection mechanism

Why does the ability to recognise and destroy tissue from other individuals of the same species exist? The phenomenon is a consequence of the immune system's need to differentiate between self and both non-self (e.g. bacteria) or perverted self (tumour or virally infected cells), allowing an organism to maintain its integrity in a hostile environment. In the case of viral infection, infected cells express on their cell surface proteins encoded by the viral genome. The resultant recognition of these proteins as abnormal/foreign by the immune surveillance system and development of a successful immune response allows the individual to eliminate infected cells thereby clearing the virus. Organ transplantation causes activation of the same process as a result of the artificial introduction of a large amount of foreign protein (antigen) which is presented to the recipient's immune system in a manner similar to viral proteins. In outbred animals and humans, unless the immune response is modified, this almost invariably results in rapid destruction of the graft usually accompanied by severe systemic toxicity. Such a dramatic

**Figure 4.1** *Antigen-processing cell (APC) offers up antigen (in the form of peptide associated with MHC antigen) to the T cell via the T cell receptor (TCR).*

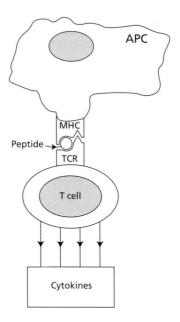

outcome can currently only be prevented by the long term use of drugs which suppress immune function in a non-specific way. Specific immunosuppression where only cells which react against donor antigens (donor reactive) are targeted for immunosuppression remains elusive. The ultimate aim of transplant immunology research is the reproducible achievement of selective immune unresponsiveness to the graft in the absence of immunosuppression. This state is termed tolerance, the recipient being tolerant of the graft, behaving as if it was 'self' rather than 'foreign'. In this way the deleterious side effects of immunosuppression such as increased infection and risk of neoplasia could be avoided.

Most of the rest of this chapter will be devoted to a description of events occurring in cell-mediated acute rejection. Conceptually the response of the immune system in acute rejection can be divided into afferent and efferent arms. During the afferent phase the presence of foreign protein (antigen) is conveyed to the immune system by specialised cells called antigen-presenting cells (APCs) which interact with T lymphocytes (those which have undergone maturation in the thymus) (Fig. 4.1). This is a complex process which has great sensitivity and specificity involving the interaction of several cell surface molecules (see section below). Having received the 'message' that foreign antigen is present, the T lymphocyte plays a crucial role in the development of the response to an allograft. Individual cells which have recognised donor antigens undergo division driven by the production of soluble growth factors called cytokines. This process is called clonal expansion as all the new cells are clones of the original donor reactive cell, their number is considerably increased and they become activated producing more cytokines which in turn activate and recruit further T cell populations (Fig. 4.2). The most important cytokine for T cell activation is interleukin-2 (IL-2) but there are

**Figure 4.2** *Conse-quences of T cell activation and release of cytokines (see text for abbreviations).*

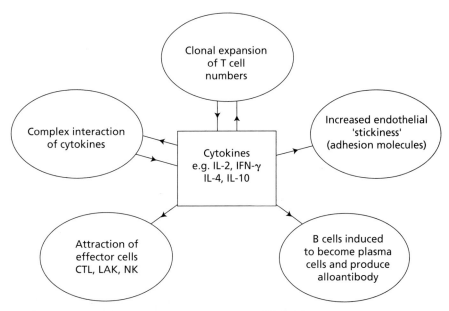

many others which affect this process. Graft infiltration by these activated lymphocytes follows, aided by activation of endothelial cells which become more 'sticky' due to cytokine-induced increased expression of adhesion molecules on their luminal surface. Recruitment of other immunocompetent cells such as natural killer (NK), lymphocyte acti-vated killer (LAK) cells and macrophages also occurs. Once the graft has been invaded by this inflammatory cell infiltrate, cell destruction takes place by a variety of mechanisms which make up the effector arm of the immune response. Most research on immunosuppression has concen-trated on the afferent arm of the response, since prevention of graft infiltration is clearly the optimal way of preventing graft damage. Each stage of this process will now be described in some detail.

## Molecular basis of self/ non-self recognition

### Major histocompatibility antigens

The molecular basis of self/non-self recognition resides in specialised cell surface molecules called the major histocompatibility antigens (MHC) which are therefore one of the main stimuli driving transplant rejection. The MHC antigens were originally discovered as a result of efforts to match tissue from different individuals which did not elicit an immune reaction, i.e. they were histocompatible. The first human MHC antigen was recognised in 1958 through work aimed at establishing serologically determined antigens in leucocytes similar to those of the red cell ABO system – hence the designation HLA, human leucocyte antigen.[7] This antigen is now known as HLA-A2. During the 1960s extensive work led to the identification of many more antigens which were codified into two allelic series designated A and B in 1968,[8] followed by a further series HLA-C, in 1970.[9] These three allelic series A, B, C are known collectively

**Table 4.1**  *Major histocompatibility antigens*

|  | Class I | Class II |
|---|---|---|
| Nomenclature | HLA-A | HLA-DR |
|  | HLA-B | (also HLA-DP |
|  | HLA-C | and HLA-DQ) |
| Distribution | Ubiquitous | Bone marrow-derived cells, |
|  | (except cornea and neurons) | not resting T lymphocytes |
|  |  | Capillary endothelial cells |

as the MHC class I antigens. In 1973, a new set of antigens was demonstrated by Van Leeuwan *et al.*[10] which were the first of the class II or D series. The class II antigens were arranged into an allelic series (DR, DP, DQ) at the 9th International Histocompatibility Workshop in Munich in 1984. This knowledge gave rise to the new discipline of tissue typing within transplantation medicine allowing a degree of HLA matching between recipient and donor and it was postulated that such matching would reduce the severity and amount of rejection (Table 4.1).

Clearly HLA antigens do not exist to make transplantation difficult. Their basic biological function became apparent in the mid 1970s when Zinkernagal and Doherty discovered that T lymphocytes would only respond to viral-derived antigens expressed on the cell surface when these were presented in association with self-MHC antigens.[11] This discovery has been the basis for much immunological research over the past 20 years and was recognised by the award of the 1996 Nobel Prize for Medicine and Physiology. Fuller understanding of this complicated system has been made possible by the development of highly inbred strains of laboratory animals (particularly mice and rats) which are genetically identical apart from specific MHC antigens. Transplantation experiments between these pure bred animals and analysis of the subsequent immune response has greatly expanded the basis of our understanding of transplant immunology. Of particular importance was the work of Snell[12] who produced many different mouse strains and showed, using both tumour and skin graft studies that rejection was dependent on many genes which varied in the strength of their response. In particular the strongest response was related to a locus on chromosome 17 which became known as the H2 or major histocompatibility (MHC) locus of the mouse. As a result of this work it became clear that the HLA antigens are the human equivalent of the mouse histocompatibility system.

In humans the genes encoding for the MHC molecules are present on the short arm of chromosome 6.[13] As mentioned previously the class I and class II regions are well characterised, the class I region being divisible into HLA A, B and C allelic series (as well as E, F, G and H)[14] of which only A and B are currently thought to be important for transplantation purposes. Class II is divided into DR, DP and DQ loci,[15] although again only DR is used for matching purposes. This area is in fact the most polymorphic region known on the human genome, presumably due to evolutionary pressure ensuring that members of a species are not immunogenetically identical and would not succumb en masse to infection with a 'super pathogen'. Between the class I and II regions is a region known as class III[13] which contains more than 70 genes encoding the various components of complement system such as C2 and C4 as well as TNF-$\alpha$ and TNF-$\beta$, Hsp 70 (heat shock protein). Also important are a number of other genes within the class II region including TAP1 and TAP2 which are genes whose combined product (a protease) controls the intracellular formation and subsequent expression of MHC molecules on the cell surface.[16]

## Molecular structure of the MHC antigens

The structure of the MHC class I molecule consists of one glycosylated 45 kilodalton (kDa) polypeptide (heavy) chain non-covalently bonded to $\beta$2-microglobulin which is a 12 kDa polypeptide.[17] The heavy chain encoded on chromosome 6 are polymorphic whereas the $\beta$2-micro-globulin gene is present on chromosome 15 and is non-polymorphic in humans; there is in fact strong conservation of its basic structure between mammalian species. The $\beta$2-microglobulin is not bound to the cell membrane but is essential for the assembly and transportation of the MHC molecule to the cell surface.

The heavy chain molecules consist of three extracellular $\alpha$ domains, a transmembrane region and a cytoplasmic tail. The $\alpha$ domain shares amino acid identity with the immunoglobulin (Ig) constant region. Many molecules associated with the immune system have elements of this same basic structure and are grouped together in the Ig superfamily.[18,19]

The three-dimensional structure of the HLA-A2 molecule has been elucidated by X-ray crystallography and was a significant advance in understanding MHC antigen function.[20,21] The outermost part of the molecule is formed by a single antiparallel $\beta$ sheet supporting two $\alpha$ helical regions creating a cleft or groove in the outward projecting part of the molecule which comes into contact with the T cell. This cleft has been demonstrated to be the site of binding of small peptides which are derived by proteases from both cellular and extracellular proteins. The presence of a peptide in this groove appears to be crucial to the stable formation of the class I antigens.[22] A specific receptor exists on all T cells (the T cell receptor or TCR) and if this binds firmly to the MHC–peptide complex, one prerequisite for T cell activation has been met. These peptides have been successfully eluted from the class I molecules and on analysis have all been found to be nine amino acids long. A similar structure has been demonstrated for HLA-B27, apart from subtle differences in the binding site which means that a different peptide will preferentially bind.[23] These findings have led to the hypothesis that each class I allele only binds a limited spectrum of peptides, all nine amino acids long which fit the specific pockets in the groove at the surface of the molecule. The specificity is produced mainly by the charge densities of the amino acids making up the sides of the groove. The combination of

**Figure 4.3** *Highly stylised drawings of MHC class I and II molecules.*

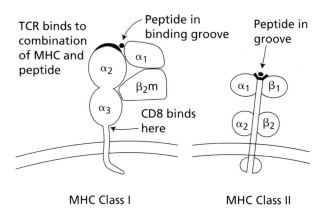

peptide/MHC confers a high degree of specificity to the MHC–TCR interaction. Class I antigens have an almost ubiquitous tissue distribution being present on almost all nucleated cells with the important exception of corneal endothelium.[24]

Structurally MHC class II antigens are non-covalently bound heterodimers consisting of $\alpha$ and $\beta$ glycoproteins, the $\alpha$ chain being 30–34 kDa and the $\beta$ chain being 26–29 kDa[25] (Fig. 4.3). There is now crystallographic evidence that the T cell binding site again contains a groove similar to that on class I molecules although it binds larger peptide fragments approximately 12–20 amino acids long.[26] Both $\alpha$ and $\beta$ chains are positioned across the membrane, with a degree of conservation in the basic structure between species, are glycosylated, have two extracellular domains and a hydrophilic intracellular domain. Their tissue distribution is much more restricted than the ubiquitous class I. They are expressed mainly on B lymphocytes, macrophages, monocytes, capillary endothelium and some epithelia especially that of the breast and the respiratory system.[27] They are also inducible, by cytokines on large vessel endothelium and in varying degrees on different cells within transplanted organs.

T cells do not recognise antigen alone, but react to the peptide/MHC complex which is presented to the T cell receptor. This occurs when processed antigen in the form of small peptides is associated with MHC molecules on the surface of the APC. Therefore, the function of the MHC molecules is to present peptides to T cell as a surveillance mechanism so that 'foreign' peptides expressed by virally infected cells, tumour cells (and unfortunately transplanted organs) are rapidly identified. There is evidence that class I molecules primarily present peptides from proteins endogenous to the cell to which they bind in the endoplasmic reticulum before reaching the cell surface via the Golgi apparatus. Class II antigens bind peptides derived from exogenous proteins in a specialised endosome/lysosome compartment.[28] Very recently the three-dimensional structure of an actual MHC/peptide complex bound to TCR has been investigated by X-ray crystallography and it confirms much of the previous theories regarding this crucial interaction.[29]

## Tissue typing and cross-matching

Tissue typing was introduced based on the hypothesis that knowing the HLA class I (A and B) and class II (DR) status of donor and recipient would allow matching of organ to recipient which would reduce the immunogenicity of the graft and therefore both the number and severity of rejection episodes. Current practice in renal transplantation is to type and match for HLA-A, B and DR which means matching for six alleles. Originally serologically based, it is now greatly refined and more accurate due to the use of monoclonal antibodies, flow cytometric analysis and polymerase chain reaction (PCR) amplification which requires only small quantities of DNA. These techniques have resulted in many of the serologically defined alleles being split into variants, although not all of these have been applied to clinical decision making (see also Chapter 3). Indeed such a policy would render clinical matching of organ and recipient very difficult. The new techniques have been valuable in giving a more accurate analysis of the effects of HLA matching on graft outcome. The importance of HLA matching in human renal transplantation is well established where large population studies such as that coordinated by Opelz[30] have shown improved long-term survival when there is a five or six antigen match. The benefit of matching for liver and cardiac transplantation is much less clear cut and currently no prospective matching (apart from ABO) for these organs takes place for practical clinical reasons. The long-term effect of HLA matching on these organs remains under debate.

The lymphocytotoxic cross-match was introduced into renal transplantation in the mid 1960s.[31] This is a method of identifying potentially damaging, pre-existing anti-HLA cytotoxic antibodies in the recipient's serum prior to transplantation by mixing cells from the donor (either splenocytes or peripheral lymph node cells) with the recipient's stored serum (for details, see Chapter 3). Evidence of cytotoxicity means that there is a significant risk of hyperacute or accelerated acute rejection and therefore a renal transplant is not performed in these circumstances. The introduction of this technique greatly reduced the incidence of hyperacute rejection in renal transplantation and fortunately it is now very seldom seen. It is noteworthy that hyperacute rejection is rare in heart[32] and almost unknown in liver transplantation despite various studies showing that 7–33% of waiting list patients have donor specific anti-HLA cytotoxic antibodies.[33] Where hyperacute rejection has occurred in liver transplantation it is usually in ABO incompatible grafts. The ability of the liver to counteract the presence of cytotoxic alloantibodies has been shown to extend to protection of a kidney graft even in the presence of a positive cross-match if combined liver and kidney transplantation is performed.[34] Transplanted alone in this situation the kidney would have a high risk of being destroyed by either hyperacute or accelerated acute rejection. The mechanism of this protection remains unknown.

## Minor histocompatibility antigens

Evidence from human living-related transplantation (mostly haplo-identical) and in bred animal transplantation (identical) has shown that even with a complete MHC match, acute rejection can still occur. This implies that there are other antigenic determinants capable of initiating an immune reaction. These are essentially peptides derived from donor proteins which are presented by class I or II MHC antigens and recognised as 'foreign' by the recipient's lymphocytes. The minor histocompatibility antigens have had much less scientific effort devoted to them than the major histocompatibility complex, partly because by being numerous, located on many different genes and generally causing less severe rejection they are not as rewarding to study as the MHC antigens. This should not lead to the idea that they are unimportant as they have been shown to cause graft failure in rodent models. One well-recognised minor antigen is the H-Y antigen which is present on the Y chromosome.[35] Another is the monocyte/endothelial antigens series which has been documented as causing rejection in both renal and cardiac transplants but always in an HLA-restricted fashion.

## T lymphocytes

Although MHC molecules are the molecular basis of rejection the pivotal cell in the immune response is the T lymphocyte[36] and in particular a subset known as T helper cells. A large amount of research has now been performed on T cells (particularly recently with respect to their role in HIV infection) so that their biology is known in great detail and would merit its own volume to do it justice. This brief account will give an outline of their structure and function as it relates to transplantation.

After initial development in the marrow from the myeloblastic common stem cell, cells destined for the lymphocyte lineage undergo further maturation, in either the thymus (T cells) or in the mammalian equivalent of the avian Bursa of Fabricius (B cells). In mammals this probably occurs in Peyer's patches and other lymphoid follicles of the small bowel. Thymic maturation of T cells is essential to their development and normal function. Mice which are born with no thymus have virtually no cellular based immunity.[37] One of the most important functions of the thymus is to ensure that while there are T cells which will be capable of reacting to a whole variety of foreign peptides, all those which would be strongly self-reactive are eliminated. This is achieved by both positive and negative selection.[38] In very basic terms T cells (termed thymocytes at this stage of their development) are presented within the thymus with self-MHC antigens. If the TCR on an individual T cell fails to bind or binds too strongly the cell dies by apoptosis. In the first instance the inability to interact with self-MHC would render the cell non-functional. In the second instance binding too strongly to the MHC may render the cell self-reactive as a result of its high affinity. Finally, those that react with medium avidity are positively selected due to the release of growth factors, mature and are eventually released into the periphery. In the thymus the DNA sequence coding for the T cell receptor, which is divided into V (variable), D (diversity, $\beta$ and $\delta$ chains only) and J (joining) regions, undergoes recombination to produce a very wide variety of TCR conformations. This results in tremendous diversity allowing interaction with presumably all potential peptide/MHC complexes that are likely to be encountered.[39]

The thymus involutes in humans in late adolescence so that theoretically no new T lymphocyte populations can mature after this age. However, recent experimental evidence raises the possibility that T cell maturation may also be possible in germinal centres of the spleen once involution of the thymus has occurred. This has been shown to occur in athymic mice in the presence of cytokine oncostatin M.[40]

The TCR is a complex molecule consisting of a trimer of T cell receptor, and associated molecules CD3 and one of two molecules from the immunoglobulin (Ig) superfamily – either CD4 or CD8 (Fig. 4.4). The actual receptor has two distinct forms one consisting of $\alpha$ and $\beta$ chains which have molecular weights ($M_R$) of 49 and 43 kDa, respectively and the other made up of $\gamma$ and $\delta$ chains with $M_R$ of 55 and 40 kDa, respectively. These chains all are members of the IgG superfamily of molecules and consist of a cytoplasmic tail and three extracellular domains. The vast majority of peripheral T cells (98–99%) are $\alpha$ $\beta$ cells although there are significant numbers of $\gamma$ $\delta$ cells in small bowel, liver and lymph nodes. CD3 consists of a complex of five polypeptide chains which are relatively invariant. To stabilise the association of the TCR/CD3 complex with the MHC molecule on the antigen presenting cell (APC) a further molecule is necessary. This varies depending on the type of T lymphocyte; for cytotoxic cells it is CD8 and for helper T cells it is CD4.[41] CD4 has five immunoglobulin (Ig)-like extracellular domains whereas CD8 is a dimer which has two isoforms, one with 2 $\alpha$ chains and one with 1 $\alpha$ and 1 $\beta$ chain, which are thought to have distinct functions; for example the $\alpha$ $\beta$ isoform has been shown to be functional in cytotoxic CD8 cells.[42] These molecules confer specificity on the type of MHC molecule bound by the TCR. CD8 binds with class I whereas CD4 binds class II. Incidentally CD4 is also the site of the receptor for retroviruses including HIV.[43] The function of CD4 and CD8 is partly to act as adhesion molecules increasing the strength of the bond between the TCR and MHC allowing activation of the T cell in the presence of much smaller amounts of antigen than is possible without this extra adhesion.[44] They also act as signal transducers in their own right.[45] Recent work suggests that the importance of the CD8 molecule to the functioning of the TCR means that it should be regarded as an intrinsic component of the TCR rather than an accessory molecule.[46]

## The mechanism of antigen presentation

### Antigen presenting cells

As previously mentioned, antigen presentation takes place by the interaction of the MHC molecule and its bound peptide on the highly specialised cell called an antigen presenting cell (APC) with the T cell receptor (TCR) on the T cell. Currently cell types proven to be efficient antigen presenting cells[47] are of the monocyte/macrophage lineage (e.g. interstitial dendritic cells, Kupffer cells), B lymphocytes and under certain conditions, endothelial cells. Dendritic cells (also called passenger leucocytes in transplanted organs because they are transferred with the organ) undergo a regular circulation between the spleen and peripheral organs performing what has been described as a 'policing' role, bringing and presenting antigens to the cells of the central lymphoid system. They seem to be particularly important in transplantation; experiments by Lechler and Bachelor have shown that passenger leucocytes transferred with kidney grafts in a rat model leave the organ within 24–48 h of transplantation and pass to the spleen where they presumably present antigen. Furthermore in certain rat renal transplant models replacement of the donor dendritic cells by cells of recipient origin prior to transplantation results in long-term acceptance of the graft without immunosuppression.[48]

Interactions between donor MHC and the recipient's TCR to enable T cells from the recipient to react directly with APCs from a donor involves a degree of cross-reaction which is dependent on the number and type of amino acid substitutions between different MHC molecules and will therefore vary considerably depending on the exact donor–recipient MHC combination.

The T cell response has also been shown to vary depending on the form of the ligand recognised. Subtle changes in the binding groove/peptide interaction can result in slightly different patterns being presented which in turn can alter the response of the T cell, for example resulting in a change in the cytokine produced[49] or even inducing anergy[50] (see below).

### Costimulation

The interaction between the TCR and MHC molecule is not sufficient for full T cell activation.[51] A second (co-stimulatory signal) is also required as the signal from the TCR alone is insufficient for T cell activation (Fig. 4.4). It is the ability to provide the second signal which is the critical requirement for a cell to be able to function as an antigen presenting cell. The most important second signal ligand pairs are CD28 (on the T cell) and B7 (on the APC) or CD40 – gp39.[52] (The first is required for full T cell activation, the second pair for activation of B cells, macrophages and endothelium.) However, in certain circumstances other adhesion molecule pairs such as CD2/lymphocyte function associated 3 (LFA3) and intracellular adhesion molecule 1 (ICAM-1)/LFA1 may also perform this function depending on the antigen presenting cell involved. These

**Figure 4.4** *Schematic diagram showing MHC/ peptide interaction with TCR complex and molecules capable of transducing second signal essential for T cell activation (see text for details).*

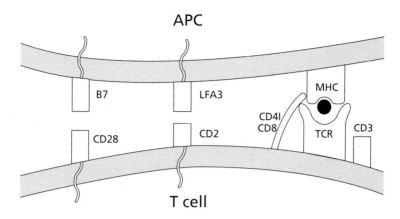

co-stimulatory molecules activate a separate pathway within the cyto-plasm providing a second signal which in combination with the signal from the TCR triggers T cell activation. There is evidence that in the absence of these additional signals engagement of the TCR by the MHC can result in a state of unresponsiveness so that the lymphocyte will not respond to further antigen stimulation.[53] This 'switched off' state is termed anergy and may be an important step in the development of graft acceptance (tolerance) by the host. This concept is particularly important for transplantation because, theoretically, selective inactivation of donor reactive T cell clones would achieve graft acceptance while leaving all other clones fully functional. In this way viral and tumour cell surveil-lance would be unaffected. Unfortunately predictable achievement of T cell anergy remains elusive in clinical practice.

Two fundamental pathways exist for antigen presentation of the transplanted tissue. Antigen may be shed from the allograft and processed by recipient APC. The antigen is 'internalised', broken down into constituent peptides and placed in association with self-MHC on the surface of the cell. This is the indirect pathway of allorecognition.[54] The direct method involves recipient T cells reacting to foreign MHC antigen and foreign peptide which has come from donor tissue.[55] Dendritic cells, present in the allograft, are probably responsible for this form of T cell stimulation. The relative importance of these two types of antigen presentation remains unclear.

The consequence of antigen presentation is T cell activation, which occurs through the TCR complex which is linked by multiple intra-cellular signalling pathways to the nucleus.[56]

Following engagement of the MHC/peptide complex with the TCR, phosphorylation occurs which in turn activates pathways leading, in association with co-stimulatory signalling, to full activation including IL2 production.[57] This results in clonal expansion of the T cell subset, followed by graft infiltration enhanced by increased endothelial activa-tion. The final result is the appearance of a lymphocytic graft infiltrate and the classical histological appearance of acute rejection. Among other cytokines produced is IFN-$\gamma$, which induces increased expression of many cell surface molecules including MHC class I and II, and various adhesion molecules on endothelium increasing the ability of T cells to migrate into the graft. The net result of this activity is that the graft is primed to act as a target for the recipient immune system.

**Adhesion molecules**

Adhesion molecules are vital to the ordered structure of a multicellular organism both for cell to cell and cell to matrix interactions. Our knowledge of these molecules has been greatly increased by the application of monoclonal antibody technology which has allowed a whole range of molecules to be discovered which function both for simple cell to cell adhesion and can also act as signalling molecules activating intracytoplasmic pathways to trigger nuclear stimulation within the target cells.

The important adhesion molecules in the rejection process mainly come from three distinct molecular families (Table 4.2). These are the Ig superfamily (described previously),[19] the integrins and the selectins.[18] Integrins are all non-covalently bonded $\alpha \beta$ heterodimers with variants within both the $\alpha_6$ and $\beta_3$ chains. Depending on which $\beta$ subunit is present three families of integrins have been recognised, the most relevant for the immune system being the $\beta_2$ integrins. There are three members of this group, lymphocyte function associated antigen (LFA-1), Mac-1 and pl50.95. All are found on leucocytes and their importance can be appreciated by a rare fatal disease called leucocyte adhesion deficiency syndrome (LAD) in which there is a single amino acid substitution in the $\beta_2$ chain resulting in a deficiency in all the $\beta_2$ integrins.[58] This results in impaired leucocyte passage across cell barriers resulting in failure of migration to sites of inflammation. It particularly affects neutrophils which do not express another adhesion molecule and therefore are completely unable to transmigrate through the endothelial cell barrier unlike lymphocytes which maintain some transmigration ability due to a degree of redundancy in their adhesion molecule expression. They also express a $\beta_1$ integrin called VLA-4 which is unique in that it is involved in both cell to cell and cell to matrix adhesion. It binds to vascular cell adhesion molecule (VCAM-1) on endothelium, macrophages and also fibronectin in matrix and is probably the reason why lymphocytes can still migrate in LAD.

**Table 4.2** *Adhesion molecules classification*

| Group name | Examples |
| --- | --- |
| Immunoglobulin superfamily | ICAM-1, ICAM-2, VCAM-1, CD2, LFA-3 |
| Integrins | LFA-1, Mac-1, VLA-4 |
| Selectins | Endothelial selectin (E-selectin) Leucocyte selectin (L-selectin) Platelet selectin (P-selectin) |

Selectins are characterised by having an N terminal lectin domain which is a protein with the ability to bind specific sugars. There are three selectins, L, E and P selectin, which are particularly involved in leucocyte trafficking. P and E selectin are involved in neutrophil adhesion to endothelium whereas L selectin is also a lymphocyte recirculation receptor especially on memory T cells. Another important molecule is CD45,[59] present on all leucocytes, hence its name of leucocyte common antigen. It has an intracytoplasmic portion with intrinsic phosphatase activity which plays a role in cell activation. On lymphocytes it is present in two distinct forms: CD45RA is a high-molecular-weight form found on naive cells, and CD45RO is a spliced low-molecular-weight form which is formed after the lymphocytes first encounter antigen. This form is characteristic of memory cells. It also acts as an adhesion molecule interacting with CD22 on B cells.

Normal efficient T cell activation requires greater adhesion than is present in the TCR–MHC ligand pair. This further adhesion is antigen independent. One of the most important ligand pairs fulfilling this role and the first to be investigated was the LFA-1 and ICAM-1 (a member of the Ig superfamily) pair.[18] LFA-1 is present on lymphocytes, as mentioned previously, and ICAM-1 on antigen-presenting cells such as dendritic cells, activated B cells, macrophages, endothelial cells and also on lymphocytes allowing lymphocyte–lymphocyte interactions. ICAM-1 expression is greatly increased by various cytokines such IL-1, IFN-$\gamma$ and TNF-$\alpha$, but this requires new protein formation and therefore only occurs over a period of hours to days. However, this ligand pair (LFA-1/ICAM-1) is responsible for the increased adhesion detectable within minutes of the TCR being activated. This increase is too rapid to be due to new protein production and has been shown to be due to a change in avidity of the LFA-1 molecules which enhances their ability to bind to the ligand. On naive cells, LFA-1 is widely dispersed over the cell surface in a low avidity state, on mature cells its distribution is clustered but still in a low avidity state. When cells are activated, this changes to a clustered high avidity state. It has been hypothesised that binding between LFA-1 with medium avidity and ICAM-1 is responsible for the initial contact between a mature T cell and target cell, but that the high avidity state only occurs if the MHC–peptide complex engages with the TCR and is recognised as immunogenic. Otherwise the T cell detaches rapidly.[60] In this way a screening/surveillance function can be performed by the T cell which only binds fully if there is antigenic material in the peptide groove. The process is controlled within minutes using changes in LFA-1 avidity but if T cell activation occurs the resultant production of cytokine leads in turn to activation of the antigen-presenting cells and increased ICAM-1 expression. Adhesion with other T cells then becomes more frequent aiding the recruitment of an inflammatory infiltrate.

Further data have shown that LFA-1 is also important for natural killer activity, B cell responses and lymphocyte adherence to endothelium both for transmigration and antigen presenting purposes. Other adhesion ligand pairs are CD2/LFA3 (CD2 on the T cell and LFA-3 on the APC) and VLA-4 which appears after a few days on activated lymphocytes and vascular cell adhesion molecule 1 (VCAM-1) to which it binds on endothelial cells. This ligand pair is possibly important in maintaining lymphocyte recruitment into the graft after the initial 24–48 hours.

## Role of endothelium

There have already been several references to the role of endothelial cells in immune responses to an allograft, and it is important to appreciate that these cells should not be regarded as simply inert cells lining blood vessels. It is now well recognised that endothelium plays an active role in inflammation through its control of local blood flow, leucocyte adhesion, transmigration and activation. Adhesion molecules expressed on the luminal side of activated endothelium include p-selectin, e-selectin, ICAM-1 (all for leucocyte adhesion) and VCAM-1 (lymphocyte adhesion). Immunohistochemistry of acutely rejecting renal allografts has shown increased expression of a variety of adhesion molecules expressed by endothelial cells as well as induction of MHC class II.[61] The actual mechanism by which leucocytes transmigrate is known in some detail. There is currently a lot of debate regarding the ability of the endothelial cell to act as an APC. The current consensus is that it probably can after activation by cytokines such as IFN-γ although the molecule which supplies the co-stimulatory signal is uncertain as endothelium does not express either form of the B7 molecule. One proposed candidate is CD2 binding to LFA-3 on the T cell.[62]

Endothelial cells can be activated by several cytokines including TNF α, IFN-γ, and IL4. IFN-γ in particular causes class II induction on EC probably resulting in its ability (albeit still disputed) to act as an antigen presenting cell.[63] Similarly GMCSF causes macrophages to acquire full stimulatory potential.[64]

## Cytokines

The role of the soluble mediators released by a variety of cells during rejection was relatively understudied for a long time because of the complexity of the interactions involved. Much new knowledge has been gained recently by applying new molecular techniques such as polymerase chain reaction (PCR) and *in situ* hybridisation to characterise the cytokines produced during rejection.

Cytokines are small soluble proteins which exert their effects by binding to specific receptors on the surface of their target cells causing functional changes usually by protein synthesis. They are involved in the activation and regulation of the immune response to any stimulus. In a transplantation context important cytokines include various interleukins (IL-1, IL-2, IL-4, IL-6, IL-9, IL-10) and interferons (e.g. IFN-γ).

One of the most important cytokines in acute cellular rejection is IL-2 which is produced by activated T cells and causes proliferation and differentiation of both T and B cells. Other immune cells such as NK and dendritic cells also express a receptor for IL-2 although the precise consequences of this interaction are not fully understood. As mentioned previously stimulation of T cells without the ability to produce IL-2 or with its effects blocked by monoclonal antibody results in a state of anergy.[50]

The pattern of cytokines produced during an immune response can have a profound effect on the outcome of infection or transplantation. In mice, infection with *Leishmania major* can result in either resistance to infection or progressive fatal disease. Which outcome occurs in a particular animal has been correlated with the particular cytokines produced, resistant animals possessing IFN-$\gamma$ secreting CD4 cells and susceptible animals IL-4-secreting cells. If the action of either cell type is blocked using specific monoclonal antibodies the disease outcome is reversed.[65,66]

Cytokines also regulate the production and function of each other which is a particularly difficult problem to unravel. IL-4 antagonises both proliferation and differentiation of B cells[67] and LAK cells[68] by IL-2. IL-10 prevents IFN-$\gamma$ and IL-2 synthesis[69] but this is an indirect effect through macrophages. This complicated cross-regulation may be helpful in controlling rejection and could even be manipulated to induce tolerance once the precise mode and site of action of the various cytokines is known.

Individual variation in the response to disease (especially between a delayed hypersensitivity (DTH) and humoral response) has now been related to different patterns of cytokine production. This was first demonstrated in the mouse where different immune responses have been linked to specific T cell clones.[70] A Th1 response is characterised by the production of IL-2, IFN-$\gamma$ and TNF-$\beta$ and is seen when DTH predominates, whereas a Th2 response is associated with IL-4, IL-5, IL-6 and IL-13 among others and is seen when antibody production is predominant. The Th1 cytokine profile has since been associated with acute rejection. In humans the picture is far less clear and the type of cytokine profile may well be the outcome of both the particular stimuli and environment of each immune event. Naive T cells certainly have the ability to produce either pattern of cytokines, so that differentiation into Th1 and Th2 subsets is not fixed in an individual cell. It appears that the method of antigen presentation and the mix of other stimulatory factors determines whether a TH1 response (mainly associated with cell-mediated immunity) or a Th2 reaction (antibody production) occurs.

The outcome of a particular transplant is also influenced by the interaction between the MHC match involved. A striking example of this has been seen in experimental rat liver transplantation where very different outcomes occur depending on the strain combination used. In DA to Lewis rat liver transplantation rapid severe acute rejection occurs, whereas Lewis to DA results in spontaneous tolerance. These pure bred strains are termed high and low responders, respectively. Farges *et al.*[71] analysed the cell infiltrate and cytokine expression in these two models but surprisingly found very little difference. The cell infiltrate in both cases was the same and the only discernible difference identified was a reduction in IL-4 production in the tolerant group.

Systemic cytokine levels are difficult to interpret because their importance lies in the local microenvironment so that systemic levels may not accurately reflect what is occurring locally. They are measured by ELISA (enzyme linked immunosorbent assay) which gives accurate serum and plasma levels in picograms. Dallman *et al.* have demonstrated a relationship between IL-2 mRNA expression and acute rejection in fine needle aspiration samples of renal grafts,[72] but in general, studies of serum levels of a variety of cytokines have failed to distinguish reliably between rejection and infection.[73] Immunosuppression can be directed to block the action of cytokines in a non-specific way. Anti-IL-2R monoclonal antibodies against the p55 chain (only expressed by activated and not resting T cells) have been used in clinical trials in combination with conventional immunosuppression with some encouraging results,[74] but the antibodies used have been mouse anti-human which have the significant disadvantage of causing a strong anti-immmunoglobulin response by the patient which diminishes the effectiveness of the treatment.

## Effector limb

The effector limb of rejection consists of the mechanisms concerned with actual graft damage and ultimate destruction once the inflammatory cell infiltrate has migrated into the graft.[75] These can be divided into specific and non-specific, the non-specific (macrophages, natural killer (NK) cells and lymphokine activated killer cells (LAK) cells) being recruited by specific T lymphocyte-based mechanisms. Cytotoxic T lymphocytes (CTL) are quite capable of significant damage by release of toxic molecules such as Fas ligand, perforins and serine esterases. However, recruitment of other cells such as leucocytes and killer cells produces the epithelial damage seen in organ transplant rejection (e.g. tubulitis) with similar inflammatory change detectable in the endothelium of the graft vasculature.

The role of B cells and antibody in acute rejection remains controversial. The humoral response is based on the production of IgM and IgG antibodies. B lymphocyte development is similar to T cell maturation but occurs from pre-B cells, as a result of processing in the Peyer's patches.[76] When naive B cells encounter antigen or cytokines such as IL-2 they develop into antibody-secreting plasma cells.

Antibodies consist of heavy and light chains, the heavy chain being encoded on chromosome 14, the $\delta$ light chain on chromosome 2 and the $\lambda$ light chain on chromosome 22. Like the rearrangement that occurs during T cell development, B genes also undergo rearrangement at D, J and V regions to produce huge variation in antibody specificities. Immature B cells produce IgM, but can switch isotype to IgG with the same binding specificity and mature B cells can express IgM and IgD antibody receptors of the same specificity. Mature cells undergo a regular circulation; if they fail to interact with antigen within a few days, they are removed by the spleen. If they meet antigen (which binds to their surface Ig receptors) they undergo differentiation, with T cell help, becoming either memory (under the influence of the cytokine IL-5) or antibody-producing plasma cells (under the influence of IL-6). If antigen cross-links the Ig receptors on the cell surface the B cells increase in size, undergo DNA synthesis and the antigen is internalised and re-expressed with a peptide in association with MHC class II. This allows the B cell to act as an antigen presenting cell.

As mentioned earlier antidonor cytotoxic antibodies can be detected in the serum of some patients before transplantation as a result of previous exposure to alloantigen either by blood transfusion or pregnancy. They can also be detected following transplantation but their role in acute rejection remains controversial. The established view is that antibody is unimportant, the dominant pathway of damage being cytotoxic T cells. However in at least one rat combination, antibody has been shown to be capable of causing acute rejection in the absence of cytotoxic CD8 T cells.[77] There have also been recent data linking antibody with a possible role in chronic rejection.[6,78]

The actual mechanism whereby grafts cells are destroyed is almost certainly multifactorial. In hyperacute rejection it is antibody deposition on the endothelium, and activation of the complement cascade and thrombosis. Cytotoxic T cells have specific methods of tissue destruction involving the production of a group of molecules called perforins[79] which form holes in membranes, followed by the release of granzyme, a protease which lyses components of cytoplasm.[80] NK and LAK cells and the cytokine $TNF_\alpha$ can also cause direct cell damage.

## Tolerance

Tolerance is defined as a state where there is no rejection of a foreign graft even in the absence of immunosuppression. The first description of tolerance was by Medawar who noted that injection of bone marrow into neonatal mice induced tolerance to alloantigen. However, the goal of producing tolerance in graft recipients remains elusive in human transplantation.

The mechanisms of tolerance are the subject of much debate and many theories have been put forward. The terms which are used in this section of immunology can be confusing; an attempt to define these terms is given in Table 4.3.

There have been a number of strategies advanced to promote the induction of tolerance in human transplantation. Non-specific presentation of antigen to a recipient prior to the transplant procedure was often performed by the process of blood transfusion. More recently, donation of antigen in the form of bone marrow, given together with immunosuppression, has been used in an attempt to produce unresponsiveness to a transplanted organ from the same donor. The site of antigen presentation to the recipient may also be important and this is reflected in experiments where donor antigen is injected into the thymus.

**Table 4.3** *Terms used in explanations of tolerance*

| Term | Explanation |
| --- | --- |
| Accommodation | Recipient does not reject graft but requires small dose of immunosuppression to maintain a functional tolerance. |
| Anergy | On presentation of antigen, failure to provide second signal (see above) results in unresponsiveness rather than activation. |
| Suppression | Transfer of cells from long-term graft recipients can carry suppressive activity to a new, similar recipient. No single 'suppressor' cell has been identified. |
| Deletion | T cell reacts with antigen and is then deleted. Probably important in controlling reaction to self-antigen. |
| Microchimerism | Low frequency of cells of donor origin found in a recipient at a site remote from the allograft. Whether the cells are 'critical' for tolerance or simply a finding in those who have become tolerant by another mechanism is debatable. |

Although this technique has been successful in animal combinations, its use in human transplantation has not yet been described. Other strategies include attempts to target molecules on the surface of important cells, particularly those molecules which are felt to be critical in the induction of T cell anergy or T cell deletion. An example is a fusion protein CTLA-4-Ig which has been designed to block the co-stimulation response (see above) and hence produce a degree of hyporesponsiveness.

Immunologically speaking the liver is a charmed organ. Spontaneous tolerance was first demonstrated in a pig liver transplant model by Calne *et al.* in the late 1960s.[81] Long-term liver transplant patients have had their immunosuppression withdrawn either as a planned part of their management or because of poor drug compliance.[82] The continued survival of the liver transplant in such patients is well described, but impossible to predict, and the criteria necessary for the survival are not known.

**Xenografts** Recently interest has increased in the potential of xenotransplantation as a means of solving the perpetual organ shortage problem. Initial research in this field was abandoned because of very poor results, but recent molecular biological advances such as gene sequencing and gene transfer techniques have created the means of developing genetically altered animals which theoretically could be bred specifically for transplantation. One of the most studied combinations is the discordant model of transplantation from pig to primate which has been chosen because of the relative ease in breeding and keeping pigs and because their similarities in terms of size to man make them an attractive source of organs.

Unmodified xenotransplantation results in rapid destruction of the xenograft within minutes of reperfusion by hyperacute rejection with activation of the complement system, endothelial damage and intravascular thrombosis. This occurs because of the presence in human blood of xenoreactive natural antibodies which are mainly directed at a disaccharide Gal $\alpha$ 1-3 Gal which is present on mammalian endothelium.[83] These IgM antibodies bind complement with consequent hyperacute rejection. However, even if complement is removed, intravascular coagulation may occur by the action of the endothelium.[84] Normal endothelial cells produce an anticoagulant which acts locally to prevent thrombosis. In the complement-depleted xenograft, retraction of endothelial cells with exposure of underlying collagen[85] and secretion of platelet activating factor endothelial cell resulting in platelet aggregation and thrombosis.[86] Complement is controlled by inhibitors such as decay accelerating factor (DAF) which is present on endothelial cells. This factor is species specific, i.e. a pig organ (with pig DAF on the endothelial cells) perfused with human blood, will not prevent human complement activation. However, it was suggested[87] that a transgenic pig with high levels of human DAF on the endothelial cells might be able to prevent the activation of the complement cascade by xenoreactive antibodies (especially if the levels of these antibodies had been reduced by plasmapheresis). Such a transgenic pig has now been bred by researchers in Cambridge and reports have been presented of the first experimental pig to baboon heart transplants showing graft survival for up to 60 days which is a significant advance over previous results in xenotransplantation.[88] Further work remains to be done before human trials with these transgenic pigs can begin. Little is known of the strength of the cell-mediated response if the hyperacute phase of rejection is overcome, although there is *in vitro* evidence to show that cell-mediated rejection would occur at a level equal to or greater than that seen with an allograft.[89]

Finally, the important issue of the potential for introducing new pathogens into the human population via transplanted animal organs needs to be addressed. The recent controversy over BSE and the origin of the HIV virus has highlighted this as a potential risk in xenotransplantation. Much more information about the pig genome (especially retroviruses embedded in the porcine DNA) will be required to satisfy public concern, before xenotransplantation involving humans can start. However, given the increasing demand for donor organs, which it is probably not possible to satisfy with human cadaveric organ donation, the need for an alternative will continue to grow.

## References

1. Medawar PB. The behaviour and fate of skin autografts and skin homografts in rabbits. J Anat 1944; 78: 176–99.
2. Gowans JL, McGregor DD, Cowan DM, Ford CE. Initiation of immune responses by small lymphocytes. Nature 1962; 196: 651–5.
3. Miller JFAP. Effect of neonatal thymectomy on the immunological responsiveness of the mouse. Proc R Soc London B 1962; 156: 415–28.
4. Billingham RE, Brent L, Medawar PB. Quantitative studies on tissue transplantation immunity III: actively acquired tolerance. Philos Trans R Soc 1956; 239: 357–414.
5. Kissmeyer-Nielson F, Olsen S, Peterson VP, Fjeldborg O. Hyperacute rejection of kidney allografts associated with pre-existing humoral antibody against donor cells. Lancet 1966; 2: 662–5.
6. Wheeler CH, Collins A, Dunn MJ, Crisp SJ, Yacoub MH, Rose ML. Characterisation of endothelial antigens associated with transplant-associated coronary artery disease. J Heart Lung Transplant 1995; 14: S188–97.
7. Dausset J. Iso-leuco-anticorps (Iso-leuko-antibodies). Acta Haematol 1958; 20: 156–66.
8. Kissmeyer-Nielson F, Svejgaard A, Hauge M. Genetics of the human HL-A transplantation system. Nature 1968; 219: 1116–19.
9. Sandberg L, Thorsby E, Kissmeyer-Nielson F, Lindholm A. In: Terasaki P (ed) Histocompatibility testing. Copenhagen: Munksgaard, 1970, pp 165–9.
10. Van Leeuwan A, Schuit HRE, Van Rood JJ. Typing for MLC (LDII) the selection of non-stimulator cells by MLC inhibition tests using ST identical stimulator cells (MISIS) and fluorescent antibody studies. Transplant Proc 1973; 5: 1539–42.
11. Zinkernagal RM, Doherty PC. Restriction of in vitro T cell-mediated cytotoxicity in lymphocytic choriomeningitis within a syngeneic or semiallogeneic system. Nature 1974; 248: 701–2.
12. Snell GD. Studies in histocompatibility. Science 1981: 213: 172–8.
13. Trowsdale J, Ragoussis J, Campbell RD. Map of the human MHC. Immunol Today 1991; 12: 433–6.
14. Koller BH, Geraghty DE, DeMars R, Duvick L, Rich SS, Orr HT. Chromosomal organisation of the human major histocompatibility complex Class I gene family. J Exp Med 1989; 169: 469–80.
15. Dunham I, Sargent CA, Dawkins RL, Campbell RD. An analysis of variation in the long-range genomic organization of the human major histocompatibility complex class II region by pulsed field gel electrophoresis. Genomics 1989; 5: 787–96.
16. Kelly A, Powis SH, Kerr LA et al. Assembly and function of the two ABC transporter proteins encoded in the human histocompatibility complex. Nature 1992; 355: 641–4.
17. Bjorkman PJ, Parham P. Structure, function and diversity of Class I major histocompatibility complex molecules. Annu Rev Biochem 1990; 59: 253–88.
18. Springer TA. Adhesion receptors of the immune system. Nature 1990; 346: 425–34.
19. Williams A, Barclay AN. The immunoglobulin superfamily – domains for cell recognition. Annu Rev Immunol 1989; 6: 381–405.
20. Bjorkman PJ, Saper MA, Samraoui B, Bennett WS, Strominger JL, Wiley DC. Structure of the human Class I histocompatibility antigen HLA-A2. Nature 1987; 329: 506–12.
21. Bjorkman PJ, Saper MA, Samraoui B, Bennett WS, Strominger JL, Wiley DC. The foreign antigen binding site and T cell recognition regions of class I histocompatibility antigens. Nature 1987; 329: 512–18.
22. Eliot T, Cerundolo V, Elvain J, Townsend A. Peptide induced conformational change of the Class I heavy chain. Nature 1991; 351: 402–6.
23. Madden DR, Gorga JC, Strominger JL, Wiley DC. The structure of HLA-B27 reveals nanomer selfpeptides bound in an extended conformation. Nature 1991; 353: 321–5.
24. Daar AS, Fuggle SV, Fabre JW, Ting A, Morris PJ. The detailed distribution of HLA A, B, C antigens in normal human organs. Transplantation 1984; 38: 287–94.
25. Kappes D, Strominger JL. Human Class II major histocompatibility complex genes and proteins. Annu Rev Biochem 1988; 57: 991–1028.

26. Rudensly AY, Preston Hurlburt P, Hong SC, Barlow A, Janeway CA. Sequence analysis of peptides bound to MHC Class II molecules. Nature 1991; 353: 622–7.

27. Daar AS, Fuggle SV, Fabre JW, Ting A, Morris PJ. The detailed distribution of major histocompatibility complex Class II antigens in normal human organs. Transplantation 1984; 38: 294–8.

28. Neefjes JJ, Stollory V, Peters PJ, Geuze HJ, Ploegh HL. The biosynthetic pathway of MHC Class II but not the Class I molecules intersects with the endocytic route. Cell 1990; 61: 171–83.

29. Garboczi DN, Ghosh P, Utz U, Fan QR, Biddison WE, Wiley DC. Structure of the complex between human T cell receptor, viral peptide and HLA-A2. Nature 1996; 384: 134–41.

30. Opelz G. HLA matching should be utilised for improving kidney transplant success rate. Transplant Proc 1991; 23: 46–50.

31. Patel R, Tersaki PI. Significance of the positive cross-match test in kidney transplantation. N Engl J Med 1969; 280: 735–9.

32. Suici-Foci N, Reed E, Marboe C et al. The role of anti-HLA matching in heart transplantation. Transplantation 1991; 51: 716.

33. Donaldson PT, Williams R. Crossmatching in liver transplantation: an overview. Transplantation 1997; 63: 1–6.

34. Fung J, Makowa L, Tzakis A et al. Combined liver-kidney transplantation: analysis of patients performed with preformed lymphocytotoxic antibodies. Transplant Proc 1988; 20 (Suppl 1): 88–91.

35. Simpson E. Immunology of the H-Y antigen and its role in sex determination. Proc R Soc London B 1983; 220: 31–46.

36. Auchincloss H Jr, Sachs DH. Transplantation and graft rejection. In: Paul WE (ed) Fundamental immunology, New York: Raven Press, 1989.

37. Pritchard H, Micklem HS. The nude (nu/nu) mouse as a model of thymus and T lymphocyte deficiency. In: Rygaard J, Povlsen CO (eds) Proceedings of the first international workshop on nude mice. Stuttgart: Verlag, 1974, pp. 127–39.

38. Kisielow P, von Boehmer H. Development and selection of T cells: facts and puzzles. Adv Immunol 1995; 58: 87–209.

39. Davis MM, Bjorkman PJ. T-cell antigen receptor genes and T-cell recognition. Nature 1988; 334: 395–401.

40. Zheng B, Han S, Zhu Q, Goldsby R, Kelsoe G. Alternative pathways for the selection of antigen specific peripheral T cells. Nature 1996; 384: 263–6.

41. Fleischer B, Schrezenmeier H, Wagner H. Function of the CD4 and CD8 molecules in human cytotoxic T lymphocytes: regulation of T cell triggering. J Immunol 1986; 136: 1625–8.

42. Moebius U, Kober G, Griscelli AL, Hercend T, Meuer SC. Expression of different CD8 isoforms on distinct human lymphocyte subpopulations. Eur J Immunol 1991; 21: 1793–800.

43. Dalgleish AG, Beverley PC, Clapham PR, Crawford DH, Greaves MF, Weiss RA. The CD4 (T4) antigen is an essential component of the receptor for the AIDS retrovirus. Nature 1984; 312: 763–7.

44. Luescher IF, Vivier E, Layer A et al. CD8 modulation of T-cell antigen receptor-ligand interactions on living cytotoxic T lymphocytes. Nature 1995; 373: 353–6.

45. Veillette A, Bookman MA, Horak EM, Bolen JB. The CD4 and CD8 T cell surface antigens are associated with the internal membrane tyrosine-protein kinase p561ck. Cell 1988; 55: 301–8.

46. Garcia KC, Scott CA, Brunmark A et al. CD8 enhances formation of stable T cell receptor/ MHC class I molecule complexes. Nature 1996; 384: 577–81.

47. Sundstrom JB, Ansari AA. Comparative study of the role of professional versus semiprofessional or non-professional antigen presenting cells in the rejection of vascularized organ allografts. Trans Immunol 1995; 3: 273–89.

48. Lechler RI, Batchelor JR. Restoration of immunogenicity to passenger cell depleted kidney allografts by the addition of donor strain dendritic cells. J Exp Med 1982; 155: 31.

49. Evavold BD, Sloan-Lancaster J, Allen PM. Tickling the TCR: selective T-cell functions stimulated by altered peptide ligands. Immunol Today 1993; 14: 602–9.

50. Sloan-Lancaster J, Evavold BD, Allen PM. Th2 cell clonal anergy as a consequence of partial activation. J Exp Med 1994; 180: 1195–205.

51. Harding FA, McArthur JG, Gross JA, Raulet DH, Allison JP. CD28 mediated signalling

co-stimulates T cells and prevents induction of anergy in T cell clones. Nature 1992; 356: 607–9.

52. Banchereau J, Bazan F, Blanchard D et al. The CD40 antigen and its ligand. Annu Rev Immunol 1994; 12: 881–922.

53. Jenkins MK, Schwartz RH. Antigen presentation by chemically modified splenocytes induces antigen-specific T cell unresponsiveness in vitro and in vivo. J Exp Med 1987; 165: 302–19.

54. Shoskes DA, Wood KJ. Indirect presentation of MHC antigens in transplantation. Immunol Today 1994; 15: 32–8.

55. Braciale TJ, Morrison LA, Sweetser MT, Sambrook J, Gething MJ, Braciale VL. Antigen presentation pathways to class I and class II MHC-restricted T lymphocytes. Immunol Rev 1987; 98: 95–114.

56. Perlmutter RM, Levin SD, Appleby MW, Anderson SJ, Alberola-Ila J. Regulation of lymphocyte function by protein phosphorylation. Annu Rev Immunol 1993; 11: 451–99.

57. Izquierdo-Pastor MI, Reif K, Cantrell D. The regulation and function of p21ras during T-cell activation and growth. Immunol Today 1995; 16: 159–64.

58. Hibbs ML, Wardlaw AJ, Stacker SA et al. Transfection of cells from patients with leukocyte adhesion deficiency with an integrin beta subunit (CD18) restores lymphocyte function-associated antigen-1 expression and function. J Clin Invest 1990; 85: 674–81.

59. Trowbridge IS, Ostergaard HL, Johnson P. CD45: a leukocyte-specific member of the protein tyrosine phosphatase family. Biochim Biophys Acta 1991; 1095: 46–56.

60. Figdor CG, van Kooyk Y, Keizer-GD. On the mode of action of LFA-1. Immunol Today 1990; 11: 277–80.

61. Gibbs P, Berkley LM, Bolton EM, Briggs JD, Bradley JA. Adhesion molecule expression (ICAM-1, VCAM-1, E-selectin and PECAM) in human kidney allografts. Trans Immunol 1993; 1: 109–13.

62. Westphal JR, Willems HW, Tax WJ, Koene RA, Ruiter DJ, de Waal RM. The proliferative response of human T cells to allogeneic IFN-γ-treated endothelial cells is mediated via both CD2/LFA-3 and LFA-1/ICAM-1 and -2 adhesion pathways. Trans Immunol 1993; 1: 183–91.

63. Hughes CC, Savage CO, Pober JS. The endothelial cell as a regulator of T cell function. Immunol Rev 1990; 117: 85–102.

64. D'Alesandro MM, Gruber DF, O'Halloran KP, MacVittie TJ. In vitro modulation of canine polymorphonuclear leukocyte function by granulocyte-macrophage colony stimulating factor. Biotherapy 1991; 3: 233–9.

65. Belosevic M, Finbloom DS, van der Meide PH, Slayter MV, Nacy CA. Administration of monoclonal anti-γ IFN antibodies in vivo abrogates natural resistance of C3H/HeN mice to infection with Leishmania major. J Immunol 1989; 143: 266–72.

66. Reiner SL, Locksley RM. The regulation of immunity to Leishmania major. Annu Rev Immunol 1995; 13: 151–77.

67. Llorente L., Crevon M-C, Karrey S, de France T, Banchereau J, Galanaud P. Interleukin (IL) 4 counteracts the helper effect of IL2 on antigen activated human B cells. Eur J Immunol 1989, 19: 765–9.

68. Spits H, Yssel H, Paliard X, Kasteleigh R, Figdor C, De Vries RJ. IL4 inhibits IL2 mediated induction of human lymphokine activated killer cells, but not the generation of antigen-specific cytotoxic lymphocytes in mixed leucocyte cultures. J Immunol 1988; 141: 29–36.

69. Mosmann TR, Moore KW. The role of IL-10 in crossregulation of TH1 and TH2 responses. Immunoparasitol Today 1991; 12: A49–A53.

70. Mosmann TR, Cherwinski H, Bond MW, Giedlin MA, Coffman RL. Two types of murine helper T cell clone. I. Definition according to profiles of lymphokine activities and secreted proteins. J Immunol 1986; 136: 2348–57.

71. Farges O, Morris PJ, Dallman MJ. Spontaneous acceptance of liver allografts in the rat. Analysis of the immune response. Transplantation 1994; 57: 171–7.

72. Dallman MJ, Larsen CP, Morris PJ. Cytokine gene transcription in vascularised organ grafts: analysis using semi quantitative polymerase chain reaction. J Exp Med 1991; 174: 493–6.

73. Colvin RB, Preffer FI, Fuller T et al. A critical analysis of serum and urine interleukin 2 receptor assays in renal allograft recipients. Trans Proc 1989; 21: 1863.

74. Kirkman RL, Shapiro ME, Carpenter CB *et al.* A randomized prospective trial of anti-Tac monoclonal antibody in human renal transplantation. Transplantation 1991; 51: 107–13.

75. Mason DW, Morris PJ. Effector mechanisms in allograft rejection. Annu Rev Immunol 1986; 4: 119–45.

76. Clark EA, Lane PJ. Regulation of human B-cell activation and adhesion. Annu Rev Immunol 1991; 9: 97–127.

77. Morton AL, Bell EB, Bolton EM *et al.* CD4+ T cell-mediated rejection of major histocompatibility complex class I-disparate grafts: a role for allo antibody. Eur J Immunol 1993; 23: 2078–84.

78. Rose ML. Role of antibody and indirect antigen presentation in transplant-associated coronary artery vasculopathy. J Heart Lung Transplant 1996; 15: 342–9.

79. Dennert G, Podack ER. Cytolosis by H-2 specific T killer cells: assembly of tubular complexes on target membranes. J Exp Med 1983; 157: 1483–95.

80. Gershenfeld HK, Weissman IL. Cloning of a cDNA for a T cell-specific serine protease from a cytotoxic T lymphocyte. Science 1986; 232: 854–8.

81. Calne RY, Sells RA, Pena JR *et al.* Induction of immunological tolerance by porcine liver allografts. Nature 1969; 223: 472–6.

82. Rao AS, Starzl TE, Demetris AJ *et al.* The two-way paradigm of transplantation immunology. Clin Immunol Immunopathol 1996; 80: S46–51.

83. Platt JL, Fischel RJ, Matas AJ, Reif SA, Bolman RM, Bach FH. Immunopathology of hyperacute xenograft rejection in a swine-to-primate model. Transplantation 1991; 52: 214–20.

84. Bach FH, Robson SC, Winkler H *et al.* Barriers to xenotransplantation. Nature Med 1995; 1: 869–73.

85. Pober JS, Cotran RS. The role of endothelial cells in inflammation. Transplantation 1991; 50: 537–44.

86. Robson SC, Candinas D, Siegel JB *et al.* Potential mechanism of abnormal thromboregulation in xenograft rejection loss of ecto ATPases upon endothelial cell activation. Trans Proc 1996; 28: 536.

87. Dalmasso AP, Vercellotti GM, Platt JL, Bach FH. Inhibition of complement mediated endothelial cell cytotoxicity by decay accelerating factor. Potential for prevention of xenograft hyperacute rejection. Transplantation 1991; 52: 530–3.

88. Schmoeckel M, Nollert G, Shahmohammadi M *et al.* Human decay accelerating factor successfully protects pig hearts from hyperacute rejection by human blood. Trans Proc 1996; 28: 768–9.

89. Pless HC, Forsythe JLR, Proud G, Taylor RM, Kirby JA. Xenotransplantation: an examination of the adhesive interactions between human lymphocytes and porcine renal epithelial cells. Trans Immunol 1994; 2: 225–30.

# 5 Immunosuppression: the old and the new

*Neil R. Parrott*

Transplantation has arguably been one of the most rapidly evolving parts of medicine over the last three decades, and there can be few examples of a clinical procedure that has gone from complete failure to outstanding success in such a short time. In the interval from the first human transplant in 1933 by Voronoy, to the time of the first successful human-to-human renal allograft in Boston by Murray in 1954, any understanding of immunosuppression and rejection was rudimentary. For the most part, there were no really effective immunosuppressive agents. It was almost certainly the evolution of immunosuppressive drugs that facilitated the successful birth of transplantation.

## The 'old' immuno-suppression

1959 was to be one of the early landmarks when Schwartz and Damashek[1] showed that 6-mercaptopurine (6-MP) was able to induce immunological tolerance in rabbits. Although 6-MP had been discovered earlier (1952) by Hitchins and coworkers,[2] it was really not until its metabolite azathioprine was elucidated that the 'modern' era of immunosuppression began.[3] The seminal work of Calne and Murray was then to illustrate that azathioprine was much more effective than 6-MP, and also less toxic. While working in Boston, Calne was able to produce long-term survivors in dog renal allografts using 6-MP and later azathioprine as an immunosuppressant.[4,5] This and subsequent work at the Peter Bent Brigham Hospital in Boston by Murray and Calne was to result in Murray being awarded the Nobel Prize in medicine.[6,7]

### Azathioprine and prednisolone

Azathioprine (Aza) is a nitroimidazole derivative of 6-mercaptopurine, and is metabolised within the liver to its active form, 6-thioinosinic acid. Azathioprine has diffuse effects on the synthesis of both DNA and RNA; it may become incorporated into the former, and result in chromosomal breaks.[8] It is presumably this fact that makes transplant patients immunosuppressed with Aza so prone to cutaneous malignancy. The catabolism of Aza is by the enzyme xanthine oxidase. It is for this reason that allopurinol (an inhibitor of xanthine oxidase) is contraindicated in the presence of Aza. The coadministration of both drugs may result in profound toxicity with marrow suppression, agranulocytosis and leucopenia. By the time that Aza had been isolated and understood, corticosteroids had long since been identified as immunosuppressive agents, so that the combination of the two drugs was quickly established as the 'gold standard' in the evolving field of transplantation. Until the discovery of cyclosporin in 1978, the combination of azathioprine and prednisolone was the mainstay of immunosuppression, and in this time, the majority of clinical research was focused on the optimal dose/combination with this double drug regimen. Early workers used very large doses of both steroid and azathioprine, so that the typical transplant recipient of the 1970s was invariably cushingoid, often leucopenic, and plagued by the other complications of the drugs, particularly steroids (Table 5.1). It was the excellent results in Belfast that showed the transplant community that the large (and damaging) doses of steroids were unnecessary, and that good or better results were possible with lower doses and fewer side effects.[9] The work in Belfast was later confirmed in Oxford[10] and in a prospective study in the USA.[11] Clearly, so long as the dose of azathioprine was reasonable ($>1.75$ mg kg$^{-1}$ day$^{-1}$ in the d'Apice[11] study), then low doses of steroids were associated with fewer side effects and acceptable graft outcome. Interestingly, the lessons learnt about steroids were to be

**Table 5.1**  *Main side effects of immunosuppression with 'conventional therapy'*

**Steroids**
- Cushingoid appearance
- Hypertension
- Hyperglycaemia and diabetes
- Steroid osteoporosis
- Avascular necrosis of bone (especially femoral head)
- Salt and water retention
- Capillary and dermal fragility
- Obesity
- Hirsutism
- Acne
- Peptic ulceration
- Pancreatitis

**Azathioprine**
- Agranulocytosis
- Leucopenia
- Hepatic dysfunction
- Malignancy (esp. skin)
- Propensity to viral warts

**Figure 5.1** *Effect of immunosuppressive regimen on late graft outcome. (From Opelz G. Effect of the maintenance immunosuppressive drug regime on kidney outcome. Transplantation 1994; 58: 443–6, with permission.)*

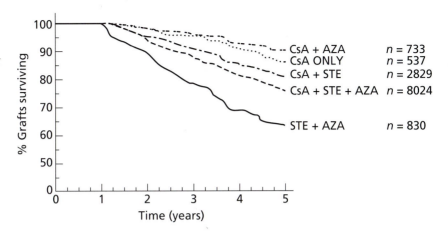

re-emphasised 20 years later, with the illustration that late graft function was mostly better in steroid-free regimes (Fig. 5.1). However, whereas 'conventional therapy' with Aza/prednisolone had undoubtedly elevated the status and success of transplantation, the one-year graft survival rates in renal transplantation were still little more than 60%. For the most part, there is no longer a justification for using azathioprine/prednisolone alone as the sole form of initial immunosuppression, and new agents have moved us far away from that regime. The next major advance was to happen in 1976.

## Cyclosporin A

The discovery by Borel *et al.*[12] of the drug cyclosporin A (CSA) in 1976 was to prove the next major advance in transplantation, and arguably the most important single contribution to transplantation since the very first human transplant by Jaboulay in 1906. Cyclosporin A is a fungal decapeptide that prevents the proliferation and clonal expansion of T lymphocytes by the inhibition of interleukin-2 at a nuclear level. The mechanism of action is discussed in more detail in the section on FK506. The early, multicentre studies of CSA in kidney transplantation showed that it was capable of reducing acute allograft rejection, and resulted in a 1-year graft survival that was between 10 and 20% better than groups immunosuppressed with azathioprine and steroids alone. In this respect, there were two major prospective randomised studies, the European Multicentre trial, and the Canadian one.[13,14] The European trial recruited 232 patients to the study, in which they were randomised to receive either 'conventional therapy' with azathioprine and prednisolone, or treatment with cyclosporin A as monotherapy. The 1-year graft survival was 52% in the control group, and 72% in the group treated with cyclosporin A. In the European study, serum creatinine was significantly elevated, and clearance reduced in the CSA arm of the study. The Canadian multicentre study recruited some 291 patients to the trial, and they were randomised to receive either cyclosporin A and prednisolone,

**Figure 5.2** *Three-month graft survival; cadaveric renal transplantation in the UK; 1978–1987.*

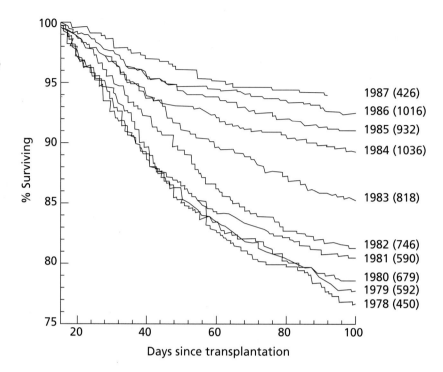

or Aza/prednisolone. After 1 year, actuarial graft survival was 77.5% and 69.8% in the CSA and 'conventional' groups respectively (*P* = 0.038). After 3 years, the graft survival was 69% and 58% in the same groups (*P* < 0.05). The authors noted that although the serum creatinine was elevated in the cyclosporin group, the graft and patient survival was greater.[15] Within a short space of time, many centres were reporting their own results with cyclosporin A, although a large number were trials with small numbers that were neither well-controlled nor randomised.[16–18] Thus CSA had become accepted as the new standard in transplant immunosuppression, and similar results were being reported for its use in heart,[19] liver[20] and pancreas transplantation.[21] Within the UK, the global results over the era between 1978 and 1987 illustrate most clearly the effect that CSA had in cadaveric renal transplantation (Fig. 5.2). Most UK transplant centres introduced CSA into their routine practice by the early 1980s. The amount of acute rejection (and therefore graft loss) was very significantly reduced as a consequence. There is a common belief that it was cyclosporin that resulted in the huge upturn in transplant numbers in the mid-1980s. For many forms of transplantation, the early success rates had not been high enough for it to be regarded as 'standard therapy' in the treatment of end-organ failure. The advent of CSA lifted many of these surgical techniques from the label of 'experimental' to 'routine', and despite the large number of side effects that have been identified with CSA (Table 5.2), it has become accepted as the new standard against which all other immunosuppressives are now judged. In 1994, CSA was released in a new formulation (Neoral

**Table 5.2**  *The side effects of cyclosporin A*

1. Nephrotoxicity
2. Hepatotoxicity
3. Diabetes/glucose intolerance
4. Neuropathy
5. Tremor
6. Gingival hypertrophy
7. Hypertrichosis

Cyclosporin) – this will be discussed under 'New immunosuppressives'. Since the introduction of cyclosporin, there have been many other new immunosuppressives, but none have yet had quite the same impact as CSA on the success of transplantation. So great has been the contribution of this drug that one-year graft survival rates of 80–90% are now reported for almost all forms of solid organ transplantation (renal and non-renal). However, the transplant community now stands at a watershed. The results of transplantation are now so good that it is impossible to improve one-year graft survival without the use of huge randomised clinical studies. The very size and cost of such studies are quite likely to deter any pharmaceutical company from investing in this market without something very special in its armamentarium. The problems of the 1990s are not therefore those of acute allograft rejection, but those of chronic graft loss. Despite the improved one-year graft survival for all transplantation, the late loss of grafts (and patients) is 3–5% per annum, and this is to some extent influenced by the immunosup-

**Table 5.3**  *Mechanism of action of the new immunosuppressive agents*

**Antimetabolites**
  *Antipurine metabolism*
    Mizoribine
    RS61443 (Mycophenolate mofetil)
  *Anti-pyrimidines*
    Brequinar sodium
    Leflunomide
**Anti-T cell agents**
    Rapamicin (Sirolimus)
    FK506 (Tacrolimus)
    Cyclosporin Neoral
**Drugs inhibiting antigen presentation**
    Deoxyspergualin
**Monoclonal antibodies**
    Anti-ICAM 1
    Anti-LFA
    Anti-Tac

pressive regime used (Fig. 5.1). This late annual loss is largely due to the devastating effects of chronic allograft rejection as well as patient death with functioning graft. It is against this background that the profession faces a barrage of new and exciting immunosuppressive agents. The purpose of the rest of this chapter is to give an overview of these new drugs, and to try and place them in perspective for transplantation in the next decade. The drugs to be described, and their mechanisms of action are summarised in Table 5.3.

**The new immuno-suppressives**

## Drugs influencing purine biosynthesis

### Mizoribine (Bredinin)
*Mechanism of action*

Mizoribine (4-carbamoyl-1-beta-D-ribofuranosyl imidazolium-5-olate) is an antimetabolite, and like both azathioprine and mycophenolate mofetil (MMF) is an inhibitor of purine metabolism. It is isolated from *Eupenicillium brefeldianum*. It was first used as a cytotoxic antibiotic and it has antiviral properties. It was noted to be immunosuppressive as early as 1976.[22] It has been used more extensively in Japan than in USA and Europe. In common with MMF, mizoribine is an inhibitor of the enzyme inosine monophosphate dehydrogenase (IMPDH), but it is a competitive inhibitor as opposed to MMF which is non-competitive.[23] The drug is able to suppress lymphoproliferation, but is ineffective in preventing the recognition phase of T cell activation or the effector phase.[24]

The drug is excreted mainly unchanged in the urine, and is therefore profoundly influenced by renal function. Serum levels peak after a mean of 2.4 h.[25,26]

*Animal studies*

The majority of animal studies have centred around rodents and dogs. Much of the early basic immunopharmacology was undertaken in rats, but the drug has been used with success as an immunosuppressant in dogs. In early animal studies, it was felt to have an immunosuppressive potency equivalent to azathioprine, but without the hepatotoxicity of the latter drug.[27]

In an early study in canine renal transplantation, the drug was found to be an effective immunosuppressant *in vivo*, but the major side effect in this model was that of erosive mucositis of the entire bowel. It was also noted that the drug caused splenic atrophy and mesenteric node atrophy.[28] In a canine renal model used by another group, mizoribine given alone was able to extend the mean survival time to 20 days. This was significantly prolonged compared to historical, non-immunosuppressed controls where mean survival time was only 8 days. Numbers were, however, small.[29]

## Human studies

Although mizoribine has been known for many years, its use in human transplantation is somewhat limited. The majority of the clinical studies have been undertaken in Japan. The early human studies were undertaken in recipients of live related transplants. In an uncontrolled, open study, mizoribine was given to 39 renal allograft recipients (21 live related, 18 cadaveric donors) in Japan. No controls were used, but the group reported 1-year graft survival of 95% for living related recipients, and 64% for cadaveric donors.[30] In 1990, a different group from Japan reported their own experience with the drug in renal transplants. At one year, there was no statistically significant difference in graft survival, but serum creatinine was lower in recipients given mizoribine compared with those on 'standard' triple therapy. Once again, this was a study that was poorly controlled, non-randomised, and with small numbers.[31] In a more recent study, the drug has been compared in an open, randomised phase II trial, contrasting triple therapy using azathioprine with triple therapy using mizoribine. The numbers are very small, and there was no significant difference in rejection, graft survival or serum creatinine in the study. The authors did, however, state that the drug was apparently well-tolerated, and safe.[32] It was suggested that the drug represents a safe alternative to azathioprine, is free of apparent hepatotoxicity, and could be given safely in patients with allopurinol (both in contrast to azathioprine).

Phase III human trials have now been undertaken with this drug. Results are not yet available for scrutiny, but are awaited with interest.

## Chronic rejection

There are no studies that have addressed this issue, and therefore no evidence to suggest it may be of benefit in patients with chronic vascular rejection (CVR).

## Summary

- An antimetabolite very similar to azathioprine
- Poor early clinical studies and little good data so far
- Little to add beyond the benefits of azathioprine
- Can be given with allopurinol, and free of hepatotoxicity

## Mycophenolate mofetil (Cellcept)

Mycophenolate mofetil (MMF) is the newest immunosuppressant to have a licence for use in human transplantation. It received a product licence in the USA in mid/late 1995, and in the UK in early 1996.

## Mechanism of action

MMF is the morpholinoethyl ester of mycophenolic acid, and is de-esterified *in vivo* to the active drug mycophenolic acid. The agent has been available for some years, but it is only relatively recently that it has gained prominence as an immunosuppressant.

MMF is an antiproliferative drug that inhibits the enzyme inosine monophosphate dehydrogenase (IMPDH), a key step in the *de novo* pathway of purine synthesis.[33] T and B lymphocytes are unique in that they rely almost entirely on the *de novo* pathway for purine biosynthesis, and, unlike most other tissues, have no salvage pathway.[34] Thus, MMF has a specific effect on lymphocytes.[35] The stages of *de novo* and salvage purine synthesis are shown in Fig. 5.3. In contrast to the effects of azathioprine, MMF selectively interrupts DNA synthesis, it inhibits just a single enzyme non-competitively (in contrast to azathioprine which inhibits many enzymes), it does not interfere with the repair of DNA, or become incorporated into it (also in contrast to azathioprine). Thus, it might be expected to be less mutagenic to DNA.

Both T and B lymphocytes rely on the *de novo* pathway, and MMF is therefore equally effective against B cells as T cells. *In vivo*, MMF is rapidly de-esterified to the active compound mycophenolic acid, which is itself glucuronated.[36] In addition to its effects on T and B cells, MMF has also beneficial effects on the synthesis of fucosylated sugars. It may, therefore, inhibit the synthesis of adhesion molecules,[37] as well as having an inhibitory effect on smooth muscle proliferation[38] and the synthesis of 'pro-fibrotic cytokines'. These factors suggest that it may have a potential role in preventing/reversing 'chronic rejection' (transplant vascular sclerosis). Unlike cyclosporin, MMF does not have any effect on early T cell activation cytokines such as interferon-γ (IFN-γ) granulocyte–monocyte-colony stimulation factor (GM-CSF), interleukin-2 (IL-2), IL-4 and IL-5.[39]

### Animals studies

MMF has been studied very extensively in a large number of animal models. To date, the published data suggest that MMF is an effective immunosuppressant in mice, rats, dogs and primates, and that the drug can prevent or reverse acute rejection in renal, islet, cardiac and small bowel models.[40–44]

### Human studies

The drug has been used extensively in humans, mainly in renal transplantation, but also in other solid organs. Some of the early studies used MMF in the treatment of refractory rejection in heart, liver[45] and kidney transplantation. In a series of 15 cardiac transplant recipients who had failed to respond to 'conventional treatment', over 90% responded to treatment with MMF.[46] In a multicentre study from the USA, 75 renal transplant recipients who were non-responsive to treatment with OKT3 or ATG, and who had biopsy-proven allograft rejection were given between 2 and 3 g/day of MMF.[47] Patients were entered into the study within 48 h of their biopsy, and continued to take cyclosporin A and steroids. Successful long-term rescue was achieved in 52 patients (69%). In 19 patients, MMF was discontinued for treatment failure, and the patient returned to dialysis. The authors found that the successful rescue was related to serum creatinine at entry

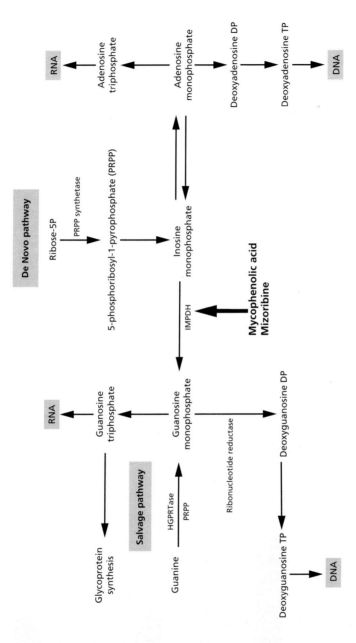

**Figure 5.3** *Pathways in purine biosynthesis.*

**Table 5.4**  *Study design and results of clinical trials with mycophenolate mofetil*

| | *n* | Number of centres | Immunosuppression | Rejection or treatment failure |
|---|---|---|---|---|
| USA | 499 | 14 | Quadruple (ATGAM) | |
| | | | Aza 1–2 mg g day$^{-1}$ | 47.6% |
| | | | MMF 2 g day$^{-1}$ | 31.1% |
| | | | MMF 3 g day$^{-1}$ | 31.1% |
| European | 491 | 20 | Triple | |
| | | | Placebo | 56.0% |
| | | | MMF 2 g day$^{-1}$ | 30.3% |
| | | | MMF 3 g day$^{-1}$ | 38.8% |
| Tricontinental | 503 | 21 | Triple | |
| | | | Aza 100–150 mg day$^{-1}$ | 50.0% |
| | | | MMF 2 g day$^{-1}$ | 38.2% |
| | | | MMF 3 g day$^{-1}$ | 34.8% |

to the study. Those with serum creatinine of greater than 4.0 mg dl$^{-1}$ had only a 52% response rate, those with creatinine values less than this had a response rate that was 79%. In the latter study, mild to moderate gastrointestinal side effects were the commonest reported, with eight cases having significant leucopenia. Two large, multicentre prospective, randomised studies of MMF in renal transplantation have now been published. A third such study, has been presented to the European Society of Organ Transplantation (Vienna, 1995), and is published in abstract form. These studies require some consideration. The published studies are from European and US centres respectively. In the European multicentre study, 491 patients were enrolled, of which 166 received CSA and placebo, 165 received CSA and MMF 2 g day$^{-1}$, and 160 received CSA in addition to MMF 3 g day$^{-1}$. Data were presented for the first 6 post-transplant months. After this time interval, 56% of the

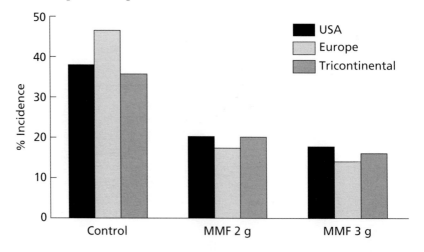

**Figure 5.4**  *The incidence (%) of biopsy-proven rejection, mycophenolate studies.*

**Table 5.5**  *Side effects of mycophenolate, from randomised studies; figures represent data from USA and European studies*

| European study | Placebo group | MMF (2 g/day) | MMF (3 g/day) |
|---|---|---|---|
| **Gastrointestinal** | | | |
| Diarrhoea | 12.7% | 12.7% | 15.6% |
| Abdominal pain | 10.8% | 11.5% | 11.3% |
| Dyspepsia | 5.4% | 3.0% | 5.0% |
| Haemorrhage (all sites) | 0 | 1.2% | 2.5% |
| All GI side effects | 41.6% | 45.5% | 52.5% |
| **Haematological** | | | |
| Leucopenia | 4.2% | 10.9% | 13.8% |
| Anaemia | 1.8% | 4.2% | 6.8% |
| Thrombocytopenia | 4.8% | 4.2% | 3.1% |
| **Opportunistic Infection** | | | |
| CMV viraemia | 13.3% | 15.8% | 15.0% |
| CMV tissue invasive | 2.4% | 3.0% | 6.9% |
| Total | 27.7% | 38.2% | 34.4% |
| **USA study** | **Azathioprine group** | **MMF (2 g/day)** | **MMF (3 g/day)** |
| **Gastrointestinal** | | | |
| Diarrhoea | 23.8% | 31.5% | 37.3% |
| Abdominal pain | not stated | not stated | not stated |
| Dyspepsia | not stated | not stated | not stated |
| Haemorrhage (all sites) | 1.2% | 4.2% | 4.2% |
| **Haematological** | | | |
| Leucopenia | 1.8% | 3.6% | 4.8% |
| Anaemia | 4.3% | 3.6% | 8.4% |
| Thrombocytopenia | 1.2% | 0.6% | 3.0% |
| **Opportunistic Infection** | | | |
| CMV viraemia | 15.2% | 14.5% | 13.3% |
| CMV tissue invasive | 6.1% | 9.1% | 10.8% |
| Total | 45.7% | 44.8% | 47.0% |

placebo group had suffered biopsy proven rejection or withdrawn from the study for any reason. In the 2 g MMF group this was 30.3%, or 38.8% in the 3 g group ($P < 0.001$). The use of second line therapy (OKT3 or ATG) was halved by the use of MMF in this study.[48] The other study currently in print is the USA multicentre study, in which patients were randomised to receive either 'standard' triple therapy, or triple therapy with 2 or 3 g day$^{-1}$ of MMF. All patients entered in to the study also received induction therapy with antithymocyte globulin (ATGAM). The primary efficacy endpoint for this and the other randomised studies was biopsy-proven rejection, or treatment failure from any cause. Rejection or treatment failure in the USA study was again significantly reduced by either dose of MMF.[49] The format of all three randomised studies are presented in Table 5.4. In each of the studies, the conclusions were broadly similar in that MMF reduced the incidence of biopsy-proven rejection by around 50%, and that the need for ATG/OKT3 to treat steroid-resistant rejection was significantly reduced to a similar degree (Fig. 5.4). The principal side effects were gastrointestinal and myelotoxic (Table 5.5). With the exception of tissue-invasive cytomegalovirus (CMV), the incidence of infection or sepsis was not raised by MMF. Thus the clinical studies confirm that MMF is a useful and powerful immunosuppressive agent, capable of reducing the incidence of allograft rejection by half. To date, the data do not show any improvement in 1-year graft survival, although the studies were not designed to demonstrate this fact. The 2 and 3 year follow-up data on these studies are awaited with interest.

### Chronic rejection

There are a number of experimental studies that suggest that MMF may be an effective agent in the treatment and prevention of graft vascular disease (GVD). All studies are derived from animal models of GVD, and are therefore merely suggestive of a possible role in humans. Using a rat heterotopic heart allograft model, Morris *et al.*[50] were able to show that MMF could reduce the arteriopathy associated with GVD, but neither cyclosporin nor FK506 were useful in this model. In a rat aortic allograft model MMF was able to reduce intimal proliferation to a significant degree, but cyclosporin and brequinar did not.[51] Using a heart xenograft model (cynomolgous monkey to baboon), it was also seen that the accelerated graft vascular sclerosis was slowed by MMF.[51]

### Summary

- Powerful immunosuppressive that is antiproliferative
- Specific and non-competitive effects on IMPDH and purine synthesis
- Extensive human studies
- Capable of halving biopsy-proven renal allograft rejection in humans
- Proven efficacy as rescue therapy
- Adjunctive to CSA or FK506
- Main side effects are gastrointestinal and haematological
- Non-nephro- or hepatotoxic

## Antipyrimidine agents

### Brequinar sodium (BQR)
#### Mechanism of action
Brequinar (6-fluoro-2-(2'-fluoro-1,1'-biphenyl-4-yl)-3-methyl-4-quinoline carboxylic acid sodium salt), like leflunomide, is one of the unique immunosuppressives, being the only agent that is an antiproliferative active against the pyrimidine nucleotides. The agent acts by inhibiting the essential enzyme dihydro-orotic acid dehydrogenase (DHODH),

essential for the *de novo* synthesis of pyrimidine in the mitochondria. The agent was originally conceived as an antitumour drug, but early phase I clinical trials in humans with solid tumours showed that the drug was quite toxic at doses greater than 300 mg m$^{-2}$. Toxic effects included severe ulcerative mucositis, dermatitis, nausea, vomiting, anorexia, diarrhoea and thrombocytopenia,[52] and in many studies, the efficacy as an antitumour agent was not great.[53,54] The drug is equally well absorbed orally or intravenously, has high bioavailability, and a long half-life permitting infrequent dosing.[52] The drug is active against both T and B cells and may have a particular role in the situation of high antibody levels (highly sensitised patients and xenotransplantation).

### Animal studies

In rats, BQR is able to reduce/prevent the rejection of heart, liver and kidney transplants,[55–57] and it acts synergistically with CSA. At a dose of 12 mg kg$^{-1}$, BQR was able to induce donor specific tolerance to both liver and kidney grafts in 50–90% of animals, but was ineffective in producing tolerance to heart grafts in this model.[56] In a LEW rat model of high sensitisation (sensitised with ACI rat skin), BQR was able to prevent accelerated cardiac allograft rejection at doses of either 3 or 12 mg/kg every 3 days.[58] Brequinar has thus shown itself to be an effective and powerful immunosuppressant not only in allograft models, but also in the more difficult setting of xenotransplantation.[59]

### Human studies

Studies in human solid organ transplantation are still few. The drug is still at an early stage of clinical development. In some early pharmacokinetic studies, Kahan[60] has shown that the oral bioavailability of Brequinar is high – 98% with only a fourfold overall pharmacokinetic variation. In preliminary data, brequinar appears to be synergistic with CSA and rapamycin, and, in phase I studies in human renal transplantation, is associated with only around 10% incidence of thrombocytopenia. There are no other currently published studies in human transplantation, and because of the very narrow therapeutic index with this agent, development of the drug has stopped at the present time.

### Summary

- Inhibitor of pyrimidine metabolism
- Effective against T and B cells
- Effective in xenotransplant models
- Synergistic with cyclosporin and rapamycin
- Severe mucositis and dermatitis in early cancer studies

## Leflunomide

### Mechanism of action

Leflunomide (HWA 486) is one of the newer agents under investigation. The drug is a synthetic compound and an isoxazol derivative. It is well absorbed orally, but metabolised into its active form A77 1726. The molecular structure is unlike any of the other immunosuppressive drugs. Initial experience with the agent was in animal models of autoimmune disease (especially arthritis), in which it was effective in preventing the disease.[61] Early work suggested that it was a potent agent, with effects on both T and B cells, and it was soon appreciated that it appeared to work somewhat later in the T cell activation process than CSA, and that its main site of action was not in the prevention of IL-2 formation, nor was it by interference with the IL-2 receptor.[62,63] Leflunomide was able to prevent the progression of rat lymphocytes through the S-phase of the cell cycle, as well as being able to inhibit human T cells from entering the G2 and M phases.[63] More recently it has been found that leflunomide acts by the inhibition of dihydro-orotate dehydrogenase (DHODH), and like brequinar it inhibits the synthesis of pyrimidine nucleotides.[64,65] As a consequence of its site of action, leflunomide has been shown to reverse experimental ongoing acute allograft rejection, some days after it has started. This is in contrast to CSA which will not reverse established acute rejection, although leflunomide is seen to act additively to CSA, and to have impact on B cells as well as T cells.[66]

### Animal studies

The effectiveness of the agent has been shown in a wide variety of animal transplant models. These include, rats, dogs, monkeys and mice.[67–70] In most of the animal models, the agent has appeared to be relatively free of side effects, but in a canine renal allograft model,[71] the drug was quite toxic at higher doses, and its therapeutic window might therefore be relatively small. Leflunomide has also been used in xenotransplant models, where it is highly effective and may be additive with CSA.[72,73]

### Human studies

To date, phase I and II human studies have been done, but none have yet appeared in the medical press. The drug has been used in phase II human studies of rheumatoid arthritis, in which it was found to be effective in doses ranging from 5 to 25 mg daily. The main side effects were gastrointestinal, along with weight loss, allergic skin reactions, and rarely hepatic dysfunction. In this large study of 402 patients, 7% withdrew from the leflunomide because of adverse events.[74]

### Chronic rejection

There are now a number of studies that suggest that leflunomide may be effective in a variety of animal models said to be representative of human chronic rejection. In a suboptimally immunosuppressed rat cardiac model, leflunomide was able to reduce arterial intimal proliferation, and although the effect was dependent on dose and timing, the drug was synergistic with CSA.[75] Its effectiveness in this situation has been shown in a number of studies, and has been suggested to be effective because of its ability to reduce smooth muscle proliferation (?by inhibiting the fibrogenic cytokines).[70,76]

## Summary

- Potent T and B cell effects, as well as active against non-immune cells
- Inhibits DHODH and pyrimidine biosynthesis
- Effective in prevention and treatment of acute rejection
- Effective in late treatment of acute cellular rejection
- Effective and promising drug in CVR
- Synergistic with CSA
- No published human trials

## Anti-T cell agents

### Rapamycin (RAPA)

#### Mechanism of action

Rapamycin (Sirolimus) is a macrolide (mol. wt 913) that was discovered in the fermentation broth of *Streptomyces hygroscopicus* which was itself from a soil sample taken from Easter Island (Rapa Nui) in the Pacific basin. Initially the drug was noted for its antifungal effects,[77] but it was later noted to be a potent immunosuppressive agent.[78,79] Structurally, it is very similar to FK506. Rapamycin is known to prevent the cytokine-dependent proliferation of T cells, but acts at a different stage of T cell activation than either cyclosporin or FK506. The latter drugs prevent the formation of interleukin-2 (IL-2). In contrast, rapamycin does not interfere with the transcription and production of IL-2, but antagonises the action of IL-2 on its receptor.[80] Similarly, RAPA does not suppress other early phase T cell activation genes such as IL-3, IL-4, TNF-$\alpha$, IFN-$\gamma$.[81] Using *in vitro* responsiveness to mitogens as a comparator, RAPA is 100 times more potent than cyclosporin.[82] Rapamycin has also been shown to inhibit the B cell mediated production of immunoglobulin, and has been suggested as a drug for use in the highly sensitised recipient. *In vitro*, the drug can suppress immunoglobulin production 1000 times more potently than cyclosporin A.[83,84] However, rapamycin binds to the same cytosolic protein as FK506, known as FKBP12 (FK binding protein 12). For this reason, rapamycin may antagonise the immunosuppressant effects of FK506 by competition with its cytosolic binding protein.[85] These data suggest that these two drugs may not be suitable for use together, although the combination of cyclosporin and rapamycin may be beneficial and possible due to the differing cytosolic binding of the two (cyclophilin and FKBP12, respectively). In a rat model, rapamycin was compared with cyclosporin A in order to contrast the toxicity of the two drugs. Rapamycin was responsible for weight loss in the treated animals. This was particularly notable in those where rapamycin was combined with cyclosporin. Rapamycin had no adverse effects on liver or renal function, but had the potential to enhance the nephro- and hepatotoxicity of cyclosporin.[86]

*Animal studies*

Rapamycin has been investigated in a large number of animal models of transplantation. In rats, RAPA is 27 times more potent than CSA in immunosuppression of heart, kidney and small bowel transplants[87] and normoglycaemia has been significantly prolonged following islet transplantation in the mouse. The effect of RAPA was dose-specific, and the drug was found to be detrimental to islet function at higher doses (1 and 5 mg kg$^{-1}$ day$^{-1}$).[88]

Rapamycin is effective and potent immunosuppressant in primates, pigs, and dogs.[89–94]

Rapamycin has been shown to be effective in combination, but also when given alone. In a recent study using monotherapy with rapamycin in a porcine renal allograft model, median survival time was significantly enhanced in animals receiving 0.5, 1.0 or 2.0 mg kg$^{-1}$ day$^{-1}$. Signs of toxicity were minimal and the drug was well tolerated. The commonest adverse event was pneumonia.[94]

The potential synergism between rapamycin and cyclosporin has been confirmed in a murine heart transplant model, where a combination of RAPA, CSA and BQR was highly effective and synergistic in prolonging survival.[95]

*Human studies*

There are only limited data on the use of rapamycin in humans. Two, phase I human studies were recently presented in USA and Professor Groth's group in Sweden have used RAPA in a study involving 16 stable renal transplant recipients. The study was randomised, double-blind, placebo-controlled. Patients were maintained on either dual therapy with CSA and steroids ($n = 10$), or on triple immunosuppression ($n = 6$). In this study, the drug was well tolerated in doses of 3 and 15 mg m$^{-2}$, and the only major adverse event was thrombocytopenia at the higher dose. There were no interactions with CSA, and the $t_{1/2}$ was 57 h.[96] In the second phase I study (also randomised double-blind, placebo-controlled) from Minneapolis, the findings were entirely similar, showing that the drug was well tolerated in a single dose between 3 and 21 mg m$^{-2}$, had a half life of 50–70 h, and that there was no interaction with CSA.[97] Preliminary data also suggested that the prophylactic use of RAPA in human renal transplants produced a significant reduction in cellular rejection. Further published data on this drug are awaited with interest, and phase II/III human studies are now being concluded.

*Chronic rejection*

Rapamycin has been shown to have potent effects against both B and T cells, but also may inhibit the production of cytokines such as platelet-derived growth factor (PDGF), and basic fibroblast growth factor (bFGF).[98] Both of these cytokines may be involved in the pathogenesis of transplant vascular sclerosis. Using a 'trauma' model of arterial damage, Gregory *et al.*[99] have shown that either mycophenolate mofetil (MMF) or rapamycin reduce intimal hyperplasia following balloon injury, but neither cyclosporin nor FK506 were effective in this role. Combined together, rapamycin and MMF were highly effective in reducing the response of smooth muscle cells to damage. In two other animal models, RAPA has been shown to be effective in reducing graft vessel disease.[100,101]

### Summary

- Very potent immunosuppressive
- Up to 100 times more potent against T cells than CSA
- Up to 1000 times more potent against B cells than CSA
- Blocks the action of IL-2, not its production
- May be synergistic with CSA
- Cannot be used in combination with FK506
- Possible effects in experimental CVR

## FK506 (Tacrolimus)
### Mechanism of action

FK506 is another of the newer immunosuppressive agents that has a licence for clinical use in Europe and the USA. It is a very potent agent and was first identified in soil samples from Tsukuba in Japan in 1984.[102] The organism producing the drug is *Streptomyces tsukubaensis*. FK506 is a macrolide antibiotic molecule of very similar structure to rapamycin.

The drug has a very similar mechanism of action to CSA but is a very dissimilar molecule (Fig. 5.5). It is soluble in methanol, ethanol and ether but very insoluble in water. Following oral absorption, the bioavailability varies between 5 and 67% (mean 27%), with time to peak concentration also being variable between 0.5 and 4.0 h.[103] FK506 is eliminated primarily by metabolism with most of the metabolites excreted in bile.[104] Less than 1% is excreted in the urine, and the absorption of the drug is not influenced by biliary diversion.[105]

Early *in vitro* tests showed that FK506 was a powerful inhibitor of human and mouse mixed lymphocyte reactivity (MLR), and that the drug was capable of suppressing cytotoxic T cell generation, IL-2, IL-3 and $\gamma$-interferon. The $IC_{50}$ values for cyclosporin and FK506 were 1.0 nmol $1^{-1}$ and 0.1 nmol $1^{-1}$, respectively. Thus, the *in vitro* studies would suggest that FK506 is 100 times more powerful than CSA.[106–108] Using T lymphoma cell lines it was shown that FK506 was able to suppress IL-2 generation in T cells, and that the likely site of action was somewhere between the cell membrane signal transduction and the mRNA transcription site for IL-2. The molecular action of FK506 is now better understood, and it is known to bind to an intracellular binding protein known as FKBP12 (FK binding protein). The drug forms a pentameric complex with calcium, calmodulin, calcineurin and FKBP which in turn is able to inhibit Calcium-dependent IL-2 generation. The pentameric complex inhibits the action of NF-AT (nuclear factor for the activation of T cells)[109] and it is the latter that binds to the gene promoter region responsible for IL-2 mRNA transcription. As more is understood

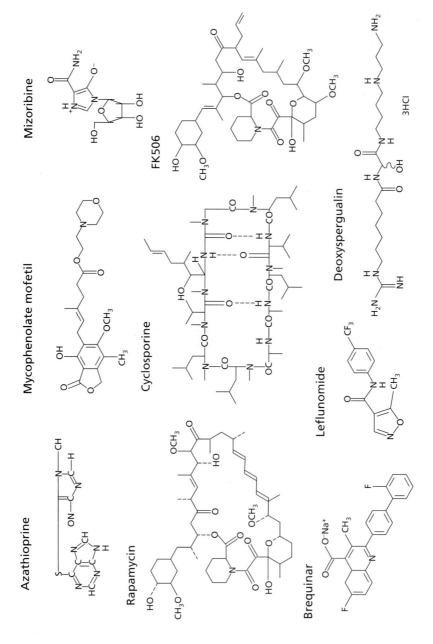

**Figure 5.5** *Structure of the main new and old immunosuppressive agents. Reprinted from reference 161 by permission of Appleton & Lange, Inc.*

about FK506, it has become apparent that it has wide-ranging effects on the immune system,[110] including effects on IL-4, IL-5, IFN-$\gamma$, and TNF-$\alpha$.

### Animal studies

FK506 has now been studied extensively in animal models. The drug is effective in prolongation of solid organ transplant survival in many animal models including transplantation of liver, kidney, heart, lung and bone marrow. The literature is extensive,[111–118] in particular the early evidence in animals suggested that previously 'forbidden' allografts such as small bowel might be feasible under FK506 immunosuppression.[111,119]

### Human studies

There are many studies attesting to the efficacy of FK506 in human transplantation, but the seminal studies are the USA and European FK506 multicentre liver studies. In the European liver study 545 patients were recruited from eight European liver centres. Patients were randomised to receive either triple therapy based on cyclosporin, or triple therapy based on FK506. The study was randomised and open. At the end of one year, the data showed very clearly that *in vivo*, FK506 was a more powerful immunosuppressant than CSA, that episodes of rejection were reduced, that the need for additional antirejection therapy was diminished, but that the one-year graft survival rates were not different between the two groups.[120] In the similar USA liver study, 478 adults and 51 children were randomised to receive either FK506 or CSA in an open label study; 263 received FK506 and 266 received cyclosporin. The primary efficacy end point was patient and graft survival at one year, with secondary end points being incidence of rejection.[121] The findings were remarkably similar to the European study, with FK506 significantly reducing acute rejection, steroid-resistant rejection, and refractory rejection. Once again, there were no significant differences in one year patient and graft survival. The outcome of the studies are summarised in Table 5.6. In both the multicentre studies, the incidence of adverse events was higher in the FK506 groups, with principle side effects being nephrotoxi-

**Table 5.6**   *Summary of multicentre studies of FK506 in liver transplantation*

| | Acute rejection (%) | P value | Steroid resistant rejection (%) | P value | Refractory rejection (%) | P value | 1-year graft survival | 1-year patient survival |
|---|---|---|---|---|---|---|---|---|
| **USA study** | | | | | | | | |
| FK506 | 58.1 | <0.002 | 16.3 | <0.001 | 2.3 | <0.001 | 82.0 | 88.0 |
| Cyclosporin | 65.0 | | 30.8 | | 12.0 | | 79.0 | 88.0 |
| **European study** | | | | | | | | |
| FK506 | 40.5 | 0.04 | | | 0.8 | 0.005 | 77.5 | 82.9 |
| Cyclosporin | 49.8 | | | | 5.3 | | 72.6 | 77.5 |

city and neurotoxicity. In other human organ transplantation, FK506 has also been shown to be an effective immunosuppressant. Much of the early work (in all aspects) was done at Professor Starzl's unit in Pittsburgh. Reporting their early experience in uncontrolled studies, Shapiro et al.[122] noted that FK506 was associated with a one- and two-year actuarial graft survival of 89% and 83%, respectively, and with 49% weaned off steroids. They reported that the side effects of nephrotoxicity, neurotoxicity and diabetogenicity were the same as in patients on CSA. Shapiro et al.[122] also reported the Pittsburgh results in paediatric renal transplantation, and showed good results in an unselected population of 43 children, and, in a separate group, showed 71% rescue from refractory rejection in a group of 24 children. There are no currently published controlled, randomised prospective studies of FK506 in renal transplantation where comparison is made to CSA. One study coming close to that objective is again from Shapiro et al.,[123] who randomised 204 adult renal allograft recipients to receive either FK506/prednisolone or FK506/prednisolone/azathioprine. The conclusion of this study was that the addition of azathioprine resulted in a reduced one-year actual graft survival (82% vs 92%, triple versus double, respectively). European and American trials comparing FK506 and cyclosporin in renal transplantation have reported in abstract form and will shortly appear in full publication. These studies are remarkably similar in result although inclusion criteria differed. Patient and graft survival did not show any improvement with FK506 use but there was a significant reduction in the incidence and severity of rejection. In the Japanese multicentre study in renal transplantation, there were no significant differences in one-year patient and graft survival comparing FK506-treated cases with historical CSA-treated controls.[124,125] In a study of 75 patients with 'refractory' rejection on CSA treatment, a salvage rate of 74% was achieved following conversion to FK506. A high percentage of the study population had received (and failed to respond to) treatment with ATG/OKT3. This study confirmed that FK506 is a powerful and useful rescue treatment in renal as well as hepatic transplantation.[126] In an small prospective randomised study of 74 lung transplants, recipients were randomised to receive either CSA-based immunosuppression or a FK506-based one. There were clear advantages to the FK506 regimen, with significant reductions in biopsy-proven rejection, and many more FK506-treated patients experiencing no rejection at all (13% rejection-free versus 3% rejection-free, $P < 0.05$).[127] Finally, the Pittsburgh group have reported a series of small bowel/multivisceral transplants under FK506 immunosuppression. It is their contention that the procedure has been facilitated by the advent of FK506, but the high rates of post-transplant lymphoproliferative disease (PTLD), and viral infections have given cause for concern.[128,129] Thus, in most human transplants, FK506 has powerful immunosuppressive effect, clinical trials have demonstrated that it produces acute and steroid-resistant rejection, but kidney data are only just appearing. There is no evidence of improved 1-year graft/patient survival, but in an analysis of the UNOS data Gjertson[130] noted an early 'trend' towards better late graft survival in renal recipients treated with FK506. Grafts treated with conventional treatment (CSA based) had a half-life ($t_{1/2}$) of 8–9 years, but with FK506 immunosuppression it reached 13 years.[130] Although this was not a statistically significant $p$ value, it means that the late results with FK506 will be looked at with keen interest.

### Chronic rejection

There is little evidence to support a potential role for FK506 in the treatment of graft vascular disease. In a small study involving rat heart transplantation, FK506 had no effect on coronary disease, and the authors concluded that it was ineffective in this role.[100]

### Summary

- Powerful agent with actions similar to CSA
- Reduces acute, and refractory rejection in humans, and need for ATG/OKT3
- Side effects similar to CSA including nephrotoxicity, neurotoxicity and diabetes
- Early results in renal allografts in comparison with CSA
- Large multicentre liver studies
- Effective salvage therapy with approx. 75% response
- Unknown (but promising) influence on late graft function

### Cyclosporin Neoral formulation

Since its introduction CSA has existed in a formulation that is less than perfect with respect to absorption and bioavailability. The molecule is lipophilic, and is slowly and incompletely absorbed in the small bowel. The drug is dispersed by bile salts and absorption may, therefore, be affected by bile flow, intestinal motility and food intake. The new formulation of CSA is known as Neoral, and is the same base molecule, but with a new 'packaging'. Neoral is a microemulsion, and its absorption is not influenced by bile flow or food. The independence from bile flow makes it potentially useful in the early post-transplant period after liver transplantation. The improved pharmacokinetics are detailed in Table 5.7, and it is clear that the bioavailability is significantly enhanced with the new formulation.[131] Neoral has now been shown to be equipotent to the parent drug, and most renal patients in the UK have been transferred to the new agent. In the setting of liver transplantation, the drug has been shown to be better absorbed, and is at least partially (but not fully) independent of bile secretion.[132,133] It is claimed that the improved bioavailability may result in reduced acute rejection, and therefore potentially the rate of chronic rejection, although the latter is speculative. In a study of Neoral in renal transplantation, 288 patients were randomised to receive either 'standard' CSA or microemulsion CSA, 3-month graft survival was no different between the two groups, but biopsy-proven acute cellular rejection was reduced very significantly

**Table 5.7** *Comparison of the pharmacokinetics of cyclosporin in its original and microemulsion formulations*

| Parameter | Cyclosporin (old formulation) | Cyclosporin (new formulation) |
|---|---|---|
| $C_{min}$ (ng/ml) | 71 ± 21 | 80 ± 23 |
| $T_{max}$ (h) | 2.2 ± 1.1 | 1.2 ± 0.3 |
| $C_{max}$ (ng/ml) | 516 ± 207 | 793 ± 230 |
| AUC (h ng/ml) | 2130 ± 585 | 2741 ± 663 |
| AUC ratio | 1.0 | 1.29 |
| $C_{max}$ ratio | 1.0 | 1.59 |

in the Neoral patients (46.4% versus 26.7%, conventional CSA versus Neoral, respectively (Mr S. Pollard, for Sandoz Pharma, personal communication)). Early data suggest that although a 1:1 changeover is recommended, the improved bioavailability may allow a 10% dose reduction.

## Drugs inhibiting antigen presentation

### *15-Deoxyspergualin (DSG)*
*Mechanism of action*
DSG (7-[(aminoiminomethyl)amino]-N-[2-[[4-[(3-aminopropyl)amino]-butyl]amino]-1-hydroxy 2-oxoethyl] is the dehydroxylated derivative of spergualin, a metabolite of *Bacillus laterosporus*. The drug was initially found to have antitumour activity,[134] but was also noted to have immunosuppressive properties. It is a semisynthetic polyamine that has what would appear to be a unique mechanism of action for it is the only immunosuppressive agent that acts 'upstream' of the T cell activation process. Although the exact mechanism of action remains to be elucidated, it would appear to be the only immunosuppressant whose main site of action is on the monocyte/macrophage series of leucocytes. Current opinion favours the view that DSG acts on antigen presenting cells (APC) – probably by interaction with heat shock protein 70 (HSP70). The drug also inhibits the translocation of NF-kappa B, necessary for the transfer of processed antigen across the cytoplasm to the nucleus in the APC. The proposed effects of DSG are illustrated in Table 5.8. The drug is 20% bound to plasma protein and is rapidly metabolised (not by the P450 system). Its bioavailability is <5%, renal clearance is low and around 10% is excreted unchanged in the urine.

*Animal studies*
In animal studies, DSG has been shown to be highly efficient in preventing rejection of islet allografts in C57BL mice, but was not able to prevent rejection in the porcine-to-mouse xenograft model.[135] The drug has been used with success in a variety of other animal transplant

**Table 5.8**  *The effects of 15-deoxyspergualin*

| | |
|---|---|
| **T cells** | Poor inhibitor of T cell responses to mitogens |
| | Inhibits mixed lymphocyte reactivity |
| | Only inhibits generation of CTL early in the initiation phase |
| **B cells** | Inhibits B cell responses to T cell dependent and T cell independent antigen |
| | Inhibits the expression of kappa light chain |
| **Monocyte/macrophage** | Blocks TNF-$\alpha$ |
| | Blocks IL-6, IL-8 |
| | Inhibits antigen presentation and processing (CD28 and B7) |
| | Inhibits NF-$\kappa$B |

models, including canine marrow transplantation,[136] heterotopic rat heart transplantation (where the drug resulted in 80% successful reversal of acute heart allograft rejection),[137] as well as in other studies of skin, heart, kidney, pancreas, liver, islets and limb allografts[138–146] (fully referenced in Yuh and Morris[147]). Animal models include mice, rats, guinea pig, pigs, dogs, monkeys and baboons.

Using a murine heterotopic heart model, Yuh and Morris[147] have extensively investigated the immunopharmacology of DSG, and found that DSG is well tolerated when given by frequent low dose (intraperitoneal) injection, with few signs of toxicity. The drug is clearly synergistic with cyclosporin A and is more potent than the latter drug. It may result in specific unresponsiveness, and timing of administration with respect to antigenic exposure may be critical for the production of unresponsiveness. Indeed, in a study by Reichenspurner *et al.*[139] in a baboon model it is possible to generate long term unresponsiveness using a combination of DSG and CSA. Thus DSG has shown itself to be a potent immunosuppressive agent in virtually all non-human animals, and to be effective in many organ transplant types. In particular, enthusiasm has been voiced for its use in islet cell transplantation[148] and, because of an ability to reduce preformed natural antibodies, it may have a useful role in xenotransplantation, or in patients with high panel reactive antibodies (PRA).[149–151]

*Human studies*
Human studies of this agent have now been undertaken in both Scandinavia and in Japan. The drug is reasonably well tolerated in humans in doses that range between 3 and 5 mg kg$^{-1}$ day$^{-1}$. The toxic effects of the drug are now well recognised and include leucopenia, thrombocytopenia, anaemia, perioral numbness, and gastrointestinal disturbances. Amemiya *et al.*[152] reported the first clinical trials (phase II) of DSG used as a rescue therapy in human renal transplantation. In 34

cases of acute rejection in 30 recipients, DSG was used in doses that ranged from 40 to 220 mg m$^{-2}$. Patients were only entered into the study if they had failed to respond to treatment with steroids, OKT3 or ATG/ALG. The overall efficacy in this 'rescue' role was 79%. The drug was given intravenously over 3 h, for a short defined course of up to 5 days. No patient had to be withdrawn because of side effects. The authors concluded that DSG was a useful agent in steroid-resistant rejection. Amemiya et al.[153] later extended their work on DSG. The results in 53 cases of acute rejection were somewhat similar to those reported in their earlier experience. In both primary treatment of acute cellular rejection (ACR) and rescue therapy, the overall response rate was 75–80%, with minimal toxicity (mainly haematopoietic). The authors concluded that 7 days treatment of 3–5 mg kg$^{-1}$ was probably the optimal treatment. In a study in the USA, DSG was used to treat steroid-resistant rejection in four cases, all of whom had biopsy-proven rejection that had failed to respond to treatment with either steroids or mono-/polyclonal antibodies. All four responded to DSG, 5 mg kg$^{-1}$ day$^{-1}$, and side effects from the treatment were minimal.[154]

### Chronic rejection

In view of the fact that DSG is unlikely to be useful in anything other than short-term use, it is doubtful whether it has any future role in treating 'chronic rejection' (transplant vascular sclerosis) of human allografts. The experimental evidence is contradictory. Gregory et al.[155] used cell culture techniques, as well as a carotid injury model in rats to show that DSG had no real effect on vascular smooth muscle proliferation *in vivo* and *in vitro*, but Nagamine[156] suggested that DSG was certainly superior to CSA in a rat cardiac allograft model, and that graft sclerosis was lower in DSG-treated rats than in CSA-treated ones. Most of the effect was attributed to changes in serum lipid profiles.

**Summary**
- DSG is highly potent, and more powerful than CSA
- Effects are mainly on APC and B cells
- Useful effects against natural (xeno-) and alloantibodies
- 70–80% effective as rescue therapy in human renal transplantation
- Not a maintenance treatment
- Particular promise for the drug in ACR, and in highly sensitised patients
- Possible use for the future in islet allo- and xenotransplantation

**Monoclonal antibodies for rejection prophylaxis**   There are no established treatment modalities in this category that are used for the prevention of allograft rejection. The use of the anti-T cell agent (anti-CD3), OKT3 is of course well known in transplantation, but use is confined to the rescue situation, where other 'first line' agents have failed. In this role it is effective,[157] but it is expensive and is associated with unpleasant side effects[158] that are mediated by cytokine release

**Table 5.9** *Some of the monoclonal antibodies used or abandoned in transplantation*

| Monoclonal | Target | Chimeric form? | Prophylaxis | Acute rejection | Comments |
|---|---|---|---|---|---|
| **Monoclonal antibodies that are currently used or under investigation** | | | | | |
| CD3 | T cell receptor | (+) | − | +++ | First dose reactions |
| CD4 | T helper cells | + | ? | − | High doses needed, effective in animals |
| CD11a | LFA-1 | (+) | ? | − | |
| CD25 | IL-2R$_\alpha$ | + | ? | − | |
| **Monoclonals abandoned from use** | | | | | |
| CD5/CD6 | T cells | − | − | − | |
| CD7 | T, NK cells | + | − | − | |
| CD45 | WBC | + | − | − | |
| CDW52 | T, B, monocytes | + | ++ | ++ | |
| CD54 | ICAM-1 | (+) | ? | ? | |

(especially TNF-$\alpha$).[159] However, it does remain a salvage treatment for many transplant centres. Finally, it has been shown that the use of this agent (as well as antithymocyte preparations) is particularly associated with post-transplant lymphoproliferative disease (PTLD) and lymphoma.[160]

A summary of some of the monoclonal antibodies, past and present is shown in Table 5.9.

**The future**  Immunosuppression is undergoing a huge change. Whereas the 1970s was a 'simple' situation, in 1996, six different drugs were available for maintenance immunosuppression (cyclosporin, new and old, FK506, azathioprine, prednisolone and mycophenolate mofetil). There is a reasonable expectation that the number will increase in the next five years, so that rapamycin, mizoribine, deoxyspergualin and leflunomide may all have product licences. It is also a reasonable expectation that it may soon be possible to have a 'steroid free' regimen – an aim that must surely reduce the long-term morbidity (and mortality) associated with steroid use. One would foresee that future immunosuppression is likely to concentrate on more 'focused' and specific immunosuppression, using multidrug therapy, in smaller doses than previously. Despite their powerful modes of action, it is unlikely that any of the new or existing drugs will be used as monotherapy. It is likely that cyclosporin neoral, FK506 or rapamycin will remain as 'core' immunosuppression, with the addition of mycophenolate or leflunomide as other maintenance agents. It is unlikely that deoxyspergualin will be used as a maintenance agent, but it is effective in acute rejection (especially antibody-mediated). There is no doubt that unfocused global immunosuppression works, as evidenced by the success of transplantation in the 1990s. However, it does so at a price. That price is malignancy and sepsis, with which we are all too familiar. For the transplant profession, the greatest danger we face is an unrealistic expectation that any of the new drugs will increase 1-year graft survival by any major degree. It is unlikely they will do so (neither mycophenolate or FK506 have shown any significant increase in one-year graft survival). We must temper our enthusiasm with patience. The major test of a new agent in the 1990s is not its effect on 1-year graft survival, but whether the drug will influence the inexorable progression of chronic graft dysfunction ('chronic rejection'), with an acceptable side-effect profile, and no increase in malignancy. This view will not meet with sympathy in the pharmaceutical industry which is unlikely to finance prolonged drug trials with a 10-year end point. However, this is one of the challenges for the future of transplantation.

# References

1. Schwartz RS, Damashek W. Drug induced immunological tolerance. Nature 1959; 183: 1682–3.
2. Elion GB, Burgi E, Hitchins GH. Studies on condensed pyrimidine systems. IX. The synthesis of some 6-substituted purines. J Am Chem Soc 1952; 74: 411–14.
3. Elion GB, Callahan S, Bieber S, Hitchins GH. A summary of investigations with 6-(iomethyl-4-nitro-5imidazolyl)(thio) purine. Cancer Chemother Rep 1961; 14: 93–8.
4. Calne RY. The rejection of renal homograft inhibition in dogs by 6-mercaptopurine. Lancet 1960; i: 417–18.
5. Calne RY, Alexandre G, Murray J. A study of the effects of drugs in prolonging survival of homologous renal transplantation in dogs. Ann N Y Acad Sci 1962; 99: 743–61.
6. Murray JE, Merrill JP, Damin GJ et al. Kidney transplantation in modified recipients. Ann Surg 1962; 156: 337–55.
7. Murray JE, Merrill JP, Harrison JH et al. Prolonged survival of human kidney homografts by immunosuppressive drug therapy. N Engl J Med 1963; 268: 1315–23.
8. Bach JF. The mode of action of immunosuppressive agents. Amsterdam: North Holland Publishing, 1975.
9. McGeown MG, Douglas JF, Brown WA et al. Advantages of low dose steroid from the day after renal transplantation. Transplantation 1980; 29: 287–9.
10. Chan L, French ME, Beare J, Oliver DO, Morris PJ. Prospective trial of high dose versus low dose prednisolone in renal transplant patients. Transplant Proc 1980; 12: 323–6.
11. d'Apice AJ, Becker GS, Kincaid-Smith P et al. A prospective randomised trial of low-dose versus high-dose steroids in cadaveric renal transplantation. Transplantation 1984; 37: 373–7.
12. Borel JF, Feurer C, Gubler HU, Stahelin H. Biological effects of cyclosporin A: a new antilymphocytic agent. Agents Actions 1976; 6: 468.
13. European Multicentre Trial Group. Cyclosporin in cadaveric renal transplantation: one year follow-up of a multicentre trial. Lancet 1983; ii: 986–9.
14. Canadian Multicentre Transplant Study Group. A randomised clinical trial of Cyclosporine in cadaveric renal transplantation. New Engl J Med 1983; 309: 809–13.
15. Canadian Multicentre Transplant Study Group. A randomised clinical trial of Cyclosporine in cadaveric renal transplantation; analysis at three years. New Engl J Med 1986; 314: 1219–25.
16. Ochiai T, Toma H, Oka T et al. Japanese Multicentre trial of Cyclosporin A in renal transplantation; overall results and analysis of the factors influencing graft survival rate. Transplant Proc 1987; 19: 2961–6.

17. Kahan BD, Kerman RH, Wideman CA, Flecher SM, Jarowenko M, Van Buren CT. Impact of cyclosporine on renal transplant practice at the University of Texas Medical School at Houston. Am J Kidney Dis 1985; 5: 288–95.

18. Albrechtsen D, Berg KJ, Bondevik H et al. Improved results using Cyclosporine in cadaveric renal transplantation. Transplant Proc 1986; 18: 92–4.

19. Emery RW, Cork R, Christensen R et al. Cardiac transplant patients at one year: Cyclosporine versus conventional immunosuppression. Chest 1986; 90: 29–33.

20. Iwatsuki S, Starzl TE, Todo S et al. Experience in 1000 liver transplants under Cyclosporine-steroid therapy: a survival report. Transplant Proc 1988; 20: 498–504.

21. Sutherland DER. Results of the International Pancreas Transplant Registry; report 1988. Diabetes 1989; 38: 46–54.

22. Mizuno K, Miyazaki T. Synthesis and cytotoxicity of Bredinin 5 monophosphate. Chem Pharm Bull 1976; 24: 2248–50.

23. Dayton J, Turka L, Mitchell BS. Depletion of guanine nucleotides selectively mediates inhibition of T-cells. Proc Am Soc Cancer Res 1990; 31: A2515.

24. Ichikawa Y, Ihara H, Takahara S et al. The immunosuppressive mode of action of mizoribine. Transplantation 1984; 38: 262–7.

25. Murase J, Mizuno K, Kawai K et al. Absorption, distribution, metabolism and excretion of Bredinin in rats. Pharmacometrics 1978; 15: 829–35.

26. Takada K, Asada S, Ichikawa Y et al. Pharmacokinetics of Bredinin in renal transplant patients. Eur J Clin Pharmacol 1983; 24: 457–61.

27. Kamata K, Okubo M, Ishigamori E et al. Immunosuppressive effects of bredinin on cell-mediated and humoral immune reactions in experimental animals. Transplantation 1983; 35: 144–9.

28. Uchida H, Yokota K, Akiyama N et al. Effectiveness of a new drug bredinin on canine kidney allotransplant survival. Transplant Proc 1979; 11: 865–70.

29. Gregory CR, Gourley IM, Haskins SC et al. Effects of mizoribine on canine renal allograft recipients. Am J Vet Res 1988; 49: 305–11.

30. Tajima A, Hata M, Ohta N, Ohtawara Y, Suzuki K, Aso Y. Bredinin, a new immunosuppressant treatment in clinical kidney allografting; experience with 39 renal transplants. Transplant Proc 1985; 17: 1320–3.

31. Kokado Y, Ishibashi M, Jiang H, Takahara S, Sonoda T. Low dose Ciclosporin Mizoribine and Prednisolone in renal transplantation: a new triple drug therapy. Clin Transplant 1990; 4: 191–7.

32. Lee HA, Slapak M, Venkat Raman G, Mason JC, Digard N, Wise M. Mizoribine as an alternative in triple therapy immunosuppressant regimes in cadaveric renal transplantation: two successive studies. Transplant Proc 1995; 27: 1050–1.

33. Allison AC, Eugui EM. Inhibitors of de novo purine and pyrimidine synthesis as immunosuppressive drugs. Transplant Proc 1993; 25 (3 suppl 2): 8–18.

34. Allison AC, Eugui EM. The design and development of an immunosuppressive drug, mycophenolate mofetil. Springer Semin Immunopathol 1993; 14: 353–80.

35. Eugui EM, Almquist SJ, Muller CD, Allison AC. Lymphocyte selective cytostatic and immunosuppressive effects of mycophenolic acid in vitro: role of deoxyguanosine nucleotide depletion. Scand J Immunol 1991; 33: 161–73.

36. Allison AC, Eugui EM, Sollinger HW. Mycophenolate mofetil (RS61443): mechanisms of action and effects in transplantation. Transplant Rev 1993; 7: 129–39.

37. Allison AC, Kowalski WJ, Muller CJ et al. Mycophenolic acid and brequinar, inhibitors of purine and pyrimidine synthesis, block the glycosylation of adhesion molecules. Transplant Proc 1993; 25: 67 (suppl 2).

38. Allison AC, Eugui EM. Immunosuppressive and other effects of mycophenolic acid and an ester prodrug, mycophenolate mofetil. Immunol Rev 1993; 136: 5–28.

39. Chang CC, Aversa G, Punnoven J, Yssel H, de Vries JE. Brequinar sodium, mycophenolic acid and cyclosporin A inhibit different stages of IL-4 or IL-13 induced IgG4 and IgE production in vitro. Ann N Y Acad Sci 1993; 696: 108–22.

40. Platz KP, Bechstein WO, Eckhoff DE, Suzuki Y, Sollinger HW. RS-61443 reverses acute

allograft rejection in dogs. Surgery 1991; 110: 736–41.

41. d'Alessandro AM, Rankin M, McVey J *et al.* Prolongation of canine intestinal allograft survival with RS-61443, cyclosporine and prednisolone. Transplant Proc 1993; 25: 1207–9.

42. Morris RE, Hoyt EG, Murphy MP, Eugui EM, Allison AC. Mycophenolic acid morpholino-ethylester (RS-61443) is a new immunosuppressant that prevents and halts heart allograft rejection by selective inhibition of T and B cell purine synthesis. Transplant Proc 1990; 22: 1659–62.

43. Hao L, Lafferty KJ, Allison AC, Eugui EM. RS-61443 allows islet allografting and specific tolerance induction in adult mice. Transplant Proc 1990; 22: 876–9.

44. Benhaim P, Anthony JP, Lin LY, McCalmont TH, Mathes SJ. A long term study of allogeneic rat hindlimb transplants immunosuppressed with RS-61443. Transplantation 1993; 56: 911–17.

45. Herbert MF, Ascher NL, Benet LZ, Roberts JP. Pharmacokinetics of oral 2-(4-morpholino) ethyl ester of mycophenolic acid (EE-MA) in liver transplant patients. Clin Pharmacol Ther 1992; 51: 131.

46. Kobashigawa JA, Renlund DG, Olsen SL *et al.* Initial results of RS-61443 for refractory cardiac rejection. J Am Coll Cardiol 1992; 19: 203A.

47. Sollinger HW, Belzer FO, Deierhoi MH *et al.* RS-61443 (Mycophenolate mofetil). A multicentre study for refractory kidney transplant rejection. Ann Surg 1992; 216: 513–19.

48. European Mycophenolate Mofetil Cooperative Study Group. Placebo-controlled study of mycophenolate mofetil combined with cyclosporin and corticosteroids for prevention of acute rejection. Lancet 1995; 345: 1321–5.

49. Sollinger HW. Mycophenolate mofetil for the prevention of acute rejection in primary cadaveric renal allograft recipients. Transplantation 1995; 60: 225–32.

50. Morris RE, Wang J, Blum JR *et al.* Immunosuppressive effects of the morpholinoethyl ester of mycophenolic acid (RS-61443) in rat and non-human primate recipients of heart allografts. Transplant Proc 1991; 23: 19 (suppl 2).

51. Steel DM, Hullett DA, Bechstein WO *et al.* Effects of immunosuppressive therapy in the rat aortic allograft model. Transplant Proc 1993; 24: 754–5.

52. Arteaga CL, Brown TD, Kuhn JG *et al.* Phase I clinical and pharmacokinetic trial of Brequinar sodium (Dup 785; NSC 368390). Cancer Res 1989; 49: 4648–53.

53. Urba S, Doroshow J, Cripps C *et al.* Multicentre phase II trial of brequinar sodium in patients with advanced squamous cell carcinoma of the head and neck. Cancer Chemother Pharmacol 1992; 31: 167–9.

54. Natale R, Wheeler R, Moore M *et al.* Multicentre Phase II trial of brequinar sodium in patients with advanced melanoma. Ann Oncol 1992; 3: 659–60

55. Cramer DV, Knoop M, Chapman FA, Wa GD, Jaffee BD, Makowka L. Prevention of liver allograft rejection in rats by a short course of therapy with Brequinar Sodium. Transplantation 1992; 54: 752–3.

56. Cramer DV, Chapman FA, Jaffee BD *et al.* The effect of a new immunosuppressive drug, brequinar sodium, on heart, liver, and kidney rejection in the rat. Transplantation 1992; 53: 303–8.

57. Cosenza CA, Cramer DV, Eiras-Hreha G, Cajulis E, Wang HK, Makowka L. The synergism of brequinar sodium and cyclosporine used in combination to prevent cardiac allograft rejection in the rat. Transplantation 1993; 56: 667–72.

58. Yasunaga C, Cramer DV, Chapman FA *et al.* The prevention of accelerated cardiac allograft rejection in sensitized recipients after treatment with brequinar sodium. Transplantation 1993; 56: 898–904.

59. Wang M, Strepkowski SM, Kahan BD. Effect of cyclosporine alone or in combination with rapamycin and brequinar on survival of hamster heart xenografts in rats. Transplant Proc 1993; 25: 2876–7.

60. Kahan BD. Concentration-controlled immunosuppressive regimens using cyclosporin with sirolimus or brequinar in human renal transplantation. Transplant Proc 1995; 27: 33–6.

61. Bartlett RR. Immunopharmacological profile of HWA 486, a novel isoxazol derivative II. In vivo immunomodulating effects differ from

those of cyclophosphamide. Int J Immunopharmacol 1986; 8: 199–204.

62. Zielinski T, Muller HJ, Bartlett RR. Effects of leflunomide (HWA 486) on expression of lymphocyte activation markers. Agents Actions 1993; 38: 80–2.

63. Cherwinski HM, McCarley D, Schatzman R, Devens B, Ransom JT. The immunosuppressant leflunomide inhibits lymphocyte progression through cell cycle by a novel mechanism. J Pharmacol Exp Ther 1995; 272: 460–8.

64. Cherwinski HM, Cohn RG, Cheung P et al. The immunosuppressant leflunomide inhibits lymphocyte proliferation by inhibiting pyrimidine biosynthesis. J Pharmacol Exp Ther 1995; 275: 1043–9.

65. Greene S, Watanabe K, Braatz-Trulson J, Iou L. Inhibition of dihydroorotate dehydrogenase by the immunosuppressive agent leflunomide. Biochem Pharmacol 1995; 50: 861–7.

66. Williams JW, Xiao F, Foster P et al. Leflunomide in experimental transplantation. Control of rejection and alloantibody production, reversal of acute rejection, and interaction with cyclosporin. Transplantation 1994; 57: 1223–31.

67. D'Silva M, Candidas D, Achilleos O et al. The immunomodulatory effect of leflunomide in rat cardiac allotransplantation. Transplantation 1995; 60: 430–7.

68. Kuchtle CC, Theones GH, Langer KH et al. Prevention of kidney and skin graft rejection in rats by leflunomide, a new immunomodulating agent. Transplant Proc 1991; 23: 1083–6.

69. He G, McAlister VC, Lee TD et al. Oral leflunomide prevents small bowel allograft rejection in the rat. Transplant Proc 1994; 26: 1613.

70. Morris RE, Huang X, Cao W et al. Leflunomide (HWA 486) and its analogue suppress T- and B-cell proliferation in vitro, acute rejection, ongoing rejection, and anti-donor antibody synthesis in mouse, rat and cynomolgous monkey transplant recipients as well as arterial intimal thickening after balloon catheter injury. Transplant Proc 1995; 27: 445–7.

71. McChesney LP, Xiao F, Sankary HN et al. An evaluation of leflunomide in the canine renal transplantation model. Transplantation 1994; 57: 1717–22.

72. Xiao F, Chong A, Foster P et al. Effects of leflunomide in control of acute rejection in hamster-to-rat cardiac xenografts. Transplant Proc 1994; 26: 1263–5.

73. Ulrichs K, Kaitschick J, Bartlett R, Muller-Ruchholtz W. Suppression of natural xenophile antibodies with the novel immunomodulating drug leflunomide. Transplant Proc 1992; 24: 718–19.

74. Mladenovic V, Domljan Z, Rozman B et al. Safety and effectiveness of leflunomide in the treatment of patients with active rheumatoid arthritis. Results of randomised, placebo-controlled, phase II studies. Arthritis Rheum 1995; 38: 1595–603.

75. Xiao F, Chong A, Shen J et al. Pharmacologically induced regression of chronic transplant rejection. Transplantation 1995; 60: 1065–72.

76. Swan SK, Crary GS, Guijarro C, Donnell MP, Keane WF, Kasiske BL. Immunosuppressive effects of leflunomide in experimental chronic vascular rejection. Transplantation 1995; 60: 887–90.

77. Sehgal SN, Baker H, Vezina C. Rapamycin (AY-22,989), a new antifungal antibiotic, isolation and characterisation. J Antibiot 1975; 28: 727.

78. Martel RR, Klicius J, Galet S. Inhibition of the immune response by rapamycin, a new antifungal antibiotic. Can J Physiol Pharmacol 1977; 55: 48.

79. Eng CP, Sehgal SN, Vezina C. Activity of Rapamycin (AY-22,989) against transplanted tumours. J Antibiot 1984; 37: 1231.

80. Kuo CJ, Chung L, Fiorentino DF, Flanagan WM, Blenis J, Crabtree GR. Rapamycin selectively inhibits interleukin-2 activation of p70 S5 kinase. Nature 1992; 358: 70–3.

81. Tocci MJ, Matkovich DA, Collier KA et al. The immunosuppressant FK506 selectively inhibits expression of early T cell activation genes. J Immunol 1989; 143: 718.

82. Dumont FJ, Starach MJ, Koprak SL, Melino MR, Sigal NH. Distinct mechanisms of suppression of murine T cell activation by the related macrolides FK 506 and rapamycin. J Immunol 1990; 144: 251–8.

83. Luo H, Chen H, Daloze P et al. Inhibition of in vitro immunoglobulin production by Rapamycin. Transplantation 1992; 53: 1071–6.

84. Luo H, Chen H, Daloze P, Chang J, Wu J. Rapamycin suppresses in vitro immuno-globulin production by human lymphocytes. Transplant Proc 1991; 23: 2236–8.

85. Sigal NH, Dumont FJ. Cyclosporin A, FK-506, and rapamycin: pharmacologic probes of lymphocyte signal transduction. Annu Rev Immunol 1992; 10: 519–60.

86. Whiting PH, Woo J, Adam BJ, Hasan NU, Davidson RJL, Thomson AW. Toxicity of Rapamycin – a comparative and combination study with cyclosporin at immunotherapeutic dosage in the rat. Transplantation 1991; 52: 203–8.

87. Strepkowski SM, Chen H, Daloze P, Kahan BD. Rapamicin, a potent immunosuppressive drug for vascularised heart, kidney and small bowel transplantation in the rat. Transplantation 1991; 51: 22–6.

88. Fabian MC, Lakey JR, Rajotte RV, Kneteman NM. The efficacy and toxicity of rapamycin in murine islet transplantation. In vitro and in vivo studies. Transplantation 1993; 56: 1137–42.

89. Collier DSJ, Calne R, Thiru S et al. Rapamycin in experimental renal allografts in dogs and pigs. Transplant Proc 1990; 22: 1674.

90. Almond PS, Moss A, Nakleh R et al. Rapamycin: immunosuppression, hyporesponsiveness, and side effects in a porcine renal allograft model. Transplantation 1993; 56: 275–81.

91. Caine RY, Collier DSJ, Lim S et al. Rapamycin for immunosuppression in organ allografting. Lancet 1989; ii: 227.

92. Morris RE, Wang J, Gregory C et al. Initial studies of the efficacy and safety of rapamycin administered to cynomolgous monkey recipients of heart allografts. J Heart Lung Transplant 1991; 10: 182.

93. Collier DSJ, Calne Ry, Pollard SG et al. Rapamycin in experimental renal allografts in primates. Transplant Proc 1991; 23: 2246.

94. Granger DK, Cromwell JW, Chen SC et al. Prolongation of renal allograft survival in a large animal model by oral rapamycin mono-therapy. Transplantation 1995; 59: 183–6.

95. Tu Y, Strepkowski SM, Chou TC, Kahan BD. The synergistic effects of cyclosporine, sirolimus, and brequinar on heart allograft survival in mice. Transplantation 1995; 59: 177–83.

96. Brattstrom C, Tyden G, Sawe J, Herlenius G, Claesson K, Groth CG. A randomised, double-blind, placebo-controlled study to determine the safety, tolerance, and preliminary pharmacokinetics of ascending single doses or orally administered Sirolimus (Rapamycin) in stable renal transplant recipients. Abstracts: Minneapolis Transplant Congress; New Immunosuppressive Drugs. Minneapolis, 27–30 August, 1995.

97. Johnson EM, Zimmerman J, Duderstadt K et al. A randomised, double-blind, placebo-controlled study to determine the safety, tolerance, and preliminary pharmacokinetics of ascending single doses or orally administered Sirolimus (Rapamycin) in stable renal transplant recipients. Abstracts: Minneapolis Transplant Congress; New Immunosuppressive Drugs. Minneapolis, 27–30 August, 1995.

98. Painter TA. Myointimal hyperplasia: pathogenesis and implications. 1. In vitro characteristics. Artif Organs 1991; 15: 42.

99. Gregory CR, Huang X, Pratt RE et al. Treatment with Rapamycin and mycophenolic acid reduces arterial intimal thickening produced by mechanical injury and allows endothelial replacement. Transplantation 1995; 59: 655–61.

100. Meiser BM, Billingham ME, Morris RE. Effects of cyclosporin, FK506 and rapamycin on graft vessel disease. Lancet 1991; 338: 1297–8.

101. Morris RE, Wang J, Blum JR et al. Immunosuppressive effects of the morphoinoethyl-ester of mycophenolic acid (RS61443) in rat and nonhuman primate recipients of heart allografts. Transplant Proc 1991; 23: 19.

102. Goto T, Kino T, Hatanaka H et al. FK506: historical perspectives. Transplant Proc 1991; 23: 2713–17.

103. Venkataramanan R, Jain A, Warty VS et al. Pharmacokinetics of FK506 in transplant patients. Transplant Proc 1991; 23: 2736–40.

104. Venkataramanan R, Warty VS, Zemaitis MA et al. Biopharmaceutical aspects of FK506. Transplant Proc 1987; 19: 30–50.

105. Furukawa H, Imuentarza O, Venkataramanan R. The effect of bile duct ligation and bile diversion on FK506 pharmacokinetics in dogs. Transplantation 1992; 53: 722–5.

106. Goto T, Kino T, Hatanaka H *et al*. FK506: historical perspectives. Transplant Proc 1991; 23: 2713–17.

107. Kino T, Hatanaka H, Miyata J *et al*. FK506, a novel immunosuppressant isolated from Streptomyces II. Immunosuppressive effect of FK506 in vitro. J Antibiot 1987; 40: 1256–65.

108. Kino T, Inamura N, Sakai F *et al*. Effect of FK506 on human mixed lymphocyte reaction in vitro. Transplant Proc 1987; 19: 36–9.

109. Granelli-Piperno A, Nolan P, Inaba K, Steinman RM. The effects of immunosuppressive agents on the induction of nuclear factors that bind to sites on the interleukin-2 promoter. J Exp Med 1990; 172: 1869–72.

110. Andersson J, Nagy S, Groth CG, Andersson U. Effects of FK506 and Cyclosporin A on cytokine production studied in vitro and at a single cell level. Immunology 1992; 75: 136–42.

111. Yoshimi F, Nakamura K, Zhu Y *et al*. Canine total orthotopic small bowel transplantation under FK506. Transplant Proc 1991; 23: 3240–2.

112. Gotoh M, Monden M, Kanai T *et al*. Tolerance induction by liver grafting and FK506 treatment in nonhuman primates. Transplant Proc 1991; 23: 3265–8.

113. Todo S, Demetris AJ, Ueda Y *et al*. Renal transplantation in baboons under FK506. Surgery 1989; 106: 444–50.

114. Kobayashi N, Sakagami K, Orita K *et al*. Effect of FK506 on abdominal organ cluster transplantation in pigs. Transplant Proc 1991; 23: 3275–9.

115. Sato K, Yokota K, Matsui T *et al*. Comparative study of FK506, cyclosporine and triple regimen immunosuppression with FK506, cyclosporine and mizoribine. Transplant Proc 1991; 23: 3296–9.

116. Katayama Y, Yada I, Namikawa S, Kusagawa M. Immunosuppressive effect of FK506 in rat lung transplantation. Transplant Proc 1991; 23: 3300–1.

117. Cooper MH, Markus PM, Cai X, Starzl T, Fung JJ. Prolonged prevention of acute graft versus host disease after allogeneic bone marrow transplantation by donor pretreatment using FK506. Transplant Proc 1991; 23: 3238–9.

118. Yamashita T, Maeda Y, Ishikawa T *et al*. Prolongation of pancreaticoduodenal allograft survival in rats by treatment with FK506. Transplant Proc 1991; 23: 3219–20.

119. Santiago SF, Fukuzawa M, Azuma T, Okada A. Effect of donor pretreatment with FK506 upon small intestine allotransplantation in rats. Transplant Proc 1991; 23: 3243–5.

120. European FK506 Multicentre liver study group. Randomised trial comparing tacrolimus (FK506) and cyclosporin in prevention of liver allograft rejection. Lancet 1994; 344: 423–8.

121. US Multicentre FK506 liver study group. A comparison of tacrolimus (FK506) and cyclosporin for immunosuppression in liver transplantation. N Engl J Med 1994; 331: 1110–15.

122. Shapiro R, Scantlebury VP, Jordan ML *et al*. FK506 in paediatric kidney transplantation – primary and rescue experience. Paediatr Nephrol 1995; 9 (Suppl): S43–8.

123. Shapiro R, Jordan ML, Scantlebury VP *et al*. A prospective randomised trial of FK506 based immunosuppression after renal transplantation. Transplantation 1995; 59: 485–90.

124. Ochiai T, Ishibashi M, Fukao K *et al*. Japanese multicentre studies of FK506 in renal transplantation. Transplant Proc 1995; 27: 50–3.

125. Ochiai T, Fukao K, Takahashi K *et al*. Phase III study of FK506 in kidney transplantation. Transplant Proc 1995; 27: 829–33.

126. Jordan ML, Shapiro R, Vivas CA *et al*. FK506 rescue therapy for resistant rejection in renal allografts under primary cyclosporine immunosuppression. Transplantation 1994; 57: 860–5.

127. Griffith BP, Bando K, Hardesty RL *et al*. A prospective randomised trial of FK506 versus cyclosporine after human pulmonary transplantation. Transplantation 1994; 57: 848–51.

128. Todo S, Tzakis A, Reyes J *et al*. Small intestinal transplantation in humans with or without colon. Transplantation 1994; 57: 840–8.

129. Todo S, Tzakis A, Reyes K *et al*. Intestinal transplantation: 4-year experience. Transplant Proc 1995; 27: 1355–6.

130. Gjertson DW. Multifactorial analysis of renal transplants reported to the United Network for Organ Sharing Registry: a 1994 update. In: Terasaki P, Cecka J (eds) Clinical transplants, California: UCLA, 1994, pp. 519–39.

131. Drewe J, Meier R, Vonderscher J et al. Enhancement of the oral absorption of cyclosporin in man. Br J Clin Pharmacol 1992; 34: 60–4.

132. Trull AK, Tan KK, Tan L, Alexander GJ, Jamieson NV. Absorption of cyclosporin from conventional and new microemulsion oral formulations in liver transplant recipients with external biliary diversion. Br J Clin Pharmacol 1995; 39: 627–31.

133. Kovarik JM, Kallay Z, Mueller EA, van Bree JB, Arns W, Renner E. Acute effect of cyclosporin on renal function following the initial changeover to a microemulsion formulation in stable kidney transplant patients. Transplant Int 1995; 8: 335–9.

134. Takeuchi T, Iinuma H, Kunimoto S et al. A new antitumour antibiotic, spergualin. J Antibiot 1981; 34: 1691.

135. Sandberg JO, Korsgren O, Groth CG, Andersson A. 15-Deoxyspergualin prolongs pancreatic islet allo- and xenograft survival in mice. Pharmacol Toxicol 1993; 73: 24–8.

136. Raff RF, Storb R, Graham T et al. What role for 15-deoxyspergualin in enhancing engraftment of unrelated histoincompatible canine marrow grafts and preventing graft-versus-host disease? Transplantation 1993; 55: 684–8.

137. Suzuki S, Kanashiro M, Watanabe H, Amemiya H. Therapeutic effect of 15-deoxyspergualin on acute graft rejection detected by $^{31}$P nuclear magnetic resonance spectography, and its effect on rat heart transplantation. Transplantation 1988; 46: 669–72.

138. Dickneite G, Schorlemmer HU, Weinmann E et al. Skin transplantation in rats and monkeys: evaluation of efficient treatment with 15-deoxyspergualin. Transplant Proc 1987; 19: 4244.

139. Reichenspurner H, Hildebrandt A, Human P et al. Does 15-deoxyspergualin induce nonreactivity after cardiac renal allotransplantation in primates? Transplantation 1990; 50: 181–5.

140. Masuda T, Shigetoshi M, Iijima M et al. Immunosuppressive activity of 15-deoxyspergualin and its effect on skin allograft in rats. J Antibiot 1987; 40: 1612–18.

141. Schubert G, Stoffregen G, Loske G et al. Synergistic effect of 15-deoxyspergualin and cyclosporin in pancreatic transplantation. Transplant Proc 1989; 21: 1096.

142. Engemann R, Gassel HJ, Lafranz E et al. The use of 15-deoxyspergualin in orthotopic rat liver transplantation: induction of transplantation tolerance and treatment of acute rejection. Transplant Proc 1988; 20 (suppl 1): 237.

143. Engemann R, Gassel HJ, Lafranz E et al. Transplantation tolerance after short term administration of 15-deoxspergualin in orthotopic rat liver transplantation. Transplant Proc 1987; 19: 4241–3.

144. Amemiya H, Suzuki S, Niiya S, Fukao K. A new immunosuppressive agent, 15-deoxyspergualin, in dog renal allografting. Transplant Proc 1989; 21: 3468–70.

145. Fukao K, Otsuka M, Iwasaki H et al. Immunosuppressive effect of deoxyspergualin on acute renal allograft rejection in dogs. Transplant Proc 1989; 21: 1090–3.

146. Amemiya H, Suzuki S, Watanabe H et al. 15-deoxyspergualin as an immunosuppressive agent in dogs. Transplant Proc 1988; 20: 229.

147. Yuh DD, Morris RE. The immunopharmacology of immunosuppression by 15-deoxyspergualin. Transplantation 1993; 55: 578–91.

148. Sutherland DE, Gores PF, Farney AC et al. Evolution of kidney, pancreas and islet transplantation for patients with diabetes at the University of Minnesota. Am J Surg 1993; 166: 456–91.

149. Jindall RM, Tepper MA, Soltys K, Cho SI. Deoxyspergualin – a novel immunosuppressant. Mt Sinai J Med 1994; 61: 51–6.

150. Yamazaki Y, Kawaguchi H, Ito K, Takahashi K, Toma H, Ota K. ABO incompatible kidney transplantation in children. J Urol 1995; 154: 914–16.

151. Gannedahl G, Ohlman S, Persson U et al. Rejection associated with early appearance of donor-reactive antibodies after kidney transplantation treated with plasmapheresis and administration of 15-deoxyspergualin. A report of two cases. Transplant Int 1992; 5: 189–92.

152. Amemiya H, Suzuki S, Ota K et al. A novel rescue drug, 15-deoxyspergualin. First clinical trials for recurrent graft rejection in renal recipients. Transplantation 1990; 49: 337–43.

153. Amemiya H, Taguchi Y, Fukao K et al. Establishment of rejection therapy with deoxysper-

gualin by multicentre controlled clinical studies in renal recipients. Transplant Proc 1993; 25: 730–3.

154. Matas AJ, Gores PF, Kelley SL *et al*. Pilot evaluation of 15-deoxyspergualin for refractory acute renal transplant rejection. Clin Transplant 1994; 8: 116–19.

155. Gregory CR, Pratt RE, Huie P *et al*. Effects of treatment with Cyclosporine, FK506, Rapamycin, Mycophenolic Acid, or Deoxyspergualin on vascular muscle proliferation in vitro and in vivo. Transplant Proc 1993; 25: 770–1.

156. Nagamine S. An experimental study of coronary arteriosclerosis after heart transplantation. Nippon Kyobu Geda Gakkai Zasshi 1993; 41: 2040–8. (English abstract)

157. Vigeral P, Chkoff N, Chatenoud L *et al*. Prophylactic use of OKT3 monoclonal antibody in cadaver kidney recipients. Utilisation of OKT3 as the sole immunosuppressive agent. Transplantation 1986; 41: 730–3.

158. Thistlethwaite JR, Cosimi AB, Delmonico FL *et al*. Evolving use of OKT3 monoclonal antibody for treatment of renal allograft rejection. Transplantation 1984; 38: 695–701.

159. Zlabinger GJ, Stuhlmeier KM, Eher R *et al*. Cytokine release and dynamics of leucocyte populations after CD3/TCR monoclonal antibody treatment. J Clin Immunol 1992; 12: 170–7.

160. Swinnen LJ, Costanzo-Nordin MR, Fisher SG *et al*. Increased incidence of lymphoproliferative disorder after immunosuppression with the monoclonal antibody OKT3 in cardiac transplant recipients. N Engl J Med 1990; 323: 1723–8.

161. Walkinshaw MD, Kallen J, Weber H-P *et al*. Immunophilin structure: a template for immunosuppressive drug design? Transplant Proc 1992; 24 (S2): 8–13.

# 6 Kidney transplantation

*John L. R. Forsythe*

Kidney transplantation is the procedure of choice for nearly all patients with end-stage renal failure. It is clinically effective, economically viable and gives good quality of life to the recipient. Targets of success such as one-year graft survival measuring 90% are regularly achieved[1,2] with the result that attention has turned to the improvement of 5-year and 10-year graft survival figures. In the cyclosporin era it is now predicted that 10-year graft survival may be in the region of 50% for living-related donor transplants and 44% for cadaver transplants. However, it has been noted that the attrition rate beyond the first year after the transplant procedure has not altered, suggesting that this is an area which now deserves greater attention.[3]

The surgeon who looks after renal patients is likely to know them for some considerable time. Surgical involvement is required in the pre-dialysis setting, around transplantation and for many years beyond. There are many more patients waiting for a kidney transplant than there are organs available and therefore it is beholden on the members of a renal transplant unit to act in a coordinated team with careful attention to detail, to make best use of a vital resource.

## Surgical preparation of the renal failure patient

It is likely that the surgeon will first meet the renal failure patient when there is a need for that patient to have access for dialysis. The decision as to which technique of dialysis should be employed is usually made by the patient after advice from nephrologists and specialist renal nurses. The final choice is often in favour of the technique which will best suit the patient's lifestyle. However, other factors may come into play which include local availability of dialysis facilities and the preference of physicians and renal nursing staff. Other medical factors which must be taken into account may lead one to encourage particular forms of dialysis, and such factors are listed in Table 6.1.

**Table 6.1** *Medical factors to be taken into account when considering dialysis*

| Encourage haemodialysis | Encourage peritoneal dialysis |
| --- | --- |
| Obesity | Poor arm veins |
| Multiple previous abdominal operations | Severe arteriosclerosis |
| Immobility or severe joint problems | Anxiety related to hospitals/needles |

### Insertion of peritoneal catheter

Chronic ambulatory peritoneal dialysis (CAPD) is the most common form of peritoneal dialysis. This requires the insertion of a silicone catheter with one tip placed inside the peritoneum, preferably in the pelvis. The catheter than passes through the layers of the abdominal wall and is led out via an exit site in the anterior abdominal wall skin around the level of the umbilicus, approximately in the mid clavicular line. Numerous methods for insertion of such catheters have been described. However, the important points are that the tip of the catheter is placed deep within the true pelvis to allow for easy filling and draining of peritoneal fluid. The silicone catheter has two cuffs of dacron, one placed so that it can become adherent to the peritoneum immediately underneath the abdominal wall musculature, and a second cuff which can be placed within the subcutaneous tunnel before the exit site. There are also many variations in catheter design, some having a preformed curl on the intraperitoneal portion of the catheter, these being preferred by many people to straight catheters because of reduction in pelvic and rectal pain experienced by the patient.

Single dacron cuff catheters are also manufactured, but are less commonly employed than the dual cuff variety. The method for placement of the catheter by laparoscopic assistance is shown in Figs 6.1 and 6.2. A direct cut-down technique in the infraumbilical area is employed

**Figure 6.1**
*Diagrammatic representation to show insertion of CAPD catheter.*

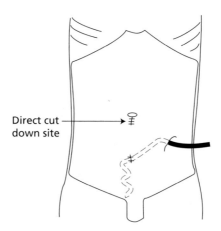

Direct cut down site

**Figure 6.2** *Cross-sectional view along pathway of CAPD catheter.*

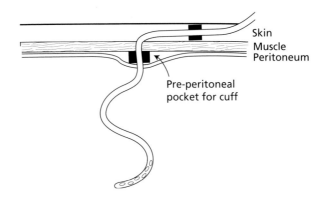

Skin
Muscle
Peritoneum

Pre-peritoneal
pocket for cuff

to gain access to the peritoneum. It is our practice to place a micro-lap port to allow a pneumoperitoneum to be created. A 3 mm micro-lap camera then gives an adequate view of the pelvis so that laparoscopy can be performed. After skin incision in the midline at the point indicated in Fig. 6.1, the catheter introducer and peel-away sheath is monitored under direct vision as entry into the peritoneum is created. The sheath can then be placed down into the pelvis, and the silicone catheter fed along the sheath until it can be seen entering the pelvis. The sheath is peeled away leaving the catheter up to the first cuff placed fully within the peritoneum. The dacron cuff is placed immediately below the rectus muscle at the level of the peritoneum. It is important that a pocket is created to allow the cuff to sit in this area so that a water tight seal can develop. The subcutaneous tunnel is created towards the exit site which has been marked before the operation by the patient and specialist renal nurse. The second dacron cuff is placed approximately half way along this subcutaneous tunnel – it must not be too close to the exit site.

Many variations of this technique have been described which include a larger primary incision with direct suture of the peritoneum to the first dacron cuff. This requires the intraperitoneal portion of the catheter to be placed by relatively blind technique, but there is still more control over the catheter than with a true percutaneous method. Both local and general anaesthesia are used by proponents of differing techniques and it is likely that the choice of placement and anaesthesia is governed by the individual performing the procedure and the local facilities available.

## Creation of arteriovenous fistula

A comprehensive description of vascular access techniques is outside the scope of this text. However, there are a number of principles which govern the vast majority of such operations. Kidney failure patients often have significant arterial vessel disease and they may have visited hospital on numerous occasions, with consequent damage to arm veins. Therefore, attention to detail and perseverance are vital to the success of the operation which aims to produce a superficial vein with high flow suitable for regular needling to allow dialysis. In general terms the more distal the arteriovenous fistula, the better. However, there is little point attempting a radiocephalic fistula with little prospect of success due to arterial or venous problems. It must also be noted that brachial fistulas may have a very high flow (up to $8\,l\,min^{-1}$) and such a shunt in the circulation may compromise a patient with pre-existing cardiac disease.

The preferred method is formation of a radiocephalic fistula at the wrist of the non-dominant hand.[4] Mobilisation of the cephalic vein allows an end-to-side anastomosis with the radial artery. Side-to-side anastomosis has no particular advantage, venous hypertension of the hand may result with no increase in the number of needling sites available.

If a forearm fistula is not possible, then a brachial to cephalic vein anastomosis would be the next choice. In the absence of good veins in the antecubital fossa, one must consider the use of the basilic vein which can be made more superficial to make needling of the vein easier. In the event that there are no suitable veins present within either arm (this is not an uncommon event in the renal patient) one must consider the placement of a prosthetic graft which may be in the form of a loop gaining inflow from the brachial artery. If no outflow is available in the upper limb, then a loop of prosthetic material may need to be placed using the femoral artery as inflow and the femoral vein at its junction with the long saphenous tributary as outflow.

### Jugular venous catheter

In those patients who are to receive haemodialysis but are not suitable for longer-term vascular access for whatever reason the option is to place a jugular venous catheter so that the tip lies in the superior vena cava or right atrium. The catheter is led out via a subcutaneous tunnel, the dacron cuff around the catheter sitting in the tunnel in order to reduce episodes of infection associated with the catheter.

## Assessment for renal transplantation

When the renal failure patient is established on dialysis, or if it is predicted that such a patient will need dialysis within the next few months, assessment for transplantation should be undertaken. Review of present medical condition can be performed and education concerning all aspects of renal transplantation can be carried out. It should be stressed that the assessment clinic is not a barrier to inclusion on the transplant list which must be overcome, rather it should be seen as a positive attempt to decide the best form of treatment for the patient. The following factors are important.

### Age

Although some units have a cut-off age above which they will not consider patients for transplantation, it is commonplace to find some patients in their 70s who are fitter than others in their 50s. Indeed a number of centres have reported good results in carefully selected elderly patients.[5] Therefore, each patient around this age should be assessed individually with the involvement of the patient, physician, anaesthetist and surgeon. However, if an elderly patient is accepted onto the transplant list, then regular review of this decision should be arranged. There seems little doubt that the older patient has less resistance to a long time on dialysis compared with a younger counterpart.

## Co-morbidity

Many renal patients also have significant vascular and respiratory disease. All attempts to palliate such co-morbidity are vital if the patient is to have a successful outcome of transplantation. Potential recipients with diabetes represent a category of patient with a higher risk since other organ systems are often affected by the underlying disease. The threshold for cardiological and vascular investigations in such patients is low.

## Cause of renal failure

### Recurring disease

It is unlikely that the patient will have been referred to the transplant assessment clinic if the risk of recurrence in a renal transplant of the primary renal disease is very high. However, it may be that patients suffering from Wegener's granulomatosis, or those with focal and segmental glomerular sclerosis, have been assessed to have a defined risk of recurrence in the transplant, but this risk is outweighed by their desire to undergo the transplant procedure. Again, the decision to place such a patient on the active transplant list must involve the whole transplant team and the patient. The best use of a scarce resource, i.e. donor kidneys, is an important consideration in such a decision.

### Urological abnormalities

Particular attention must be paid to those patients who have experienced renal failure due to upper and lower urinary tract problems. It is important to ensure that the primary problem will no longer be present to damage the transplant kidney, e.g. bladder dysfunction or recurrent urinary tract infection. The eradication of an infective focus is also vital. Complex problems may require urological expertise.

### Polycystic kidney disease

In this complaint the kidneys may be enormous and affect the side chosen for subsequent renal transplantation. In exceptional cases polycystic nephrectomy may be necessary, simply to make room for a transplant. Polycystic nephrectomy may also be necessary to eradicate infection or recurrent haemorrhage as a problem in these patients.

### Urological

If there is any suggestion of bladder dysfunction then full cystometrogram and urodynamics may be required. If it is felt that techniques such as intermittent self-catheterisation will be necessary following a renal transplant, the patient should be told of this decision and training begun. In exceptional cases, where a urinary diversion is felt to be the only solution to the lower urinary tract problems, the conduit should be fashioned either by a renal transplant surgeon or by a urologist who recognises the peculiar circumstances of placing a transplant ureter across the peritoneum and into the conduit. It is inadvisable to leave the conduit to be performed at the same time as the renal transplant itself. This increases the chance of morbidity from either operation.

### Peripheral vascular disease

Renal failure is a potent initiator of vascular disease on its own. When combined with smoking over a long time period, there are very few patients who have no signs of vascular disease. Part of the assessment process must include searching for evidence of such disease, both from history and examination. Any significant problem should be investigated further by exercise tests and Doppler wave form analysis, or in severe cases angiography may be necessary.

### Infection

Any focus of infection must be sought out and eradicated prior to acceptance onto the transplant list. This includes urological causes as well as infection associated with a CAPD catheter or a long-term dialysis central venous catheter. In addition dental examination is advised to deal with any intraoral caries or overt infection.

### Chronic infections such as hepatitis B, hepatitis C and HIV (AIDS)

HIV is an absolute contraindication to transplantation because any patients who have been HIV positive and undergone transplantation have fared badly.[6] The status of patients with hepatitis B and hepatitis C remains controversial. There is evidence to suggest that both hepatitis B and C may become more aggressive following transplantation with the immunosuppression that is necessary. There is no uniform policy for these circumstances and individual units now define their own policy after cooperation between the transplant team and hepatologists.

### Cancer

The presence of previous malignancy is a relative contraindication to transplantation. Immunosuppression, which is mandatory, will tend to increase the aggressive nature of any cancer. Patients who have had locally invasive tumours completely resected are an exception to this rule. Some centres accept patients with tumours of a less aggressive nature after an arbitrary period of disease-free survival. In such cases the risks of immunosuppression causing earlier return of disease should be discussed with the patient.

### Blood transfusion

Before cyclosporin, the positive effect of blood transfusion was such that patients were routinely transfused in order to improve graft survival. With the advent of cyclosporin, the potential benefit of this practice is no longer present and the dangers of sensitisation and antibody production are great.

## The call-up for a renal transplant

The potential recipient should be seen as soon as possible following admission and a full history and examination undertaken.

### History

Any change in the patient's condition since the time of transplant assessment should be sought. In particular, history of recent infection will be important in the decision as to whether the transplant can go ahead. Review of any urinary problems is also advisable at this stage. The type of dialysis used by the patient and the time of last dialysis should be noted as this will help decide whether a further episode of dialysis is needed prior to operation.

Recipient blood group, tissue typing and virology must be recorded in the notes. In addition the following donor details should be included for later ease of reference:

- age
- cause of death
- blood group
- tissue typing
- virology

### Examination

Full examination should be performed to ensure that the patient is fit for general anaesthesia and surgery. Particular attention should be paid to previous abdominal surgery, site of vascular access and signs of peripheral vascular disease.

A critical appraisal of the patient's fluid status must be performed. All patients will have been rendered nil by mouth from admission to the transplant unit and dialysis patients may well be relatively fluid deplete, especially those undergoing haemodialysis. Once all results are known and it is accepted that the patient is going ahead to transplant, then any obvious fluid depletion should be corrected by intravenous therapy.

## Investigations

The investigations which should be performed immediately prior to the operation are as follows:

- Full blood count
- Urea and electrolytes with creatinine
- Baseline calcium/liver function tests
- Random blood glucose
- Clotting screen
- Cross-match for 2 units of blood
- Lymphocytotoxic cross-match
- FACS cross-match
- Virology (CMV, HIV, Hep B, Hep C)
- Chest X-ray, ECG
- Urine culture (if possible)

Of these the full blood count should be examined to note the level of anaemia and any indication of occult infection. The biochemistry indicates whether dialysis is necessary and particular attention must be paid to the potassium level as dialysis in the postoperative phase for hyperkalaemia alone should be avoided.

The lymphocytotoxic cross-match should be sent off as soon as possible as this is often the time-limiting factor for the transplant to go ahead. A serum sample should be sent to the relevant laboratory to be paired with lymph nodes and spleen taken at the time of retrieval. Units vary in policy, but all would wish for a lymphocytotoxic cross-match to be available prior to operation and most would wish to see the result of a FACS cross-match (see Chapter 3).

## Prophylaxis

### Deep venous thrombosis prophylaxis

The rate of deep venous thrombosis (DVT) which requires treatment is low following the renal transplant procedure, in the region of 2%.[7] However, these figures are mainly from a time when the patients were more anaemic with little use of erythropoietin. Therefore, many units suggest the use of anti-DVT prophylaxis, either in the form of graduated compression stockings or subcutaneous heparin injection. In either case these measures should be instituted before induction of general anaesthesia.

### Antibiotic prophylaxis

Renal patients are immunosuppressed by their disease and further depleted by antirejection drugs. Therefore, a single dose of prophylactic antibiotic at the time of surgery is indicated. The choice of drugs varies between units, but should include cover against skin organisms as well as those found within the urinary tract which is opened during the surgical procedure.

### Prophylaxis against rejection

Formerly, patients were preloaded with quite large doses of background immunosuppressive agents prior to the transplant operation. Nowadays, it is more common to limit the use of agents such as cyclosporin or tacrolimus, introducing these in the postoperative phase when the level of primary renal function has been assessed. However, most units continue to give a large bolus of steroid (e.g. 500 mg methylprednisolone) at the time of the operation so that this large dose of steroids is present on revascularisation of the graft.

When all results of the investigations have been completed and it is accepted that the patient is receiving a renal transplant, consent for the operation should be obtained. The following points should be mentioned to the patient.

1. Procedure: a brief description of the procedure, the length of time taken for the operation and 'attachments' to the patient postoperatively (catheters, drains, IV lines) should be described. As noted below it is our routine to place a ureteric stent at the time of transplantation. This event should also be mentioned to the patient.
2. Delayed graft function: it is important at this stage to mention to the patient that the kidney does not always function straight away. This short explanation will greatly allay anxiety in the postoperative phase, should delayed graft function occur.
3. Rejection: to the patient, rejection may be synonymous with loss of graft. The fact that this is not the case should already have been explained, but reinforcement at this time is good policy.
4. The transplant kidney: it is reasonable to tell the patient of the degree of match which the kidney represents for them. Any unusual problems could also be mentioned at this stage, e.g. abnormal anatomy which may make the operation more difficult than the routine.

The patient then proceeds to induction of anaesthesia in the operating room. At this time a central venous line should be placed to allow for monitoring of central pressure in the immediate postoperative period.

A size 18 FG urinary catheter should be inserted after induction of the anaesthesia. Any smaller catheter is likely to increase the number of problems with haematuria-induced retention of urine after the operation. At this stage, the bladder should be filled with saline and the catheter spiggoted, or an attachment left in place to allow such filling to occur at the time of ureteric implantation. This step facilitates definition of the bladder which can be quite difficult in patients who have been oligo-anuric for some time.

**Transplant operation**

## Preparation of the donor kidney

Around the same time as the patient leaves the ward for the operating theatre, back table dissection of the kidney should commence. This gives an adequate time for this important manoeuvre. Good preparation will ensure an adequate length of vessels with good haemostasis at the time of clamp release. Bad preparation can result in a difficult anastomosis and release of clamps may induce significant blood loss.

The kidney should be orientated as it is in the body. The renal vein should be picked up and dissection carried out back towards the kidney. Small branches and the gonadal and adrenal branches should be ligated and divided. A balance must be struck between mobility of the vein, which will be gained by dissection up towards the hilum, and risk of damaging the vascular supply to the renal pelvis. The renal vein is now folded over the kidney and the artery dissected out from any adherent fat. Care must be taken to identify any abnormal anatomy, given that this is a common finding. Again, the artery should not be followed too deeply into the renal hilum. The ureter is now dissected free with great care to leave a small amount of tissue around the ureter since this will protect the blood supply to this structure.

Once all of these vital elements of the kidney have been identified and dissected out, the fat which has been left around the kidney at the time of retrieval can be removed. The adrenal gland has often been taken together with the kidney at the time of organ procurement – this should be removed with the perinephric fat and any vasculature not already dealt with should be ligated and divided.

The renal vein and artery should be left full length until the recipient vessels have been fully evaluated. However, it is quite acceptable to form the aortic and IVC patch on the renal vessels in preparation for later anastomosis. It is our practice at this stage to flush the renal artery with 100–200 ml of kidney perfusion fluid. Care must be taken at the time of this cannulation of the renal artery to avoid any intimal damage, but it is felt that this manoeuvre may help remove products of metabolism which have built up during the cold ischaemic period. It is also useful in detecting small defects in the artery or vein which have gone unnoticed in the dissection process.

## Incision

It is conventional wisdom that a left kidney should be transplanted to the right iliac fossa and a right kidney to the left iliac fossa. However, there is little doubt that the right-sided iliac vessels are a little more superficial and, provided the orientation of the transplant kidney is checked, there is no problem in transplanting either kidney to the right side. Obviously, it is sensible to avoid previous abdominal incisions and this factor, as well as any asymmetry in peripheral vascular disease, should be a factor in dictating the side of choice for operation. The incision is curvilinear with its lowest portion placed a few centimetres above the pubic symphysis and extending just to the midline. The upper portion of the incision should pass approximately 4 cm medial to the anterior superior iliac spine.

Muscles are divided by diathermy and dissected in layers. Great care must be taken to avoid entering the peritoneum. This is particularly the case in CAPD patients as any need for dialysis in the postoperative phase may be jeopardised. The inferior epigastric artery will be encountered beneath the rectus muscle. This should be ligated and divided. The round ligament should be treated in a similar fashion in the female. The spermatic cord should be controlled and any adherent tissue removed. This allows good mobility in the medial part of the wound which is important both at the time of the venous anastomosis and during the ureteric anastomosis. Dissection is carried down to the iliac vessels and exposure should be engineered from the common iliac artery down to the external iliac artery underneath the inguinal ligament. Early in the procedure, it is advisable to examine the bifurcation of the common iliac artery as there is often a plaque of atherosclerosis present at this point. A significant plaque would tend to preclude the use of the internal iliac artery as in-flow to the kidney. Similarly, if the patient has had a previous renal transplant on the other side with use of the internal iliac artery, it would be advisable to use common or external iliac for a repeat transplant to avoid buttock claudication and sexual dysfunction which may result from distal internal iliac ligation.[8] Small lymphatic vessels running in the same orientation as the arteries should be dissected out and if necessary, ligated and divided. In children and sometimes in older women, the external iliac artery may be of acceptable size when first approached, but arterial spasm causes significant diminution of diameter. In this case it is advisable to consider use of the common iliac artery since even with measures to overcome spasm, use of such an external iliac artery may prejudice good renal transplant blood flow.

Attention is then turned to the venous system and the external iliac vein should be mobilised from its origin to the level of the inguinal ligament. Sometimes there are small branches passing directly back from the external iliac vein which must be treated with great respect as damage to these branches can be very troublesome. It is very rare to need division of the internal iliac vein to allow for complete mobilisation. However, it is useful to gain mobility of the tissues medial to the vein as this potential space is occupied by the transplant kidney when it is manoeuvred into position and creation of space facilitates performance of the venous anastomosis, especially with a short renal vein. Time spent in reconnaissance of the iliac vessels is rarely wasted and should make the vascular anastomosis as easy as possible.

It is considered highly desirable to have a self-retaining retractor system, e.g. Omnitract retractor, once the dissection has been carried out. Although such retractor systems can be expensive, the operative field is held in good position and held still which allows the surgeon to concentrate on the vascular anastomoses which are to be undertaken.

### Vascular anastomosis

Systemic heparinisation is rarely required in renal patients because of underlying haematological abnormalities. However, history of previous clotting abnormalities or the presence of almost normal haematological indices in certain patients should encourage review of this general policy.

The iliac vein is cross-clamped and a venotomy carefully planned to allow the arterial anastomosis to be slightly staggered which aids the performance of the anastomosis. The venotomy is size matched with the renal vein of the graft. It is better to have the venotomy slightly too small than slightly too large. Double-ended 5/0 prolene sutures are placed at either end of the venotomy and it is advisable to place a stay suture at each side of the vein. This attempts to avoid the complication of inclusion of the opposite wall of the venous anastomosis whilst one side is being performed.

The kidney is removed from the ice at this stage, but should be carefully packed in order to keep the temperature around the kidney as low as possible. The two end sutures already present in the iliac vein are now passed through either end of the renal vein and the venous anastomosis completed by a continuous suture down either side of the vein.

There are two major types of arterial anastomosis. The first is an end-to-side anastomosis between the renal artery and the common iliac artery or the external iliac artery. It is likely that the aortic patch will be preserved for this type of anastomosis, but it is very important that the resultant renal artery is not much longer than the renal vein, causing severe kinking of the vessel. Clamps must be carefully applied to the recipient vessels as renal failure patients often have significant atherosclerosis, even in the absence of other risk factors. After formation of an arteriotomy in the selected vessel, 5/0 or 6/0 prolene is used to form a continuous anastomosis between donor and recipient vessels. If recipient vessels are particularly atheromatous then interrupted sutures may be used, only tying the sutures once the whole side of the anastomosis has been completed. This enables careful placement of the suture needle to avoid intimal damage.

The second type of anastomosis is an end-to-end anastomosis to the internal iliac artery. This is the most satisfactory haemodynamic type of anastomosis and often allows the kidney to lie in a very good position with little kinking of vessels at the end of the operation. Surgeons may employ an interrupted suturing technique for this type of anastomosis. An alternative is to use a continuous suture tying the knot of the suture at a short distance from the arterial wall producing a 'growth factor' as described by Starzl.[9] The object of either of these techniques is to avoid later anastomotic strictures.

At this point clamps are released – the venous clamp first. The kidney should fill rapidly and change colour quickly. Any bleeding around the anastomosis should be controlled as quickly as possible and it is preferable to avoid reclamping. Such warm ischaemia following cold ischaemia tends to impair later graft function.

## Vascular abnormalities

Anomalies of the renal artery or renal vein are very common, amounting to 30% of kidneys retrieved. Figure 6.3 shows some of the more common anomalies and suggested anastomotic techniques. If all the renal vessels come off the aorta within a short distance, it is ideal that a single aortic patch is used for anastomosis. However, if this is not possible then the second artery should be protected by anastomosis separately, or by end-to-side linkage to the main renal artery. This obviously needs to be performed on the back table prior to transplant

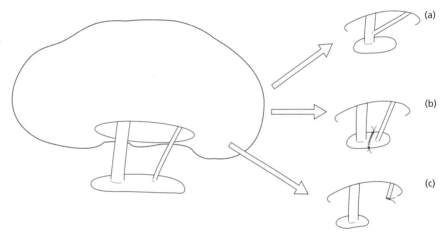

**Figure 6.3**   *Common arterial abnormalities with possible solutions. (a) End-to-side anastomosis of small to larger renal artery; (b) shortening of the aortic patch with resuture; (c) tieing off a renal artery is to be avoided, especially if the extra artery is to the lower pole as it supplies blood to the upper ureter.*

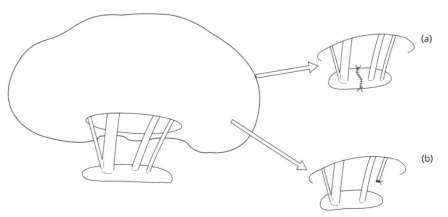

**Figure 6.4**   *Common vein abnormalities with possible solutions. (a) The renal vein may be anastomosed using a long patch, but rarely the patch requires to be shortened; (b) small renal veins may sometimes be tied off to leave a more manageable length of IVC patch.*

procedure. Every attempt must be made to revascularise all renal arteries. This is especially true of a lower pole vessel since the blood supply to the ureter may be dependent on continuity of this structure. Venous abnormalities are less common (Fig. 6.4). Most of these can be dealt with by anastomosis of the complete IVC patch to the iliac vein. On occasions this may produce a long patch but it is very rare that the patch requires to be shortened.

When the arterial and venous clamps have been removed and the kidney is seen to have a satisfactory blood supply, there is a natural tendency for all in the operating theatre, including the surgeon, to anticipate the end of the operation. However, the ureteric anastomosis is yet to be completed and inattention to detail in this part of the procedure is as much a potential disaster as in the vascular anastomoses.

Retraction should be adjusted to focus on the lower end of the wound. Distension of the bladder by fluid introduced via the urinary catheter aids the dissection of the bladder in preparation for anastomosis with the transplant ureter. In the male, it should be remembered that the ureter is best placed underneath the spermatic cord on its course to the bladder.

There are two major types of anastomosis used by transplant surgeons.

### The extravesical ureteroneocystostomy

This is the author's preferred method, it was first described as an antireflux procedure[10] and was then adapted as the external ureteroneocystostomy.[11] This is easy to perform, causes less problems with haematuria postoperatively and is no better or worse than other techniques at preventing ureteric reflux.[12] The bladder muscle is divided in layers until the mucosa balloons out over a length of approximately 5 cm. The mucosa is then opened at the distal end of the bladder wound. The ureter is cleaned of adventitial tissue and care is taken to avoid ischaemia of the tip. The ureter is spatulated and may be anastomosed using polydioxinone suture as a continuous or interrupted technique. The muscle layers are then closed over the transplant ureter so that it runs in a muscular tunnel before entry into the bladder.

### Leadbetter/Politano technique

The most common procedure is a variation of the technique described by Politano and Leadbetter in 1958.[13] This technique requires a formal anterior cystotomy to gain access to the interior of the bladder. A separate stab incision is made in a more posterolateral plane and the ureter is led along a submucosal tunnel before its opening into the mucosa of the bladder. The transplant ureter is spatulated and fixed to the mucosa of the bladder using interrupted polydioxinone sutures. A separate closure of the cystotomy is performed in two layers using interrupted sutures.

### To stent, or not?

The use of a ureteric stent in renal transplantation is still controversial. The author preferred not to employ the use of a stent before being involved in a trial which enlisted 300 patients and indicated a significant advantage to those who were randomised to stent insertion.[14] A double J stent placed at the time of operation can be removed at 8–12 weeks after the transplant by fibreoptic cystoscopy under local anaesthesia. This seems a small price to pay for the consequent reduction in all ureteric complications.

The operation is only complete when haemostasis has been checked carefully. It is of note that reoperation for haemorrhage is rarely necessary for anastomotic problems since the surgeon is very careful about this aspect of the operation. More often the hilum of the kidney is the site of a small persistent bleed and this fact should aid prevention rather than cure. A closed suction drain is then placed into the retroperitoneal space and the wound is closed in layers with polydioxinone suture. The placement of the kidney is vital. A good operation can be spoiled by bad positioning of the kidney with resultant kinking of the vessels. Care must be taken to avoid any such complication and the colour of the kidney must be re-examined repeatedly as the wound is closed. If a large kidney is being placed within a small recipient, a peritoneal pocket can be fashioned which will aid satisfactory positioning of the kidney.

## The early postoperative phase

The presence or absence of primary function in the early postoperative phase is very important. Although one may try to reassure the patient that the absence of good transplant function is of little concern, there is no doubt that the patient becomes more difficult to manage and that there is a definite effect on graft survival even measured many years after the transplant.[15] These two facts may well be connected.

### Primary function

Primary function should be expected with nearly all living donor transplants and most cadaveric donor procedures. The urine output of the patient may represent a slight increase over preoperative levels but it may also be many litres in 24 h. Monitoring of fluid balance is vital with no substitute for repeat observations. The situation may change over a few hours and should be monitored accordingly. A state of polyuria does not always mean that electrolyte imbalance is being corrected immediately. Therefore biochemical monitoring is also important.

The patient with primary renal transplant function may exhibit all of the complications of those with delayed function which are mentioned below. However, such complications may be easier to detect particularly by routine review of the patient and attention to details such as those listed in Table 6.2.

**Table 6.2** *Aspects for regular review following kidney transplantation*

| | |
|---|---|
| **Fluid balance** | Vital signs and central venous pressure |
| | Urinary output |
| | Daily weight |
| | Regular examination |
| **Immunosuppression** | Cyclosporin levels |
| | Tacrolimus levels |
| | Haematology |
| | History (tremor etc.) |
| **Renal failure** | Urinary output |
| | Biochemical screening |
| | Creatinine clearance |

## Delayed graft function

An early postoperative check in this condition reveals that the patient is passing little urine and certainly no more than was their baseline urine output before the transplant procedure. Immediate management is aided by attention to the following questions.

1. Is the patient bleeding? This should be obvious by reference to vital signs, drain fluid and examination of the wound. Unless bleeding comes under control quickly, the best policy is re-exploration as increased pressure in the confined space around the kidney may have dire consequence.
2. Is the catheter working? A simple mechanical problem with the catheter may cause urinary retention causing unwanted stress on the recent ureteric anastomosis. Haematuria may be a problem and this can require a gentle bladder washout to be performed. On very rare occasions the patient may need to return to theatre to have cystoscopic removal of a clot within the bladder.
3. Is the patient hypovolaemic? The answer to this problem needs to be checked and rechecked. Regular measurement of the vital signs, central venous pressure and repeat examination of the patient are mandatory. If it is truly felt that the patient is hypovolaemic, then a small fluid challenge should be given and the effect on fluid status monitored.
4. Is there a vascular complication? The incidence of vascular complication is approximately 4%[16] and this complication is always uppermost in the mind of the operating surgeon. If the above questions have been answered satisfactorily, a duplex scan should be obtained at the first opportunity. This modality detects a vascular abnormality effectively[17] therefore providing reassurance when a normal result is obtained. Any abnormal findings should be checked by re-exploration which unfortunately often results in transplant nephrectomy.

If the patient is in a euvolaemic state with a well-draining urinary catheter and a normal duplex ultrasound report, then the cause of delayed graft function is likely to be acute tubular necrosis. This state may continue for several days and requires continued close observation to rule out any other complications. Good fluid balance must be maintained with the oral fluid intake strictly controlled as the need for intravenous therapy reduces. Dialysis may need to be reinstituted with the patient returning to the form of renal replacement therapy used prior to the operation. However, peritoneal dialysis may need to be restricted if the peritoneum was breached at the time of the transplant procedure. The need for dialysis should be carefully explained to the patient; many see this necessity as a sign of imminent transplant failure.

Aids in the assessment of the renal graft during this difficult time include drug level monitoring, repeat ultrasound of the graft as well as regular haematological and biochemical checks. There are no immunological markers of proven value so that reliance has fallen on the core biopsy and histology. Fine needle aspiration cytology has been practised for many years in Scandinavia[18] and other centres throughout Europe. However, this technique has not gained the same popularity in the UK or the USA. Perhaps this is because the core biopsy is known to be a sensitive indicator of graft dysfunction and is safe.[19] The safety level has been enhanced by the recent use of ultrasound guidance and a spring-loaded biopsy gun for the performance of the procedure.

The common complications which may affect the allograft are discussed below.

### Drug toxicity

Both cyclosporin and tacrolimus are toxic to the kidney. Minor degrees of drug toxicity are very common requiring alteration of dose. More major dysfunction may be detected by regular drug level monitoring. If these levels are seen to be very high then a dose of cyclosporin or tacrolimus should be omitted. Given that the half-life of tacrolimus is longer than that of cyclosporin, two doses may need to be omitted. In addition to drug toxicity due to the common immunosuppressive agents, the use of non-steroidal anti-inflammatory drugs and antibiotics which are nephrotoxic may produce transplant dysfunction. The use of drugs which alter the levels of cyclosporin and tacrolimus must be carefully monitored.

### Urological problems

Ureteric leak or obstruction may occur because of poor surgical technique, distal ureteric ischaemia or immunological damage to the ureter.[20] Ureteric leak tends to happen in the early postoperative phase whereas stenosis and consequent obstruction occurs later.

Urinary leak is likely to present as increased pain experienced by the patient in the region of the wound. Ultrasound may detect fluid around the kidney which if aspirated will be found to have a high creatinine level. Antegrade nephrostomy and nephrostogram will help delineate the problem. Placing a double J stent across the defect may be sufficient to allow healing. However, further surgery with renewal of the anastomosis using healthy tissue may be necessary.

Ureteric obstruction may result in few symptoms or signs. Reduction of urinary output or graft function may give a clue to the diagnosis but routine ultrasound is likely to show a dilated collecting system and perhaps a dilated ureter to the level of obstruction. Nephrostomy relieves the immediate problem and gives access for imaging and definitive diagnosis. The vast majority of these problems can be managed by endoscopic measures usually requiring the introduction of a double J stent across the stricture.

### Rejection

The greatest risk of graft rejection occurs in the first two weeks after the transplant procedure. This problem may present with the patient complaining of malaise, increased tenderness in the wound area and joint pains whilst exhibiting pyrexia, hypertension, graft tenderness and reduction of function. Unfortunately the ease of such a diagnosis is rare. Each patient may have a few of the above symptoms of rejection but many have none. Most centres have developed a policy of early graft biopsy in the face of any diminution of function. In those cases where there is little or no transplant function, a system of protocol biopsies may be developed to detect smouldering occult rejection. For example many units would plan a biopsy in patients suffering delayed graft function at day 4 or 5 after the transplant operation and then again 5 days later if no improvement had occurred.

The treatment of rejection is mainly by the use of high-dose intravenous steroids, e.g. 500 mg methyl prednisolone daily given on three consecutive days. Most rejection episodes respond to this treatment but where the response is poor or rejection returns quickly, the diagnosis of steroid-resistant rejection is made and this may be treated by the use of polyclonal antibody products such as antithymocyte globulin (ATG) or monoclonal antibody preparations such as OKT3. Recently, the addition of new immunosuppressive agents to the armamentarium have allowed rescue treatment with products such as tacrolimus and mycophenolate mofetil.[21,22] Due to all of these agents, irreversible rejection is now very uncommon (see Chapter 5).

### Lymphocoele

This complication rarely occurs in the first few days after transplantation and is more likely to be seen in the period from two weeks to many months after the transplant operation. The cause of the lymphatic collection is leakage from recipient lymphatics dissected out at the time of vessel manipulation. This fluid can build up to a large quantity and a surprisingly high pressure within a closed cavity. This pressure is certainly sufficient to cause compression of the renal transplant with ureteric obstruction. Diagnosis is by ultrasound and aspiration of the fluid which has a creatinine level similar to that in the blood. Aspiration may also be sufficient for emergency treatment causing reduction in pressure on the transplant. However, permanent treatment is likely to require surgery. The procedure of choice is fenestration of the perito-neum which overlies the lymphocoele, allowing drainage of the lympha-tic fluid into the peritoneum where it is then absorbed. A $4 \times 4$ cm window should be created to prevent sealing by intra-abdominal contents. This operation is ideally suited to laparoscopic surgery[23] and laparoscopic ultrasound may be useful in avoiding any damage to vital structures while the window of peritoneum is removed.

**Longer-term problems**

Many of the above complications may occur months or years after the renal transplant operation. However, these problems do become less common with the emphasis switching to other factors which threaten the recipient and his graft.

### Hypertension

Successful kidney transplantation removes renal failure as a cause for hypertension. However, new risk factors appear such as the use of immunosuppressive therapy, renal transplant arterial stenosis, the effect of native failed kidneys and the consequence of allograft rejection. Indeed, there is experimental evidence that transplantation of a kidney from a hypertensive donor into a normotensive recipient can cause hypertension in the recipient.[24] Therefore hypertension is common but should lead to a search for trigger factors.[25] Several antihypertensive drugs may be required to achieve good control.

### Lipid problems

The combination of renal disease, steroids[26] and cyclosporin[27] is a potent mix for hyperlipidaemia. The incidence of such problems is relatively high within the renal transplant population. The realisation of this problem in many centres has come quite late with the result that corrective action has not been taken as early as possible. Dietary advice, review of immunosuppression and finally the use of lipid-lowering agents represents the management of most patients in the renal trans-plant follow-up clinic.

### Cardiovascular disease

The foregoing information demonstrates that the renal transplant patient is at risk from accelerated vascular disease, hypertension and hyper-lipidaemia. Added to this, at least 30% of the patients are diabetic. It is little wonder then, that cardiovascular disease is the major cause of mortality in patients who have received a renal transplant.[28] It is this fact that has encouraged a holistic approach to the care of the patient in the renal transplant clinic. Obviously the function of the graft is very important but reduction in some of the risk factors mentioned above must be the target if improvement in patient survival is to be obtained.

### Chronic rejection

Before use of this term, it is important to define its meaning. In the past, chronic rejection referred to most cases of reduction in graft function where none of the obvious complications such as acute rejection, cyclosporin nephrotoxicity and urological problems could be proven. Nowadays, chronic allograft dysfunction is the overall diagnosis given to such cases. Careful investigation of these patients reveals many causes for the deterioration in graft function. These include advancing vascular disease, cardiac disease, hypertension, recurrent urinary tract infection, late acute rejection and drug toxicity. After removal of this group of problems, one is left with a true chronic damage due to immunological action. This is characterised by vascular occlusion seen in conjunction with glomerulopathy on core biopsy of the renal graft. Chronic rejection has no treatment and this is why it is very important to differentiate this diagnosis from any other cause of graft function deterioration. It is hoped that some of the newer agents being developed for transplantation may help the problem of chronic allograft rejection (see Chapter 5).

### Renal artery stenosis

The incidence of this complication ranges between 3 and 5% across all published data. The problem is likely to present from months to years after the renal transplant was performed. Hypertension associated with a deterioration in renal function should prompt investigation initially by duplex ultrasonography. If this modality supports the diagnosis then angiography should be organised. Angioplasty is the most common form of treatment and is especially valuable for non-anastomotic strictures. Surgery is rarely necessary but may be more successful than angioplasty in preventing recurrence. The surgery is difficult because of fibrosis in the region of the vasculature and there is significant risk of graft loss.

## Choice of immuno-suppression

Cyclosporin (in the form of Neoral) remains the backbone of immunosuppression for renal transplantation. In the past, many units began cyclosporin in a loading dose prior to the operation but now, most centres rely on high dose steroids (e.g. methyl prednisolone 500 mg) given at the time of transplant and a further dose 24 h later, to begin the process of immunosuppression. Thereafter, the decision between various forms of background immunosuppression needs to be made. Some units still employ cyclosporin monotherapy based on the fact that there is no strong evidence for the addition of steroids when looking at crude survival data only.[29] In the same manner evidence for use of 'triple therapy' is not very strong when comparison is made with the use of cyclosporin and steroids alone.[30] Yet triple immunosuppression using azathioprine, prednisolone and cyclosporin together produces good results with rejection-free patients in nearly 40% of renal transplants.[31] This factor is a powerful argument for the use of triple therapy, given that the major cause of late graft loss is chronic rejection.[32] It appears that the prior occurrence of acute rejection is an important factor in the development of chronic allograft immune damage.[33] The reduction of acute rejection episodes plus the fact that triple therapy is very easy to use, make it the most popular form of background immunosuppression in Europe.

The place of tacrolimus and mycophenolate mofetil (MMF) in the treatment of renal transplant patients is yet to be fully established. Most centres are now using these agents in those patients who are considered to be at high risk of immune activity. Results from multicentre trials show that tacrolimus-based triple therapy or cyclosporin, steroid and MMF have no patient or graft-survival benefit at one year but do show a further reduction in acute rejection episodes.[34,35] The argument that it is important to avoid chronic rejection by reducing acute rejection, may therefore increase the use of these new drugs. Survival figures for two and three years after transplant using these agents are keenly awaited.

**The future**

Results of renal transplantation are so good that this procedure has evolved in a few years from a research curiosity into a routine treatment for the patient with renal failure. This success has encouraged more patients to be included on the waiting list for a transplant, although the organ donor numbers are decreasing. In the United Kingdom and the Euro transplant region, there are 15 000 people on the waiting list for renal transplantation with only 4000 transplant procedures per year.[36]

An increase in the age of the population with a consequent rise in the incidence of renal disease makes matter worse. Such problems have brought about difficult ethical issues concerning encouragement of organ donation which have been responded to by different approaches in differing countries (see Chapter 1). The interest in xenotransplantation is also driven largely by the lack of organ donors. Until xenotransplantation becomes a reality we will have to deal with present problems and one of the possible solutions is to increase the living donation of kidneys.

There is a large discrepancy between countries in the rate of living donation. For example, Norway has a percentage of 40% whereas the United Kingdom (not the lowest European figure), has a living donation rate of 5%.

Many centres have a policy of always discussing living donation with each possible recipient. Good education and counselling is vital to ensure proper donor selection. It is reasonable to tell the recipient and the prospective donor that the results of living donation transplant are very good with little risk to the donor. However, the donor should have all possible risks fully spelt out so that a proper informed decision can be

**Table 6.3** *Investigations to be carried out in a potential living donor*

| Haematology | Clinical chemistry | Virology | Clinical bacteriology |
|---|---|---|---|
| ☐ FBC | ☐ Us and ES | ☐ Hep B | ☐ TPHA |
| | ☐ LFTs | ☐ Hep C | |
| | ☐ Glucose | ☐ HIV | |
| | ☐ Uric acid | ☐ CMV | |
| | ☐ Calcium | | |
| | ☐ Phosphate | | |
| | ☐ Total protein | | |
| ☐ MSU | ☐ Urinalysis | ☐ Chest X-ray | ☐ ECG |
| ☐ 24 hour urine protein and creatinine (with bloods) | | | ☐ angiography |
| ☐ Renal U/S | ☐ IVP | ☐ Blood pressure – erect/supine | |

made. Any living donor transplants that are performed in the UK are living-related transplants with very few exceptions. In other countries the use of living-unrelated donors is much greater and although this is a very controversial area, the results recently published from the United States[37] are very good indeed, providing evidence which has further fuelled the debate regarding living donation.

Table 6.3 shows an example of the investigations which a potential living donor should undergo. There is still considerable variation between centres in the work-up for donation.[38] It is of note that in the UK, the Human Organ Transplant Act (1989) requires proof of relationship between the donor and recipient or if this proof does not exist then special dispensation needs to be sought from a committee set up for the purpose. This is in addition to the transplant clinicians satisfying themselves that the donation is a true gift with no coercion or commercial award.

The welcome reduction in road traffic accident deaths and mortality from intracerebral haemorrhage has significant implication for the growing number of patients accepted onto dialysis lists. It is likely that the number of living donor transplants will increase over the next few years unless another answer to the organ donor crisis can be found.

## References

1. Cecka JM, Terasaki PI. The UNOS Scientific Renal Transplant Registry. In: Terasaki PI, Cecka (eds) Clinical transplants 1994, Los Angeles: UCLA Tissue Typing Laboratory, 1995; pp. 1–18.
2. Connolly JK, Dyer PA, Martin S, Parrott NR, Pearson RC, Johnson RWG. Importance of minimising HLA-DR mismatch and cold preservation time in cadaveric renal transplantation. Transplantation 1996; 61: 709–14.
3. Hostetter TH. Chronic transplant rejection. Kidney Int 1994; 46: 266–79.
4. Koo Seen Lin LC, Burnapp L. Contemporary vascular access surgery for chronic haemodialysis. J R Coll Surg Edin 1996; 41: 164–9.

5. Ost L, Lundgren G, Groth CG. Renal transplants in the older patient. In: Progress in transplantation Vol 2. Edinburgh: Churchill Livingstone, 1985, pp. 1–15.
6. Lang P, Niavolet P, Groupe Cooperatif de Transplantation d'Ile de France. HIV infection in renal transplant patients. In: Louraine JL (eds) Transplantation and clinical immunology Vol. 23. Amsterdam: Excerpta Medica 1991, p. 221.
7. Allen RD, Michie CA, Murie JA, Morris PJ. Deep venous thrombosis after renal transplantation. Surg Gynecol Obstet 1987; 164: 137–9.
8. Billet A, Dajner JF, Queral LA. Surgical correction of vasculogenic impotence in a patient after bilateral renal transplantation. Surgery 1982; 91: 108–11.
9. Starzl TE, Iwatski S, Shaw BW. A growth factor in fine vascular anastomoses. Surg Gynecol Obstet 1984; 159: 164–5.
10. Lich R, Haverton LW, David LA. Recurrent urosepsis in children. J Urol 1961; 86: 554–9.
11. Calne RY. Color atlas of renal transplantation. Oradell, NJ: Medical Economic Books, 1984.
12. Thrasher JB, Temple DR, Spees EK. Extravesical versus Leadbetter–Politano ureteroneocystostomy: a comparison of urological complications in 320 renal transplants. J Urol 1990; 144: 1105–9.
13. Politano VA, Leadbetter WF. An operative technique for the correction of vesicoureteral reflux. J Urol 1968; 79: 932–9.
14. Pleass HCC, Clark KR, Rigg KM, Reddy KS, Forsythe JLR. Urological complications after renal transplantation. Transplant Proc 1995; 27: 1091–2.
15. Belitsky P, MacDonald P, Gajewski J et al. Significance of delayed function in cyclosporin-treated cadaver kidney transplants. Transplant Proc 1987; 19: 2096–7.
16. Jones RM, Murie JA, Ting A, Dunnill MS, Morris PJ. Renal vascular thrombosis of cadaveric renal allografts in patients receiving cyclosporine, azathioprine and prednisolone triple therapy. Clin Transplant 1988; 2: 122–4.
17. Johnson CP, Toley WD, Gallagher-Lepak S, Roza AM, Adams MB. Evaluation of renal transplant dysfunction using color Doppler sonography. Surg Gynecol Obstet 1991; 173(4): 279–84.
18. von Willebrand E. Fine needle aspiration cytology of human renal transplants. Clin Immunol Immunopathol 1980; 17(3): 309–22.
19. Huraib S, Goldberg H, Katz A. Percutaneous needle biopsy of the transplanted kidney: technique and complications. Am J Kidney Dis 1989; 14(1): 13–17.
20. Loughlin KR, Tilney NL, Richie JP. Urologic complications in 718 renal transplant patients. Surgery 1984; 95(3): 297–302.
21. Jordan ML, Shapiro R, Vivas CA, Scantlebury VP, Rhondhawa P, Cartieri G. FK506 rescue for resistant rejection of renal allografts under primary cyclosporine immunosuppression. Transplantation 1994; 57: 860–5.
22. Sollinger HW, Belzer FO, Deierhoi MH et al. RS-61443 rescue therapy in refractory kidney transplant rejection. Transplant Proc 1993; 25: 698–9.
23. Khauli RB, Mosenthal AC, Coushaj PF. Treatment of lymphocoele and lymphatic fistula following renal transplantation by laparoscopic peritoneal window. J Urol 1992; 147: 1353–5.
24. de Wardener HE. The primary role of the kidney and salt intake in the etiology of essential hypertension. Clin Sci 1990; 79(3): 193–200.
25. Luke RG, Curtis JJ, Jones P, Whelchel JD, Diethelm AG. Mechanisms of post transplant hypertension. Am J Kidney Dis 1985; 5(4): A79–84.
26. Appel G. Lipid abnormalities in renal disease. Kidney Int 1991; 39(1): 169–83.
27. Kasiske BL, Tortorice KL, Heim-Dothoy KL et al. The adverse effect of cyclosporine on serum lipids in renal transplant recipients. Am J Kidney Dis 1991; 17(6): 700–7.
28. Wing AJ, Broyer M, Brunner EP et al. Combined report of regular dialysis and transplantation in Europe 1984. Proc Eur Dial Transplant Assoc 1985; 21: 2–65.
29. Johnson RWG, Wise MH, Bakran A et al. A four year prospective study of cyclosporine in cadaver renal transplantation. Transplant Proc 1985; 17: 1197–8.
30. Hardie IR for the Australian Collaborative Trials Committee. Optimal combination of immunosuppressive agents for renal transplantation: first report of a multicenter, randomized trial comparing cyclosporine and prednisolone with cyclosporine and azathioprine and with triple therapy in cadaver renal

transplantation. Transplant Proc 1993; 25: 583–4.

31. Jones RM, Murie JA, Allen RD et al. Triple therapy in cadaver renal transplantation. Br J Surg 1988; 75(1): 4–8.

32. Bassadonna GP, Matas AJ, Gillingham KJ et al. Relationship between early vs. late acute rejection and onset of chronic rejection in kidney transplantation. Transplant Proc 1993; 25: 910–11.

33. Almond PS, Matas A, Gillingham K et al. Risk factors for chronic rejection in renal allograft recipients. Transplantation 1993; 55: 742–7.

34. van Hoof for the European multi-centre trial comparing Tacrolimus and Cyclosporin in the prevention of renal allograft rejection. Abstract presented at XVI Congress of the International Society of Organ Transplantation 1996.

35. Pichlmayer R for the European mycophenolate mofetil Co-operative Study Group. Placebo-controlled study of mycophenolate mofetil combined with cyclosporine and corticosteroids for prevention of acute rejection. Lancet 1995; 345: 1321–5.

36. New W, Solomon M, Dingwall R, McHale J. A question of give and take. London: Kings Fund Institute, 1994, p. 16.

37. Terasaki PI, Cecka JM, Gjertson DW, Takenoto S. High survival rates of kidney transplants from spousal and living unrelated donors. N Engl J Med 1995; 333: 333–6.

38. Bia MJ, Ramos EL, Danovitch GM et al. Evaluation of living renal donors. Transplantation 1995; 60: 322–7.

# 7 Liver transplantation

*John A. C. Buckels*

**Introduction**  The last 15 years have seen dramatic changes in the practice of liver transplantation. In 1980 in Europe, fewer than 30 liver grafts were performed compared with over 3000 in 1995. During this period liver transplantation has evolved from a rare undertaking performed in terminally ill patients as a last-ditch emergency, with not surprisingly poor results, to a semi-elective operation with current predictable success rates of around 90% in non-fulminant cases.

**Indications**  Initially liver transplantation was reserved for patients with end-stage chronic liver disease or unresectable primary liver malignancy. In recent years there has been a considerable broadening of the accepted indications to include fulminant hepatic failure as well as patients with non-cirrhotic liver-based inborn errors of metabolism. Improving results have led to a semi-elective approach with not only quantity of life but also quality of life a major concern. Thus patients who may not be in immediate danger of death but have poor quality of life due to severe lassitude or pruritis, might now be considered candidates.

Broadly, the current indications can be classified into four groups: chronic liver failure, acute liver failure, primary hepatic malignancy not treatable by conventional surgical resection techniques and inborn errors of metabolism due to a liver-based enzyme defect but without parenchymal liver disease (Table 7.1).

### Chronic liver failure

This is the most common indication for liver replacement. Chronic liver failure can be caused by a wide variety of diseases including auto-immune, viral, congenital and alcohol induced.

Primary biliary cirrhosis (PBC), an autoimmune disease mainly affecting middle-aged and elderly women of Northern European descent, is the commonest indication for liver transplantation in the UK. Despite numerous clinical trials, no medical therapy was available until recently when ursodeoxycholic acid was shown to have benefit.[1] Though this study demonstrated an improvement in cholestasis, as yet there is no definite evidence that the need for transplantation will be prevented or

**Table 7.1** *Commoner indications for liver transplantation*

| | |
|---|---|
| **Chronic liver failure** | Primary biliary cirrhosis |
| | Primary sclerosing cholangitis |
| | Autoimmune chronic active hepatitis |
| | Alcoholic cirrhosis |
| | Cryptogenic cirrhosis |
| | HBV or HCV cirrhosis |
| | Biliary atresia |
| | $\alpha_1$-antitrypsin deficiency |
| | Budd–Chiari syndrome |
| **Acute liver failure** | Viral hepatitis (non-A non B, HBV, HAV) |
| | Drugs, e.g. paracetamol, antituberculosis therapy, halothane |
| | Toxins and solvents |
| **Primary hepatic malignancy** | Unresectable HCC in non-cirrhotic liver |
| | Smaller HCC in cirrhotic liver |
| **Inborn errors of metabolism** | Crigler–Najjar type 1 |
| | Proprionic acidaemia |
| | Primary oxalosis |
| | Urea cycle defects |

even deferred. Several studies on survival in PBC have led to the development of a prognostic index which is helpful in planning the timing of liver replacement.[2]

Primary sclerosing cholangitis (PSC) is a condition associated in most patients with inflammatory bowel disease. Progression of PSC is less predictable than PBC though a prognostic index has also been developed which may help timing of transplantation. Up to 30% of PSC patients will ultimately develop cholangiocarcinoma which is usually incurable at diagnosis. Thus earlier referral and consideration for grafting would seem appropriate for these patients.

Chronic active hepatitis (CAH) is less common than the above but should be mentioned as immunosuppressive therapy will often delay progression of the disease. Caution must be exercised as excess immunosuppression prior to transplantation may increase morbidity and mortality so that judging the optimal time for grafting can tax the skills of even the most experienced hepatologists.

An increasing number of viruses are known to cause chronic liver disease. The hepatitis B virus (HBV) is a major world health problem with an estimated 300 million carriers. In Western Europe and North America the carrier rate is low (0.5%) and is mainly confined to high risk groups including intravenous drug users, homosexuals and immigrants from high prevalence areas. Nevertheless HBV is a significant problem because of the risks of early recurrence after grafting. Patients who are HBV-DNA positive at time of grafting develop rapid recurrence with early death and the results of current trials of antiviral therapy using agents such as lamivudine prior to transplantation are awaited. Hepatitis

C virus (HCV) is the commonest post-transfusion hepatitis and most patients gained the disease due to transfusion (especially haemophiliacs), or from intravenous drug abuse. The development of cirrhosis is slow and insidious but with a significant risk of subsequent hepatocellular carcinoma development. Recurrence of HCV after transplantation is common but not usually problematic in the early years.

Alcoholic liver disease (ALD) is the commonest cause of cirrhosis in many parts of the western world though early on few were accepted for transplantation. Many transplant physicians were initially reluctant to consider liver grafts in patients with ALD because of risks of recurrent drinking and public attitudes. With time it has been shown that, in the alcoholic who can prove abstinence prior to grafting, the results are equivalent to other indications and that recidivism is uncommon. As a result there has been increasing pressure to accept reformed drinkers and an increasing proportion of such individuals are now being grafted.

### Childhood chronic liver disease

The commonest cause of chronic liver failure in children is biliary atresia. This causes rapid development of cirrhosis and death within the first two years of life. If diagnosed early (within 8 weeks) and treated surgically with a portoenterostomy (Kasai operation), the progression of liver disease is delayed and a proportion will survive long term. However, many are not referred in time and others still develop end-stage liver disease and die within the first few years of life if not transplanted. In addition to the signs of chronic liver disease in adults, failure to thrive is common and should be considered an indication for grafting.

### Acute fulminant liver failure

Acute fulminant hepatic failure (AFHF) is defined as the development of hepatic encephalopathy within eight weeks of onset of symptoms in a patient without previous liver disease.[3] A slower form, subacute or late onset hepatic failure, has also been recognised with encephalopathy developing between eight weeks and six months of onset of symptoms. The commonest causes of AFHF in the UK include drugs and toxins (e.g. paracetamol overdose, antituberculous drugs, halothane and solvents), viral hepatitis (hepatitis A, B, and non-A and non-B) and miscellaneous causes including Wilson's disease, fatty liver of pregnancy and Budd–Chiari syndrome. The progression of AFHF leads to cerebral oedema with risks of coning as well as hepatorenal failure. With intensive treatment in specialised centres some patients may recover but it is important to recognise those who will not. Patients with viral hepatitis (usually hepatitis B and non-A non-B) who develop increasing encephalopathy plus worsening coagulation, require consideration of grafting. Specific prognostic factors for spontaneous recovery have been published and these are helpful in decision-making about transplantation.[4]

Patients who present with acidosis after paracetamol poisoning are also at high risk and, providing there is no long-term psychiatric problem, should also be listed for emergency transplantation.

### Inborn errors of metabolism

There are an increasing number of inborn errors of metabolism with a deficiency of a single hepatic enzyme which are being treated by liver transplantation, even though the liver is otherwise structurally and functionally normal (Table 7.1). It is important to balance the risks of the underlying abnormality against the risks of the operation and subsequent lifelong immunosuppression. Timing is important in that transplantation should be performed before irretrievable damage is done to other organs such as renal impairment in primary oxalosis or cerebral damage in Crigler–Najjar syndrome.

### Primary hepatic malignancy

Hepatocellular carcinoma (HCC) is the commonest primary liver malignancy. This is rare in the UK but is one of the commonest cancers worldwide. Most cases occur in a cirrhotic liver which is one risk factor for the development of HCC, as are the presence of HCV or HBV. Patients with large symptomatic HCC in cirrhotic livers do badly with high rates of recurrence after transplantation though patients with small incidental lesions fare as well as patients grafted for benign conditions. It has been recommended that transplantation be restricted to patients with HCC who have lesions up to 3 cm and up to three in number.[5] HCC occurring in a non-cirrhotic liver are rare and tend to present with advanced disease. Conventional resection is the treatment of choice, though if this is not possible, transplantation can be considered. Recurrence occurs in the majority and given the shortage of donor livers, transplantation should perhaps only be considered for younger patients. Other rarer primary hepatic tumours that are unresectable but might be considered for transplantation include epithelioid haemangioendothelioma, sarcomata and cholangiocellular carcinoma. Hilar cholangiocarcinomas almost invariably recur early after grafting and are no longer considered appropriate candidates.

Liver transplantation for metastatic disease has been performed with very poor results except in rare cases of metastatic neuroendocrine tumours which are slow growing and in which pharmacological control of hormonal syndromes was not possible, or in patients with painful bulky disease. In such cases eventual recurrence does supervene but often many years later with a reasonable quality of life in the intervening period.

## Timing of referral

For both chronic and acute liver failure, timely referral is necessary if a successful outcome is to be achieved. Many patients with chronic liver disease can remain stable for long periods then suddenly decompensate. This is often due to a complication such as variceal bleeding, portal vein thrombosis, development of hepatic malignancy or spontaneous bacterial peritonitis. The ability to intervene before any major deterioration is dependent on the recognition of early indicators of disease progression. For cholestatic conditions such as PBC and PSC the level of bilirubin is an obvious indicator of the underlying disease and is likely to lead to an early referral for specialist opinion. For many liver conditions the appearance of jaundice is a very late feature and other clues to liver deterioration such as failing synthetic function as shown by a falling albumin or rising prothrombin time, can be found.

Variceal haemorrhage is perhaps one of the most dangerous and frightening complications of cirrhosis. Repeated sclerotherapy has often been effective in controlling acute bleeding episodes but is not without risks. Oesophageal perforation, ulcers and strictures have all been recorded and may delay or even prevent subsequent liver replacement. Recently transjugular intrahepatic portosystemic shunts (TIPSS) placed by the radiologist have proved very useful in controlled acute variceal bleeds and enable the patient to be prepared for subsequent grafting in an optimal state.

For children, the presence of serious liver disease can lead to failure to thrive which if resistant to nutritional correction is itself a good indication for liver replacement. Inborn errors of metabolism are more likely to present in childhood. Conditions which produce an unacceptable quality of life rather than an imminent risk to life, such as Crigler–Najjar syndrome, should also be considered for liver replacement.

## Patient assessment

Patients are best assessed by a joint team of hepatologists and transplant surgeons. Initial attention is to the diagnosis of the primary liver disease. This will require a careful review of the medical and surgical history of the patient together with an evaluation of antibody results and viral hepatitis markers. Liver biopsy has often been performed at an earlier stage and this will normally be reviewed by a specialist pathologist at the transplant centre. In some patients the underlying diagnosis may be occult and in such patients the cirrhosis is termed cryptogenic, though the incidence has fallen with the identification of the marker for hepatitis C. Often patients who drink moderate amounts of alcohol are labelled as having alcoholic liver disease. This may be incorrect and an open mind approach for these cases should be encouraged, remembering that modest alcohol intake may uncover other liver conditions such as $\alpha_1$-antitrypsin deficiency or haemochromatosis. Any possible medical therapy such as immunosuppression of autoimmune liver disease or penicillamine therapy in Wilson's disease should be considered if transplantation might be deferred. In the majority of cases, however, referral is late and patients may need to be placed on the transplant waiting list shortly after initial evaluation.

Assessment for transplantation includes both physical fitness for major surgery as well as psychological evaluation and counselling. Involvement of the transplant anaesthetist at this stage is mandatory and detailed evaluation of the cardiorespiratory system may be required in some patients. This may require anything from simple exercise ECG tests in patients with possible ischaemic heart disease to Swan–Ganz catheterisation for those with evidence of raised right-sided cardiac pressures or suspected major pulmonary shunts as seen in the hepato-pulmonary syndrome.[6]

Specific requirements for the surgeon are patency of the portal vein and, if this is not detected on Doppler ultrasound, then further imaging such as angiography, spiral computed tomography (CT) or magnetic resonance imaging (MRI) scans should be performed to establish the venous anatomy. An absent portal vein is not a contraindication if a patent superior mesenteric vein or large coronary vein can be identified which would be suitable for anastomosis to the donor portal vein, with or without a length of interposition graft.[7]

Patients with primary hepatocellular carcinoma require detailed investigation for evidence of disease outside the liver which would be an absolute contraindication to liver grafting. This would include laparoscopy to detect peritoneal disease or transcapsular spread, isotope bone scanning and computed tomographic studies of the abdomen and chest. As stated earlier, hilar cholangiocarcinomas are not considered suitable for transplantation but in patients with PSC it may be difficult to differentiate between malignant and benign hilar strictures. We have found that malignancy was present in one-quarter of patients with significant biliary dilatation but that pretransplant diagnosis was difficult and may rely on operative biopsy and frozen section in cases of doubt.

Cirrhosis associated with significant respiratory problems can pose major problems. Patients with $\alpha_1$-antitrypsin deficiency tend to have either predominantly liver or pulmonary involvement. Some patients with advancing liver disease do have respiratory problems but there is evidence that timely liver replacement may halt the progression of the lung disease. Cystic fibrosis can cause end-stage liver disease before pulmonary failure and transplantation can be successful. However, cases with advanced lung disease might require combined pulmonary-liver replacement. The hepatopulmonary syndrome requires careful assessment with the help of the respiratory physician and anaesthetist and should be suspected in patients with breathlessness, clubbing or cyanosis. Cardiac catheterisation studies and measurements of intrapulmonary shunting may be needed to establish the patient's fitness to withstand liver replacement together with the identification of potentially reversible changes.[6]

Patients with advanced muscle wasting pose major problems for recovery after liver replacement. This occurs in both children and adults and might be helped by enteral feeding in the pretransplant phase. Weaning from the ventilator after surgery is likely to be difficult in severe cases but full recovery is possible and muscle wasting alone should not be considered an absolute contraindication to liver replacement.

Late presentation of end-stage liver disease is often accompanied by renal impairment due to hepatorenal failure. This syndrome is characterised by rising serum creatinine and a low urinary sodium. Liver transplantation will usually reverse the renal failure though dialysis is often needed for one to two weeks postgrafting and inevitably the mortality in this group is higher.

In many cases a number of the above risk factors coexist and the decision to proceed with liver transplantation requires careful evaluation. With the increasing demand for liver replacement, it is likely that patients with predictably poorer outcomes will be excluded from transplantation in the not too distant future, given the limited donor pool. In such difficult circumstances, it is important that transplant doctors are responsible for the allocation of livers. Decisions should not be left to well-meaning committees who do not have full insight into the clinical problems.

**Liver donors**
The topics of organ donation and retrieval are covered in a separate chapter but a few points particular to the liver are worth emphasising. First, successful outcome is possible even in haemodynamically unstable donors and in those with abnormal liver function tests.[8] Assessment of the liver by an experienced transplant surgeon at time of retrieval is a useful guide to subsequent function. In cases of doubt, particularly if there is evidence of fatty change, a frozen section histological assessment prior to implantation can be helpful. When considering a marginal donor liver it is worth emphasising that a relatively fit recipient can often cope with a less than perfect graft. Conversely a poor risk recipient will need a graft which immediately functions well for the best chance of survival.

Size matching of donor and recipient is attempted when selecting a patient for a particular liver. Attempting to place a large graft in a small recipient can cause major technical problems. Patients with cholestatic disease such as PSC and particularly PBC often have large livers and will accept grafts from significantly larger donors as can patients with marked ascites.

**Basic operation**
The surgical details of liver transplantation have been well described and will not be repeated, though a diagram of the anastomoses used is given in Fig. 7.1. This text will focus on important recent developments and improvements in our understanding of the pathophysiological changes during surgery. Undoubtedly many factors can be identified which have contributed to the improved early outcome after liver replacement, not least of which is elective day-time operating. An awake and alert surgical/anaesthetic team is much more likely to produce the best technical results, a lesson learnt long ago in the airline industry. The

**Figure 7.1** *Whole liver graft depicting standard anastomoses.*

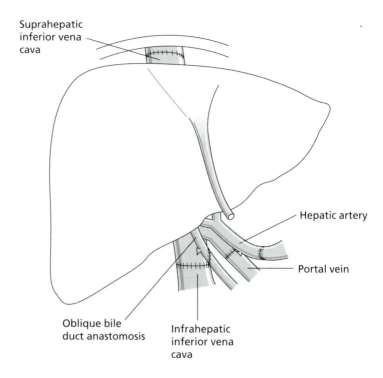

Suprahepatic inferior vena cava

Hepatic artery

Portal vein

Oblique bile duct anastomosis

Infrahepatic inferior vena cava

ability to store livers long enough to allow daylight operating came from the development of University of Wisconsin preservation fluid which allows satisfactory immediate graft function for storage periods of 18 h or more.

Meticulous attention to haemostasis is needed and conventional means of haemostasis are aided by recent developments in diathermy such as the argon beam coagulator and the use of fibrin glue. The monitoring of coagulation parameters, usually by the anaesthetists in the operating room with the help of the thromboelectrogram (TEG), essentially means that blood coagulation is optimised and that predictable deteriorations in clotting which often occur on reperfusion can be anticipated and minimised. The TEG measures the quality of blood clot allowing a dynamic evaluation of the coagulation status of the patient in the operating room and the selection of the most appropriate clotting factors, whether fresh frozen plasma, platelets or cryoprecipitate. The role of antifibrinolytic agents such as Aprotinin (Trasyslol) is uncertain from clinical studies.

Patients with end-stage liver disease often exhibit significant haemodynamic instability, even in the absence of excess operative blood loss. We have recognised a frequent syndrome of high cardiac output with low systemic vascular resistance (SVR) that in many ways resembles sepsis or septic shock. Often the SVR will progressively fall during surgery, particularly after reperfusion. This can usually be reversed with an infusion of adrenaline or noradrenaline, though continuous monitoring of the haemodynamic parameters with a Swan–Ganz cathether by the anaesthetists is necessary for accurate control.

## Advances in operative technique

The introduction of venovenous bypass for the anhepatic phase was a significant milestone in the evolution of liver transplantation. This produced a significant stabilisation of haemodynamic parameters during portal vein and caval clamping with a clear reduction in transfusion requirements. A more recently proposed alternative to bypass is to preserve the vena cava at the time of hepatectomy and anastomose the back of the donor vena cava to the front of the recipient cava (piggy-back technique).[9] Both preservation of caval flow during the anhepatic phase by partial clamping and access to the anastomosis, if the donor liver is large, can be difficult. Thus many units currently utilise bypass in preference to the piggy-back technique. Not all patients require bypass and a minority of units still perform liver replacement without either technique.

One of the most significant developments in surgical technique, particularly for paediatric recipients has been the use of anatomically reduced grafts (Fig. 7.2). The shortfall in size-matched grafts for small children led to the development of reduced grafts in the mid 1980s and such grafts now account for the majority of transplants in children under three years of age. The most commonly used technique is to transplant the left lateral lobe (segments II and III) with venous outflow based on

**Figure 7.2**

*Anatomically reduced graft employing segments II and III. Venous drainage via left hepatic vein anastomosed to retained recipient vena cava. When part of split-liver technique, venous graft may be anastomosed to left portal vein branch to provide adequate length.*

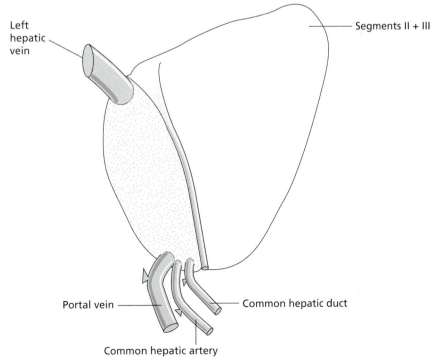

Left hepatic vein

Segments II + III

Portal vein

Common hepatic duct

Common hepatic artery

the left hepatic vein which is anastomosed to the retained recipient vena cava.[10] In this way grafts from adult donors can be used for children. Though weight ratios as high as ten-to-one between donor and recipient have been recorded, in most units weight ratios of four to six are sought. Transplants for very small children will therefore need livers cut down from larger child donors. One aspect of the reduced graft approach for small children is the low incidence of hepatic artery thrombosis compared with whole grafts from small donors. In the last five years the reduced graft technique has been taken further, in that instead of discarding the rest of the liver, the right lobe is grafted, usually into an adult recipient (split-liver). Because of the need to provide vascular inflow to both lobes, some form of vascular graft is needed to allow satisfactory anastomoses in the recipient. The details vary between units but the author's preference is to keep the main hepatic artery with the left lateral segment but the main portal vein with the right lobe. Usually it is necessary to utilise a donor iliac artery graft to extend the right hepatic artery for the right lobe and a donor iliac vein graft segment to lengthen the left portal vein for the left lateral graft. The liver is divided in the line of the falciform ligament and the vena cava retained with the right lobe (Fig. 7.3). In practice, segments I and IV are removed and discarded. Vessels at the cut surface are carefully ligated and the raw area sprayed with fibrin glue (Tiseel, Immuno, Vienna).

The risk of death on the waiting list has led some units to undertake living related liver transplantation. This is clearly technically more demanding and potentially more dangerous than living related renal donation. Nevertheless, excellent early results are being obtained by

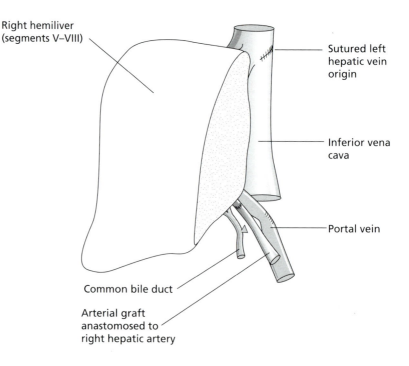

**Figure 7.3** *Right lobe derived from split-liver technique. Segments II/III taken as separate graft, segments I and IV discarded to retain segments V–VIII. Vena cava, main portal vein and common bile duct retained with hemiliver, arterial graft anastomosed to right hepatic artery branch.*

Right hemiliver (segments V–VIII)

Sutured left hepatic vein origin

Inferior vena cava

Portal vein

Common bile duct

Arterial graft anastomosed to right hepatic artery

several units and in the longer term, given the increasing demand for liver grafting, this is likely to become common and established practice. The usual situation is for donation of the left lateral lobe to a child from one of the parents. Careful preoperative evaluation is needed of both donor size and anatomy as well as psychological aspects. Hopes that the close compatibility between donor and recipient would reduce rejection and therefore risks of immunosuppression have not been realised.

The biliary anastomosis has often been described as the Achilles' heel of liver transplantation. Early techniques utilising the donor gall bladder as a conduit between the donor and recipient ducts have been abandoned because of the almost universal development of stones in the conduit which prove very difficult to remove by endoscopic approaches. The currently performed end-to-end duct anastomosis is followed by stricture formation in up to 10% of cases and techniques of anastomosing the ducts obliquely with the ends spatulated or by utilising a side-to-side anastomosis are gaining wider acceptance.[11] The use of a T-tube has been abandoned by most units and postoperative investigation of the biliary tract is discussed later in the complications section. Patients with absent (biliary atresia) or diseased (PSC) bile ducts have a biliary–enteric anastomosis performed onto a Roux-en-Y jejunal loop. Clinical experience suggests that patients undergoing regrafting should perhaps also have a duct to jejunal anastomosis due to the high incidence of stricture formation if the duct-to-duct anastomosis is repeated.

**Immuno-suppression**

The drugs used in immunosuppression are the subject of Chapter 5. However, as recognised from early animal liver transplant experience, the liver appears to behave differently from other organs in that late rejection is uncommon. Moreover, the expected life-span of a liver graft is likely to be considerably longer than the mean of 10 years seen with renal and cardiac transplants. As a result most patients can be maintained long term on relatively low doses of immunosuppressive drugs and, unique to liver patients, a significant number of patients have stopped their immunosuppressive drugs without necessarily incurring graft loss. The observation that the Kupffer cells in the grafted liver change from donor to recipient within a few months suggests that the graft is in effect a chimera and may explain the differences in rejection when compared with other organs. This subject is currently being studied intensively in an attempt to understand how graft tolerance might be achieved as well as the identification of which patients will manage without immunosuppression.

Most liver transplant centres use triple therapy as baseline immunosuppression, based on cyclosporin or tacrolimus. Cyclosporin is now available as the microemulsion form Neoral, which has more predictable, bile-independent absorption from the gastrointestinal tract. Such properties are also seen with tacrolimus with the result that both these drugs may be administered via nasogastric tube and rarely require parenteral dosage. Azathioprine is given at a level around $2\,\mathrm{mg\,kg^{-1}}$, at first by the intravenous route, changing to conventional treatment when the recipient can tolerate oral fluids. Steroid therapy begins at the parenteral equivalent of 20 mg oral prednisolone and is kept at this level in the immediate postoperative period, unless acute rejection supervenes (see below). The author practises rapid reduction of oral steroid as there are significant, well-documented disadvantages of long-term steroids and this course of management has no deleterious effect on graft survival.

## Complications

These can be classified as immediate (intensive care phase), early (during first three months) or late (Table 7.2).

**Table 7.2**   *Complications after liver transplantation*

| | |
|---|---|
| **Immediate** | Primary non-function |
| | Haemorrhage |
| | Acute renal failure |
| **Early** | Primary poor function |
| | Acute renal failure |
| | Acute rejection |
| | Hepatic artery thrombosis |
| | Biliary leakage/obstruction |
| | Cholangitis |
| | Chronic rejection |
| | Bacterial and opportunistic infection (fungal and viral) |
| **Late** | Biliary |
| | Chronic rejection |
| | Post-transplant hepatitis |
| | Malignancy |

### Immediate complications after surgery

The immediate complications following liver transplantation include primary non-function, haemorrhage and acute renal failure. The incidence of these are significantly influenced by the quality of the donor liver and the conduct of the transplant operation itself.

#### Primary non-function

This is a syndrome where the newly implanted liver fails to work. This may be due to pre-existing but occult problems in the donor, poor retrieval or preservation, or injury caused by reperfusion (post-reperfusion syndrome). After reperfusion of the liver with blood the clinical picture is a patient who develops a progressive acidosis, coagulopathy, renal failure and all the features of acute fulminant hepatic failure. Haemodynamic instability and death rapidly follow unless urgent regrafting can be undertaken. Fortunately primary non-function is rare, though primary poor function occurs in 5–10% of cases. In such cases some features of acute liver failure such as reduced clotting and high transaminases are seen but supportive treatment is usually successful while the liver recovers, improvement often being seen within two weeks. Graft biopsy in these cases often reveals microvesicular or even macrovesicular fat or perivenular necrosis (so-called preservation injury). These patients often remain cholestatic for many weeks and other causes of this need to be excluded by ultrasound and graft biopsy.

### Haemorrhage

Routine cases without previous surgery may require minimal or no transfused blood. However, patients with severe portal hypertension and previous major upper abdominal operations can pose a major surgical challenge and extensive bleeding can occur. Meticulous haemostasis, venovenous bypass for decompression during the anhepatic phase, warming of blood and blood products and strict control of coagulation parameters (see Basic operation section earlier) will usually be effective. The reperfusion stage is often associated with a worsening of coagulation which can be anticipated and hopefully prevented. Patients with ongoing bleeding have a very high mortality but occasionally the use of packs or abdominal binders can salvage a seemingly hopeless situation, if the new liver functions and produces clotting factors. Usually, such patients will need to return to the operating theatre for lavage some 48–72 h after grafting to remove stale blood and clots, when unexpectedly few will have signs of ongoing bleeding.

### Renal failure

Many patients undergoing liver replacement already have impaired renal function due to the hepatorenal syndrome (see Patient assessment). A combination of factors including preoperative hypotension and haemorrhage, vena caval clamping and postoperative nephrotoxic drugs produce renal dysfunction in a significant number of patients. This problem will respond to optimal hydration and an infusion of dopamine in most patients. However, some will develop anuria and require renal replacement therapy, particularly if initial graft function is poor as characterised by high serum transaminases in the immediate postoperative period. This is best performed as continuous venovenous filtration or haemodialysis and most patients will produce a diuresis within 2 to 3 weeks. Acute renal failure is more common in patients with acute fulminant hepatic failure, many of whom will be dialysis dependent prior to grafting. Again the prognosis is good with return of renal function within 2 to 3 weeks.

## Early complications after surgery

The number of potential complications is large and varied leading to a long learning curve for the liver transplant team. With experience, many problems can be pre-empted by the early recognition of clinical patterns and potential disasters avoided. Those most commonly encountered are rejection, infection, biliary complications and graft ischaemia and these will be dealt with in turn.

### Rejection

Acute rejection will be found in around 80% of cases biopsied at the end of the first week. There is increasing acceptance that these changes do not require additional immunosuppression if other parameters of graft function, particularly the liver function tests and prothrombin time are improving. Biopsies showing features of severe cellular rejection are usually treated in the same way as less severe forms associated with significant biochemical abnormalities. Most units use intravenous high-dose steroid though the oral route is probably as effective and most patients respond to either regimen. The fact that units using higher overall doses of baseline immunosuppression encounter as many problems with rejection as units using much lower regimens suggest that it is the change in dosage to achieve resolution which is the critical factor. Steroid-resistant rejection will sometimes respond to other agents including monoclonal (OKT3) or polyclonal antibodies (ATG) or switching to tacrolimus. Patients with ongoing rejection despite these therapeutic changes can often be salvaged by retransplantation, though severe recurrent rejection in the new graft can be a problem.

Chronic or irreversible rejection in the liver is chiefly an epithelial rather than a vascular phenomenon in contrast to other organ transplants. The small bile radicals are destroyed (vanishing bile duct syndrome, VBDS) and this process is usually irreversible.[12] This can occur very early on after grafting and if progressive leads to loss of the liver transplant. In this situation, urgent regrafting is the only option though recurrent VBDS does occur in some cases. There is some evidence that lower chronic rejection rates are seen with immunosuppressive regimes based on tacrolimus rather than cyclosporin, and that patients with early chronic rejection on cyclosporin who are switched to tacrolimus may have graft function salvaged. The overall chronic rejection rates are between 5 and 10%. It is unique to the liver that chronic rejection is so infrequent compared to the almost inevitable long-term changes which occur in other solid organ grafts.

One final immunological complication seen after liver grafting is graft-versus-host disease when livers from ABO blood group-compatible but non-identical donors are used. Thus if a blood group 'O' donor liver is grafted into any other blood group or an 'A' or 'B' donor grafted into an 'AB' recipient, anti-A or anti-B antibodies are produced by the liver causing an acute haemolytic anaemia accompanied by a significant rise in the bilirubin. This is usually a mild and self-limiting process occurring between one and two weeks postoperatively. It is important to recognise this and correct any anaemia with donor-specific group blood. Further transfusion with recipient group blood is likely to worsen the haemolysis with risks of coagulopathy and even renal impairment. Cases with a rapid rise in bilirubin should always be investigated for possible haemolysis and a direct Coomb's test will usually be positive.

### Infection

The topic of infection is covered in Chapter 12 but infectious problems specifically related to liver transplantation are discussed here. The main potential septic problems relate to the lungs and biliary tract. The combination of a large painful upper abdominal wound, postoperative ventilation and the high incidence of pleural effusions lead to a significant risk for postoperative chest infections. Adequate pain control, good physiotherapy and early extubation should prevent under ventilation and the risk of secondary pulmonary infection. Pleural effusions if restricting ventilation should be tapped promptly.

Biliary infections are probably less common since the omission of T-tubes and the diagnosis of cholangitis is often presumptive and made after other causes of infection are excluded, particularly if there is a change in the liver function tests. Bile leaks or obstruction need to be excluded by ultrasonography or endoscopic retrograde cholangiography (ERCP) (see Biliary complications).

Serious cytomegalovirus (CMV) infections tend to be primary (transmitted by the donor liver) rather than reactivation infections and should be avoidable if CMV-matched donors are used. Clinical infection usually presents at 4–8 weeks with fever and leucopenia. This will respond well to a combination of reduction in baseline immunosuppression and gancyclovir therapy. Serological tests vary between centres and often take time. Recently developed PCR tests provide rapid results, as does tissue biopsy (liver biopsy or rectal or gastric biopsy in patients with gastrointestinal symptoms). Asymptomatic seroconversion does not require treatment. Some units routinely use prophylaxis with gancyclovir though a high index of suspicion with surveillance enable prompt treatment with negligible mortality.

Fungal colonisation is common in patients with chronic liver failure and prophylaxis with oral agents will reduce oral and oesophageal infection. Diagnosis of invasive fungal infection is often made late and patients should be treated on suspicion with full antifungal therapy. Patients with AFHF who often have a prolonged time in intensive care have a higher incidence of fungal infections and should be given systemic antifungals prophylactically.

### Biliary complications

Biliary complications continue to be a significant problem in most units undertaking liver replacement. These include bile leaks, anastomotic strictures, non-anastomotic strictures of the donor bile duct and sludge formation. The overall incidence in adults is around 10% but it is higher in children. The use of T-tubes to splint the biliary anastomosis, popular for many years, is falling out of favour. Though there is no published difference in the incidence of strictures between cases with or without a T-tube, there is a small but significant morbidity from bile leaks after T-tube removal. The theoretical advantage of being able to check on the biliary anatomy as part of the postoperative investigation of liver dysfunction seems less necessary with the ability to image the biliary tree effectively using ultrasound, MRI cholangiography, endoscopic retrograde cholangiography (ERCP) or percutaneous transhepatic cholangiography (PTC) even in the absence of dilated ducts.

With all suspected biliary complications, patency of the hepatic artery should be checked with Doppler ultrasound as hepatic artery thrombosis will cause ischaemia and necrosis of the biliary tree. Simple bile leaks are usually diagnosed early postoperatively either by the presence of bile in the drain fluid or in the percutaneous aspirate of fluid found on ultrasound. In all but the most minor cases, ERCP is recommended to identify the site of and amount of the leak and for the possible insertion of an internal stent which may allow healing. The presence of a major biliary disruption or an associated biliary obstruction is an indication for an urgent reconstruction using a Roux-en-Y jejunal loop. Biliary obstruction without leakage will usually be evident from simple ultrasound and can be confirmed by ERCP or PTC. Balloon dilatation may be possible though it is not recommended for early obstruction (within the first two or three weeks due to possibility of anastomotic disruption) and such cases should also undergo formal biliary reconstruction. Biliary strictures involving the confluence are a rare but serious complication that were once attributed to prolonged preservation times. Even quite complicated strictures can be resolved by a skilled radiologist using a PTC approach though a small number of cases might require regrafting if this fails.

### Graft ischaemia

Hepatic arterial thrombosis (HAT) can be a devasting complication after liver transplantation. This occurs most frequently in the first postoperative month leading to graft necrosis, intrahepatic abscess or biliary necrosis and bile leakage. The onset of HAT is often heralded by a massive rise in transaminases, particularly in the first few days after grafting. Later presentations may be less acute with evidence of Gram negative sepsis or bile leakage. In all suspected cases, patency of the artery should be checked with Doppler ultrasound and confirmed by angiography. Urgent thrombectomy has been successful in some cases though the majority of early cases will need regrafting. Late arterial thrombosis may be occult and if asymptomatic can probably be ignored. Rates of HAT in the early series approached 10% in adults and over 20% in children. Current rates in most units are significantly lower at approximately 5% in adults and 10% in children and this is probably a learning curve effect. Though technical problems account for most cases, overtransfusion at time of surgery to produce high haematocrit has been reported as a risk factor.[13]

## Late complications

### Biliary

The late biliary complications seen after transplantation are usually manifest as obstruction with possible secondary sepsis and cholangitis. Patients may be jaundiced with intermittent fevers though a number are anicteric but have abnormal liver function tests, particularly a raised alkaline phosphatase. All suspected cases should undergo ultrasound examination which will detect duct dilatation. The commonest cause is an anastomotic stricture, with or without stone or sludge formation in the proximal dilated biliary tree. Late non-anastomotic strictures are rare as is duct dilatation due to sphincter of Oddi dysfunction. In all suspected cases with a duct-to-duct anastomosis, ERCP should be performed. This will provide a precise road map of the biliary tree and may allow duct clearance and even dilatation of any stricture. Unfortunately most strictures will recur and therefore, unless the patient is unfit, a formal biliary reconstruction using a Roux-en-Y jejunal loop is recommended. If the patient had a duct-to-jejunal anastomosis or if an ERCP was not possible then a PTC should be performed. Again dilatation of any stricture is possible but recurrence is common and surgical correction may be required.

### Chronic rejection

Chronic rejection (introduced under early complications) can occur at any stage but, despite its name, is usually seen within the first 12 months after grafting. The two main diagnostic histological features are the vanishing bile duct syndrome and an obliterative vasculopathy affecting large and medium-sized arteries. In the Birmingham series, _de novo_ features of chronic rejection have rarely been seen after the first 12 months post-transplant[14] though many other series do report late chronic rejection. One major difficulty is the differentiation from other late patterns of graft damage, particularly chronic hepatitis which is discussed in the following section. It should be stressed again that chronic rejection, which seems inevitable with other solid organ transplants affects the liver in only a minority of patients.

### Chronic post-transplant hepatitis

It is now recognised that histological examination of the transplanted liver in stable long-term patients shows frequent abnormalities.[15] A detailed pathological account is not possible in this review but the main findings will be briefly discussed. The commonest histological abnormalities are non-specific inflammation and chronic hepatitis, and differentiation between these and both chronic rejection and recurrent disease in the grafted liver (i.e. PBC or PSC) can be difficult. The causes of the histological changes are unknown though unrecognised viral infections may be responsible for some cases. The importance of documenting such changes is that any histological abnormality must be interpreted in conjunction with both the clinical state of the patient as well as the liver function tests. Thus mild abnormalities found on a biopsy in a symptomatic patient must be compared with those seen in asymptomatic patients with normal liver biochemistry and do not automatically constitute an indication for change in therapy.

### Malignancy

Malignancy is well recognised as a potential complication of long-term immunosuppression and this is dealt with in Chapter 12. Two brief points specifically relating to the liver should be stressed. First, longer survival is seen with the liver compared with other solid organs and therefore the time exposed to the risk of malignancy is greater. Given that a significant proportion (20–25%) of liver recipients are paediatric, it is important to share this risk with the parents so they have reasonable knowledge of late potential problems, particularly as the risks of the most common malignancy seen, namely skin cancer including melanoma, can be avoided by a strict policy of avoiding excessive sun exposure.

A second aspect of liver grafting is the tendency for patients grafted for primary liver malignancy to develop recurrence within the grafted liver. This might seem a paradox as the only part of the body definitely free from cancer at the time of surgery is the new liver graft. The predilection for circulating malignant cells to return and then grow in the liver is now well recognised and emphasises the need to identify some therapy which would destroy such cells around the time of the transplant operation.

**Retrans-plantation**  Some 10–15% of patients will suffer graft failure and need transplanta-tion, the incidence being higher in children than adults. Broad indica-tions for regrafting are given in Table 7.3. With hepatic artery thrombosis and primary non-function rates falling, chronic rejection is the most common cause. Early retransplantation is technically straightforward though if the graft has failed acutely the patient may be less well than at the time of the initial transplant. With the shortage of donor organs, every regraft is potentially another patient dying without a chance of a transplant and thus every attempt must be made to avoid graft loss. Patients who repeatedly reject (so called 'liver eaters') probably should

**Table 7.3**  *Indications for retransplantation*

Primary non-function
Early hepatic arterial thrombosis
Drug-resistant severe acute rejection
Established chronic rejection

not be offered repeated transplants. Late regrafting, usually for chronic rejection, can be difficult and dangerous due to dense adhesions around the liver.

**Survival and quality of life**

One-year survival rates for elective transplant in patients with benign disease now exceed 90% in many centres, with predicted 10-year survivals rates around 70%. Patients grafted for acute fulminant hepatic failure fare less well with higher early death rates usually related to cerebral complications due to raised intracranial pressure and multi-organ failure. Nevertheless one-year survival rates of 70–80% have been obtained by experienced centres and, like patients grafted for benign chronic liver disease, the survival curves are relatively flat. The outcome in children is equally good, even in high risk groups such as children aged under 1 year, in whom donor organ shortage might prevent grafting at the optimal time.[16]

Survival rates for patients grafted for primary liver cancer (HCC) are less good, particularly if the tumours are large. However, patients transplanted for asymptomatic lesions up to 3 cm in diameter occurring in a cirrhotic liver have survival rates close to those seen in patients grafted for benign disease.[5]

In the early days of liver replacement with most patients dying, it was the excellent quality of life in the survivors which was the inspiration for the pioneers to persist in their endeavours. This improvement in well-being is very obvious in patients grafted for chronic liver failure. Patients transplanted for AFHF usually cannot recall the later stages of their illness and life with a new liver and long-term medication will not be an improvement on their memories of their pretransplant stage. These patients require additional counselling and understanding in order to come to terms with such a major change in life style.

**The future**

The most serious issue currently facing liver transplant physicians is the major shortfall in donor organs needed to meet an ever-increasing demand. Though some of this deficit will be met by living related donation and organ splitting, this is only likely to have a significant impact for paediatric recipients. For adults needing liver replacement, allocation is likely to be on the basis of predicted long-term survival and thus patients with a poorer predicted outcome will be denied access to donor livers. Increasing the overall number of donors might have some impact though attempts have so far been largely unsuccessful (differing organ retrieval rates in different countries suggests potential for change). The use of genetically modified xenografts, a potential major breakthrough for heart recipients, is unlikely to benefit liver failure patients due to the diverse nature of enzyme and clotting systems between species. Thus liver xenografts are unlikely to be possible for the foreseeable future.

## References

1. Heathcote EJ, Cauchdudek K, Walker V *et al.* The Canadian multicenter double-blind randomised controlled trial of ursodeoxycholic acid in primary biliary cirrhosis. Hepatology 1994; 19: 1149–56.
2. Hughes MD, Rasthino C, Pocock S. Predictor for short term survivors with an application in PBC. Stat Med 1992; 11: 1731–45.
3. Trey C, Davison CS. The management of fulminant hepatic failure. In: Popper H, Schaffner F (eds) Progress in liver disease. New York: Grune & Stratton, 1970; pp. 282–98.
4. O'Grady J, Alexander GJM, Hayllar KM *et al.* Early indicators of prognosis in fulminant hepatic failure. Gastroenterology 1989; 97: 439–45.
5. Bismuth H, Chiche L, Adam R *et al.* Liver resection versus transplantation for hepatocellular carcinoma in cirrhotic patients. Ann Surg 1993; 218: 145–51.
6. Kuo PC. Pulmonary hypertension: considerations in the liver transplant candidate. Transpl Int 1996; 9: 141–50.
7. Kirsch JP, Howard TK, Klintman GB *et al.* Problematic vascular reconstruction in liver transplantation. Part II. Portovenous conduits. Surgery 1990; 107: 544–8.
8. Mirza D, Gunson BK, Da Silva RF *et al.* Policies in Europe on 'marginal quality' donor liver. Lancet 1994; 344: 1480–3.
9. Belghiti J, Panis Y, Sauvanet A *et al.* A new technique of side to side caval anastomosis during orthotopic liver transplantation without inferior caval occlusion. Surg Gynecol Obstet 1992; 175: 271–2.
10. Strong R, Ong TH, Pettay P *et al.* A new method of segmental orthotopic liver transplantation in children. Surgery 1988; 104: 104–7.
11. Keck H, Langrehr JM, Knoop M *et al.* Reconstruction of the bile duct using the side to side anastomosis in 389 orthotopic liver transplants. Transplant Proc 1995; 27: 1250–1.
12. Hubscher SG, Buckels JAC, Elias E *et al.* Vanishing bile-duct syndrome following liver transplantation – is it reversible? Transplantation 1991; 51: 1004–10.
13. Buckels JAC, Tisone G, Gunson BK *et al.* Low haematocrit reduces hepatic artery thrombosis after liver transplantation. Transplant Proc 1989; 21: 2460–1.
14. Hubscher SG. Histological findings in long term survivors following liver transplantation. In: Neuberger J, Lucey MR (eds) Liver transplantation practice and management. London: British Medical Journal 1994; pp. 292–306.
15. Hubscher SG. Chronic hepatitis in liver allografts. Hepatology 1990; 12: 1257–8.
16. Beath SV, Brook GD, Kelly DA *et al.* Successful liver transplantation in babies under 1 year. BMJ 1994; 307: 825–8.

# 8 Pancreas transplantation

*Richard D. M. Allen*

**Introduction**

At the end of 1996, clinical pancreas transplantation had a 30-year history in which an estimated 9000 procedures had been performed for the treatment of insulin dependent diabetes (IDDM). Nevertheless, it remains a controversial treatment option for diabetics. Proponents point to the unequalled glucose control provided by the procedure and the improved quality of life for the recipient, and claim that it is the treatment of choice for appropriate patients with diabetic nephropathy. Opponents, however, make counterclaims of unstoppable surgeons with an emotional commitment to provide an unphysiological procedure for which assessment by controlled data is unavailable. The reality is somewhere between these two polarised views, with vascularised pancreas transplantation offering a viable therapeutic option for a minority of insulin dependent diabetics at the wrong end of the spectrum of presentation of complications that occur secondary to diabetes. The procedure is clearly worthy of continuing evaluation in units with a major interest in experimental and clinical aspects of transplantation as a means of treating diabetes. Furthermore, the pancreas transplant procedure in its current form provides a standard of glucose control against which alternative therapeutic options of intensive insulin therapy, islet transplantation and the future prospect of gene therapy must be compared.

**Rationale**

The discovery and subsequent use of insulin in 1926 was, and continues to be, a life-saving measure for patients with juvenile onset or Type I insulin-dependent diabetes mellitus. In most instances, the condition is diagnosed before the age of 20 years and is associated with absence of circulating insulin. Untreated, death occurs as a result of ketoacidosis. The lack of insulin is most likely the effect of a chronic autoimmune process selectively destroying the insulin-producing beta cells within the million or so islets which comprise the endocrine portion of the pancreas. The initiating event and development of the autoimmune response against the beta cell is poorly understood, although identified circulating autoantibodies in Type I diabetes include those directed against the beta cell surface antigens and insulin. When more than 80% of the beta cells have been destroyed by the autoimmune process, the characteristic presentation of hyperglycaemia and ketoacidosis results.

For most Type I diabetics, subsequent treatment with exogenous insulin is life saving and the disease becomes principally one of inconvenience, with insulin requirements varying according to dietary intake and the amount of prolonged vigorous exercise undertaken. However, for about 40% of patients, major and often life-threatening complications occur as a result of presumed imperfect blood glucose control. The development of these chronic complications is of major concern to all informed diabetics for they may lead to either death from cardiovascular disease and renal failure or debilitating symptoms produced by damage to retinae and nerves. They tend to be more common in patients with poor glycaemic control and often follow a recognisable clinical pattern. Diabetic nephropathy severe enough to cause renal failure usually occurs at 20–30 years after the diagnosis of Type I diabetes and is preceded by microalbuminuria, proteinuria and hypertension before eventual uremia. It is almost invariably associated with both severe proliferative retinopathy and neuropathy affecting both the autonomic and peripheral nervous systems. Type I diabetics have a mortality rate about five times greater than the general population.

An additional 90% of diabetics become hyperglycaemic at a mature age as a result of the poor response of target cells to circulating insulin. These Type II diabetics initially have increased levels of circulating insulin and can be managed by restriction of dietary intake of carbohydrate and the use of oral hypoglycaemic agents. The incidence of renal failure in Type II diabetics is less than for Type I, but associated hyperinsulinaemia may be the reason for the increased incidence of peripheral vascular disease in this group of patients.

Although the pathogenesis of the two types of diabetes is different, the complications are similar and support the theory that the common problems of metabolic dysfunction and high blood sugar levels are the cause of the long-term complications of diabetes.[1] Hence, the goal for treatment of diabetes is to normalise blood sugar levels. This is supported by mounting objective evidence that good glycaemic control both delays the onset and modifies the progression of secondary complications. Two recently published trials, one in Stockholm and the other in the United States, have demonstrated the advantages of intensive insulin therapy on the incidence of nephropathy, retinopathy and neuropathy.[2,3] Intensive insulin therapy includes greater attention to patient education, measurement of blood glucose level and administration of insulin two to four times daily and frequent interaction between patient and the diabetes management team. The benefit of such therapy has been a declining incidence of diabetic nephropathy due to Type I diabetes and has been elegantly demonstrated in a regional study in the south-east of Sweden.[4,5] Diabetic nephropathy remains the commonest cause of renal failure, in developed communities. Until the

**Figure 8.1** *Number of new patients presenting in the 10 year period from 1985 in Australia requiring treatment for end-stage renal failure as a result of diabetic nephropathy. The solid bar represent patients with Type I diabetes. (Data are provided by ANZDATA Registry.)*

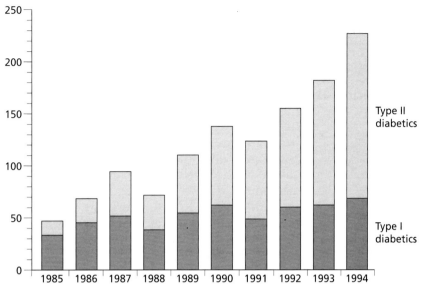

early 1980s, Type I diabetes was the predominant cause of diabetic nephropathy. However, the experience in Australia, which mirrors that of other developed countries, is that Type II diabetes has become the commonest cause (Fig. 8.1).

Such is the success of intensive insulin therapy that one could question if a role exists for pancreas transplantation. However, there is a down side to intensive insulin therapy. The frequency of hypoglycaemia is significantly increased, with resultant risk of central nervous system damage and even death from accident. The life style of the diabetic becomes increasingly restricted and is not easily tolerated, particularly by adolescents. Furthermore, despite the intensive therapy, control of hyperglycaemia as measured by haemoglobin $A^{1C}$ levels remains less than perfect. It, therefore, may be reasonable to suggest that the extent of nephropathy will persist with patients presenting at a later time. The potential advantage of pancreas transplantation is that it is the only treatment option available to Type I diabetics that normalises haemoglobin $A^{1C}$ levels. It is able to do so by continuous adjustment of insulin secretion in response to circulating glucose levels. This minute to minute control for 24 h per day can not be achieved by intensive insulin therapy. Hence, the decision to offer a patient a pancreas transplant is not based on its ability to save lives as is the case for heart, liver and lung transplantation, but on its ability to improve the recipient's quality of life by removing the restrictions of intensive insulin therapy. Therefore, the assessment of the value of pancreas transplantation must be more subtle than the question of life and death and is based on the risk of the procedure versus the benefit. Although there remains a need for conventional immunosuppression, the procedure will be of limited appeal to the great majority of insulin-dependent diabetics and their caring physicians.

**Recipient categories**

An essential criterion for pancreas transplantation is that the recipients have Type I IDDM. There is little to be gained from transplanting the hyperinsulinaemic Type II diabetic, even if they have become insulin dependent. The grey area is the patient aged about 30–40 years who becomes insulin dependent after a short period of time, perhaps only a few months after initially coping with oral hypoglycaemic agents. If they subsequently develop secondary complications of diabetes 10–20 years after commencing insulin, they may appropriately be classified as Type I (or perhaps Type I$\frac{1}{2}$) diabetics. If, however, the patient develops secondary complications within a few years of becoming insulin dependent, they are more likely to be Type II diabetics with peripheral resistance to insulin. The presence of circulating C-peptide may be a more objective way of differentiating these patients.

There are three recipient categories of pancreas transplantation that are defined by the timing of pancreas transplantation. In turn, the time of transplantation is determined by a combination of risk factors acceptable to the patient and surgeon, transplant unit policy and the availability of organs. In the United States, the health insurance status of the patient may also be a factor. The categories are pancreas transplantation alone (PTA), simultaneous pancreas kidney transplantation (SPK) and pancreas transplantation after previous successful kidney transplantation (PAK). To this, could be added a fourth category of relevance to the Type I diabetic with nephropathy, namely kidney transplantation alone (KTA).[6,7]

The Department of Surgery at the University of Minnesota in Minneapolis has deservedly become the Mecca of pancreas transplantation. Pioneering clinical pancreas transplantation, the department with names of Lillehei, Najarian, Simmons, Sutherland, Matas, Dunn and Gruessner, has for more than 30 years set the pace in clinical pancreas transplantation.[8–10] Perhaps unstoppable, they can not be described as unthinking as they have set out to challenge the management of the uraemic diabetic patient, the patient that neither the diabetologist nor the nephrologist is keen to take care of. After several years of preservation and implantation technique experiments in large animals, the Minneapolis group undertook clinical experimental studies in patients who to quote Lillehei, 'must have reached a point where conventional therapy had nothing to offer them'. Lillehei reasoned that uraemic patients with diabetes would not be able to endure the rigours of a kidney transplant without correction of the metabolic defect produced by insulin deficiency. Hence, the initial experience in patients with advanced complications of diabetes was understandably poor because of technical problems, rejection and perhaps poor patient selection. The programme was temporarily halted in 1974 to concentrate on clinical islet transplantation. In the mean time, the group had also demonstrated that KTA was a very viable option for

**Figure 8.2** *Primary pancreas graft survival by recipient category for bladder drained cadaver pancreas transplants performed in the United States between January 1987 and May 1995 (SPK = simultaneous pancreas kidney transplants, PAK = pancreas after kidney transplants, PTA = pancreas transplantation alone). From IPTR Newsletter 1996, edited by D E R Sutherland.*

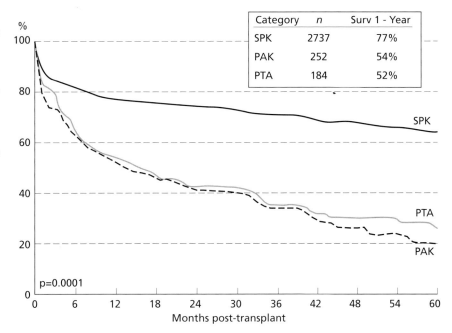

| Category | n | Surv 1 - Year |
|----------|------|------|
| SPK | 2737 | 77% |
| PAK | 252 | 54% |
| PTA | 184 | 52% |

diabetes with kidney failure.[6] The rationale for adding a pancreas transplant at that time was to augment the improvement in quality of life achieved by correcting uraemia. Because of the perceived need to reduce the magnitude of the operative procedure of SPK, the Minneapolis group undertook pancreas transplantation as a solitary procedure, initially for those with previously successful kidney transplants and then in non-uraemic patients with emerging complications of diabetes or labile diabetes.

The Munich meeting of the European Transplantation Society in November 1985 helped to define more clearly the role and indications for pancreas transplantation. Other groups working in the field of pancreas transplantation from Lyon, Munich, Stockholm, Oslo and Madison reported encouraging results with pancreas one-year graft survival of 50–60% after SPK.[11–15] There were several major reasons for the improved pancreas graft survival. First, graft loss from rejection was reduced by the use of cyclosporin and the ability of the kidney to provide an implied diagnosis of rejection. Secondly, careful cardiovascular screening of the patients to reduce graft loss from patient death was shown to be important. Thirdly, the Madison group demonstrated the technical advantage of urinary bladder drainage of the exocrine output of the pancreas.[15] Thereafter, the number of pancreas transplants performed in Europe and the USA, including Minneapolis, increased exponentially. More than 95% were associated with exocrine bladder drainage. Recent pancreas graft survival figures for each category is demonstrated in Fig. 8.2. The differential graft survival in favour of SPK can be explained by graft loss from rejection (Fig. 8.3).

**Figure 8.3** *Graft loss for immunological reasons in technically successful bladder drained cadaver pancreas transplants performed in the USA between January 1987 and May 1995 (SPK = simultaneous pancreas kidney transplants, PAK = pancreas after kidney transplants, PTA = pancreas transplantation alone). From IPTR Newsletter 1996, edited by D E R Sutherland.*

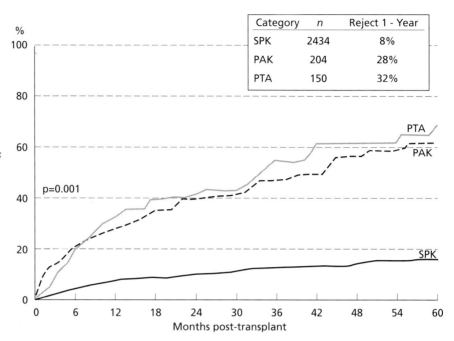

| Category | n | Reject 1 - Year |
|----------|------|-----------------|
| SPK | 2434 | 8% |
| PAK | 204 | 28% |
| PTA | 150 | 32% |

## Pancreas transplantation alone

Despite more than 200 PTA procedures in Minneapolis, this procedure has yet to find an established role acceptable to other units.[10] Potential indications for PTA may include aggressive neuropathy, hypoglycaemia unawareness, early nephropathy evidenced by proteinuria and resistance to subcutaneous insulin. In recent years, however, convincing evidence has accumulated to demonstrate the safer treatment option of intensive insulin therapy is also capable of modifying the progression of secondary complications, particularly if undertaken early in the natural history of these complications. Equally, retinopathy is well managed by laser photocoagulation and careful ophthalmologic surveillance. Hence, it is difficult to recommend to the pre-uraemic diabetic patient that they swap the risks of intensive insulin therapy for those associated with long-term non-specific immunosuppression necessary for a procedure that at best has a success rate of 60% at one year. A further complicating factor is that most of these patients have biopsy evidence of diabetic nephropathy. Native renal function in this situation is further affected adversely by the nephrotoxic effect of cyclosporin, often halving the glomerular filtration rate (GFR) within a month of transplantation.[16] Thereafter, however, renal function tends to remain stable.

## Simultaneous pancreas and kidney transplantation

Proteinuria, hypertension and declining GFR are the hallmarks of almost inevitable progression to renal failure. For this group of patients, renal transplantation is otherwise necessary at some stage, and there is little additional risk to the patient as a result of long-term immunosuppression. Unfortunately, the majority have advanced neuropathy and retinopathy and to an extent that glycaemic control provided by transplantation of the pancreas may be unable to modify. Hence, the important question for this group of patients is whether simplification of diabetes management is worth the risk of technical complications associated with the pancreas transplant procedure. Even the argument that the pancreas transplant would reduce the risk of graft loss from recurrent nephropathy is real but not strong, for after 10 years, graft loss for this reason after KTA is in the order of 4%.[6,17] Nevertheless, there are additional arguments to support SPK which are discussed later in this chapter, including the protective effect of the pancreas on transplant kidney function, axonal regeneration of peripheral nerves and improved cardiac function.

Timing of SPK is important. Diabetic patients with symptoms of autonomic neuropathy, particularly impaired gastric emptying, do not cope well when symptoms are compounded by the cachexia and the lethargy of uraemia. These patients rapidly lose their independence and self-esteem when overcome by mounting medical problems. Family life is stressed by the inability to maintain employment and emotional support for these patients is often difficult to achieve. Hence, the optimum time to offer a patient SPK is before the need for dialysis, when the serum creatinine is in the region of 300–400 $\mu$mol l$^{-1}$ and the GFR is 15–20 ml min$^{-1}$ The patient is nutritionally better able to cope with the rigours of SPK and more likely to be able to return to the work force if transplanted before a prolonged period of unemployment.[18] This can only be achieved if the patient is transplanted preferentially and without the probable delay necessary for well-matched HLA grafts.

In the short to medium term, it would seem that use of poorly matched kidney grafts has not had an adverse effect on patient and kidney graft survival.[19,20] Comparative assessment of kidney graft survival is made difficult by the lack of appropriate control groups. Centres undertaking pancreas transplantation tend to offer SPK to fitter patients and KTA to the less fit who in turn are more likely to have graft loss as a result of patient death.

## Pancreas after kidney transplantation

An alternative approach and one favoured by the Minneapolis group, is to push for living-related kidney transplantation followed by cadaver pancreas transplantation 6–12 months later.[10] Almost half the renal transplant procedures performed by this group are living related. This approach is based on the perceived need to maximise the use of available cadaver kidneys as well as the appreciation that the diabetic patient's life is saved by the renal transplant and not a pancreas. Furthermore, if uraemia is corrected, patients will be able to cope better with the rigours of the pancreas transplant procedure. Until very recently, the major disadvantage of this approach has been the inferior pancreas graft survival after PAK. However, the 1996 Newsletter of the International Pancreas Transplant Registry (IPTR) demonstrated dramatic improve-

**Table 8.1** *Pancreas after kidney graft survival figures for USA cadaveric pancreas transplants*

| Years | Number of transplants | 1-year graft survival (%) |
|---|---|---|
| 1987–1989 | 59 | 51 |
| 1990–1991 | 52 | 57 |
| 1992–1993 | 62 | 61 |
| 1994–1995 | 66 | 79 |

ment of PAK grafts in the United States in 1994 and 1995 with a 79% one year graft survival achieved (Table 8.1). This result is dependent on protocol pancreas biopsies and quadruple immunosuppression which often includes tacrolimus and mycophenolate mofetil.[21] The success of PAK, however, is offset by the increased risk of major infection.

## Criteria for patient selection

Careful screening of diabetic patients before placement on a waiting list for pancreas transplantation is an essential ingredient for success and criteria are highlighted in Table 8.2.[22] Of these, absence of significant uncorrectable cardiac disease is perhaps the most important.[23] Management of coronary artery disease in diabetic renal transplant candidates is controversial as most patients do not have symptoms of angina. Up to 40% of these patients when screened by coronary angiography have a stenosis of greater than 75% in one or more coronary arteries. Whereas routine coronary angiography is advocated by some units, others consider persantin thallium scanning to be an appropriate screening test. Demonstrated coronary artery blood flow abnormalities are then further investigated by coronary angiography. The threshold for performing the latter should be low because coronary revascularisation in IDDM patients with renal failure has been shown to decrease the cardiac morbidity and mortality following renal transplantation.

The level of GFR before acceptance onto a waiting list varies between units and may be one of the reasons why units with the more generous

**Table 8.2** *Criteria for pancreas transplantation*

| | | |
|---|---|---|
| **Absolute** | 1. | Type I diabetes mellitus |
| | 2. | End-stage renal failure (GFR $\leqslant$ 20 ml min$^{-1}$) |
| | | or |
| | | Functioning renal transplant |
| | 3. | Absent, insignificant or surgically corrected coronary artery disease |
| | 4. | Age <50 years |
| | 5. | Non-smoker |
| **Relative** | 6. | Bodyweight <125% of ideal |
| | 7. | No psychiatric illness |

values of up to 45 ml min$^{-1}$ have better results than units accepting patients near to or after commencing dialysis. Determining an absolute age is problematic but 50 years would seem to be an appropriate compromise age limit. Those presenting over the age of 50 years tend to have had diabetes for a longer period of time, have more secondary complications and a greater incidence of coronary artery disease. The relative contraindications of obesity and psychiatric illness may be considered more important if other criteria are questionable. The decreased pancreas and renal graft survival in obese patients corresponds to decreased patient survival.[24] Using similar advertised criteria to those in Table 8.2, the Omaha group interviewed 205 perspective diabetic patients, evaluating three quarters of them, and eventually placing half on the waiting list.[25]

**The donor pancreas**
Retrieving the donor pancreas and preparing it for subsequent transplantation is the most challenging and technically difficult part of the surgical procedure of pancreas transplantation.[26] It is made more difficult by the obvious priority that must be given to the patient requiring a liver transplant and because the need for donor organs is greater than the supply. The pancreas transplant surgical team have essentially become the 'poor cousins' of the solid organ transplantation community. Furthermore, pancreas transplantation represents only a small part of transplantation activities in national and regional transplant organisations. For example, Eurotransplant in 1994 reported 892 liver transplants and only 95 pancreas transplants from 1500 donors.[27] A cooperative approach between the liver and pancreas transplant teams is therefore essential and made easier if the one team performs the whole donor retrieval procedure.

The need to prioritise the liver transplant recipient is most apparent at the time of separation of the pancreas from the liver. The two organs have shared arterial supply and the venous drainage of the pancreas is part of the principal blood supply to the liver. In the 1980s, liver and pancreas transplants were performed in comparatively small numbers and the need to share organ donors was not as great as the need a decade later with the existence of many more transplant units and the widening of indications for liver transplantation. By preference, the pancreas transplant surgeon would prefer the coeliac trunk with intact splenic and gastroduodenal arteries, and the superior mesenteric artery with its inferior pancreaticoduodenal branches and a full length of portal vein. Concomitant liver retrieval, however, leaves the donor pancreas with the stump of splenic artery, a ligated gastroduodenal artery and the superior mesenteric artery.

The generous liver transplant surgeon will provide the pancreas with a 2–3 cm portal vein but more commonly, it is only 1 cm or so long. Without the need to retrieve the pancreas, a liver transplant surgeon is able to divide the pancreas in half at the level of the portal vein, maximising the length of that vein and facilitating subsequent portal vein perfusion. To this extent, the need to retrieve the pancreas is of nuisance value to the liver retrieval surgeon. The pancreas surgeon, however, is prone to be upset if his requirements are not catered for at the retrieval procedure.[27]

The feasibility of transplantation of the pancreas after ligation of the gastroduodenal artery is made possible by the rich blood supply to adjoining organs provided by an anastomotic system involving the coeliac and mesenteric arteries. Inherent with this anastomotic system is considerable variability, and in one study of 400 dissections of the abdominal vasculature, no two specimens were the same.[28] In another study, 76% of donors had a single hepatic artery from the coeliac trunk.[29] In 13% of cases, the right hepatic or the main hepatic artery came off the superior mesenteric artery. In other words, at one in eight combined donor procedures, the decision must be made as to whether there is sufficient blood supply to the head of the pancreas to allow for subsequent safe pancreas transplantation. If the aberrant right hepatic artery branches off the superior mesenteric artery close to its origin, safe pancreas transplantation is usually possible. However, more distal branching of the right hepatic artery from the superior mesenteric artery usually involves one or more prominent branches to the head of the pancreas and duodenum and subsequent pancreas transplantation is not advisable.

### Donor age

The donor age has been described by the Minneapolis group as the single most important factor in the success of pancreas transplantation.[30] Older donors are associated with an increased technical failure rate as well as reduced graft and patient survival rates. This is reflected in IPTR data with the majority of donors being aged between 20 and 40 years. Large studies from individual institutions report mean ages in the vicinity of 25 years. There are few data on the lower age limit although a reasonable donor guideline would be about 5 years, height of 100 cm and weight of 20 kg.[31]

### Retrieval technique

The restrictive age range for pancreas donation is such that the liver will nearly always be retrieved at the same time. Described techniques vary from detailed dissection of the pancreas and separation from the liver *in situ* to en bloc techniques involving removal of the liver, pancreas and kidneys with subsequent bench top separation of the organs.[27,32,33] The compromise technique undertaken by most involves en bloc removal of the liver and the pancreas, with advantages of providing shorter donor surgery time, the opportunity to carefully sort out variations in vascular anatomy[34] and probable better preservation of both the pancreas and the liver. *In situ* separation of the two organs may lead to spasm of the arterial supply. It is nevertheless important to note that the multiorgan retrieval procedure, which includes retrieval of the pancreas, has had no deleterious effect on liver transplant outcome and continues to provide excellent pancreatic graft performance.[32] Retrieving the pancreas with the liver certainly adds to the donor surgical procedure time, perhaps as much as 30 min. Technical considerations include the advantage of careful dissection of the tail of the pancreas off the stomach and use of the spleen as a handle, thus minimising trauma to the pancreas from handling. The duodenum is stapled and divided at the level of the pylorus and at the ligament of Treitz. There may also be an advantage in irrigating the duodenum with aqueous betadine solution prior to stapling.

## Other donor selection factors

Obesity in the donor is by itself not a contraindication for pancreas retrieval. Nevertheless, a pancreas heavily infiltrated by adipose tissue is not an attractive option. If the donor is at the upper age limit and has atherosclerotic major vessels, use of such a pancreas is inadvisable. Elevated serum glucose levels are frequently seen in healthy brain dead donors and are considered a benign finding caused by increased sympathetic activity, use of steroids and large volume fluid replacement with dextrose containing solutions.[35,36] In an obese patient, however, it may also mean Type II diabetes and a donor glycosylated haemoglobin level may be of assistance. Elevated serum amylase levels are also seen in donors with cerebral trauma and do not influence pancreas graft survival. Associated blunt abdominal trauma may, however, result in a transection of the pancreas, a finding which will be found at time of donor surgery and preclude pancreas retrieval.

Matching of donors and recipients is usually limited to ABO blood group matching, negative lymphocytotoxicity cross-match and perhaps considerations for size of the donor and the recipient. Placement of the pancreas and the kidney from a large donor can provide difficulty in a small recipient. Matching for human leucocyte antigens (HLA) is an attractive option to improve graft survival of PAK and PTA and is possible in large organ sharing organisations that exist in the United States and Europe. Generally, however, the comparatively small number of patients on waiting lists for pancreas transplantation are such that it is unlikely that a chance matching of more than one or two DR antigens will occur.

## Pancreas preservation

Because of multiorgan donation and priority given to the liver recipient, whatever is good for the liver, will be good for the pancreas. The exception to this statement is the choice of preservation fluid. The most commonly used fluid, University of Wisconsin (UW) solution was initially developed for pancreas transplantation. It allowed safe cold storage times for the pancreas of up to 72 h in dogs and subsequently also became the preservation fluid of choice for liver preservation.[37,38] However, this solution is viscous because of its high potassium content and therefore perfuses slowly. Hence, some liver programmes prefer to cool the liver rapidly with cold crystalloid solutions and then use UW solutions. Care should be taken for exessive amounts of crystalloid solution have been shown to be deleterious to pancreas graft function, being associated with an increased incidence of graft pancreatitis and venous thrombosis.[39]

The common practice for cold perfusion of the donor organs is a combination of aortic and portal vein flushing. When the liver and the pancreas are retrieved en bloc, the portal perfusion cannula is inserted via the superior mesenteric vein or via the divided portal vein. The latter is technically more difficult and both are probably unnecessary and could be replaced by aortic perfusion alone, as adequate portal perfusion can be achieved by arterial perfusion of the mesenteric and coeliac arteries alone. With satisfactory cold storage time of the pancreas of up to 24 h, back to back donor and recipient procedures are not necessary. As donor surgery tends to be a nocturnal pursuit, the recipient procedure can be undertaken in daylight hours which is probably safer for the recipient and physiologically more acceptable for the surgical team.

## Techniques of recipient surgery

The aim of the surgical procedure is to provide normal glucose haemostasis for the recipient. This requires a maximum number of islets and at present, the unnecessary transplantation of the exocrine portion of the pancreas which makes up 99% of the bulk of the pancreas. The decisions to be made by the transplanting surgeon are first, how much of the pancreas to transplant, and secondly, how to manage the exocrine function of the pancreas. Options are segmental or whole transplantation with duct occlusion, enteric drainage or bladder exocrine drainage.[11,15,40] By 1992, 98% of pancreas transplants performed in the United States were whole pancreases with bladder exocrine drainage. Before 1985, the favoured technique involved a segmental transplant which was either duct occluded, enteric drained or bladder drained. The Madison group popularised the bladder drainage technique, initially with a pancreas segment,[15,41] and later by the whole pancreas with a duodenal button and eventually with a duodenal segment. The latter provided for easier anastomosis to the bladder with decreased technical complications, particularly compared to that of the enteric drainage technique which was popularised by the Stockholm group.[40] Attempts to evaluate the two techniques in a prospective manner by several groups were short lived because of increased morbidity associated with enteric fistulae. The ability to protect the duodenum-to-bladder anastomosis with a bladder catheter was therefore seen as advantageous as was the ability to monitor pancreas graft function by measurement of amylase in the urine. Proponents of the enteric technique counter this claim by providing percutaneous pancreatic duct drainage.[41] This permitted absolute measurement of amylase production and cytology of pancreatic juice.[42]

The disadvantage was an increased incidence of pancreas infections and enteric fistulae.

Choices also exist for the position of pancreas and the site of vascular anastomoses. Earlier experience with placement of the pancreas in an extraperitoneal position, not dissimilar to that for the kidney, caused local wound problems from digestive pancreatic enzymes and infection.[43,44] The peritoneal cavity is better able to cope with enzymes released from the pancreas in the initial days after transplantation and is now the position of choice. The use of the iliac vessels for vascular anastomosis however remains a contentious issue. The result is non-physiologic systemic delivery of insulin. In the past, elaborate attempts have been made to provide portal venous drainage with a recipient anastomosis to the mesenteric circulation.[45] Venous thrombosis rates were high and this form of anastomosis failed to gain popularity. Nevertheless, the technique has been revisited by the Memphis, Chicago and Pittsburgh groups.[46–48] They anastomose the portal vein to the side of the superior mesenteric vein distal to at least one major branch, and then transplant duodenum to a Roux-en-Y limb in a side-to-side manner. They reported equivalent graft survival to the more conventional bladder drained technique with less incidence of reflux pancreatitis, and claim advantages of avoidance of metabolic acidosis and a reduction in fasting hyperinsulinaemia.[46] One can anticipate that the portal venous and enteric drained pancreas transplant procedure will gain greater popularity in coming years provided the results in terms of graft survival and patient morbidity are better or at least the same as the bladder drained technique. For PAK and PTA, however, in the absence of a simultaneously transplanted kidney, enteric drainage has a major disadvantage of not permitting monitoring of pancreas graft function by measurement of urinary amylase.

## Bench top preparation

The most critical and technically demanding part of the pancreas transplant procedure is the preparation and reconstruction of the vascular anatomy of the pancreas prior to transplantation. It is performed at the recipient hospital and invariably takes two hours or more. During this time, if the surgeon is confident that the pancreas can be subsequently transplanted, a separate surgical team can begin the recipient operation, performing a laparotomy and preparing the iliac vessels for subsequent vascular anastomosis. In some centres, probably the minority, the kidney is transplanted before the pancreas.

Being presented with a pancreas after separation from the liver can be a daunting experience, particularly if it has been retrieved from an obese donor. The pancreas is pale and not dissimilar in colour to the fat in the region of the splenic hilum, bowel mesentery and the tough thick tissue (which includes neural, lymphatic and fibrous components) surrounding the origin of the superior mesenteric artery. The divided end of the

**Figure 8.4** *When the pancreas is retrieved in conjunction with the liver, it is necessary to reconstruct the arterial supply and venous drainage of the pancreas using donor common iliac artery and its bifurcation and common iliac vein respectively. The end of the donor external iliac artery is anastomosed to the stump of the superior mesenteric artery and the internal iliac artery to the stump of the splenic artery.*

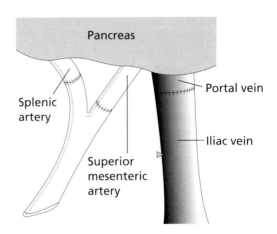

splenic artery and the stump of the portal vein are usually only apparent because of attached prolene marker sutures. The common bile duct and the gastroduodenal artery will have been ligated at the time of retrieval. The temptation is to remove all non-pancreatic tissue and reduce the duodenal segment to about 10 cm in length. This is reasonable at the tail end of the pancreas but excessive dissection, particularly around the third and fourth parts of the duodenum and the bowel mesentery is likely to increase the risk of impairing the blood supply to the head of the pancreas and the duodenum. In this respect, nothing replaces surgical experience.

The donor common iliac artery and its two major branches are used to reconstruct the arterial supply to the pancreas.[49] About 1.5 cm length of internal iliac artery is anastomosed end-to-end to the splenic artery. A short length of external iliac artery is anastomosed to the shortened end of the superior mesenteric artery just before it enters the pancreas substance (Fig. 8.4). Alternative techniques have been described including use of a segment of distal superior mesenteric artery to fashion an interposition graft between the superior mesenteric artery and the end of the splenic artery, or using the distal end of the superior mesenteric artery, and passing it anteriorly over the pancreas to the upper border where is anastomosed to the end of the splenic artery.[50,51]

Extension of the portal vein is controversial with many surgeons claiming that it is unnecessary provided extensive mobilisation of the right iliac vein is undertaken. Worse, it has been suggested that it leads to an increased risk of venous thrombosis. Proponents of a vein extension graft, using 2 or 3 cm of donor common iliac vein, claim avoidance of the frequently difficult division of the recipient internal iliac veins and ability to place the pancreas in a more anterior position where it can be readily palpated and biopsied using a percutaneous technique. The duodenal segment is usually 10–15 cm long and stapled at either end at the time of the retrieval procedure. Stapling alone, however, is associated with leaks from the duodenal segment, particularly at the mesenteric border at the distal end of the duodenum. For this reason both staple lines are buried with a continuous absorbable suture.

## The recipient procedure

The advent of HLA typing and lymphocytotoxicity cross-matching with donor peripheral blood often allows the potential recipient to be informed of the availability of a pancreas, before retrieval of the pancreas. Many potential recipients are chronically constipated and appropriate bowel preparation on admission facilitates subsequent surgery and makes for easier postoperative management. An insulin infusion is commenced together with a steady-rate infusion of dextrose to obtain blood glucose levels of 12–15 mmol $l^{-1}$ at time of induction of anaesthesia.

Before anaesthesia, multilumened central venous access and peripheral arterial access are obtained. Postoperative analgesia is made easy by insertion of an epidural cannula to cover the T8 dermatome and below. Broad spectrum antibiotics to cover Gram positive and Gram negative bacteria, as well as fluconazole for candida prophylaxis, are given intravenously. The potential source of candida can be either the duodenal segment or the patient's own flora.

A midline incision is made from midway between the xiphisternum down to the pubic tubercle, passing to the left of the umbilicus. The caecum is mobilised, as is the bifurcation of the right common iliac artery lateral to the ureter and gonadal vessels. The external iliac vein is then mobilised and, depending on the mobility of the vein and the presence of an extension portal vein graft, the internal iliac veins are ligated and divided with great care. Similarly, the sigmoid colon is mobilised and the external iliac vessels mobilised lateral to the left ureter. Invariably, the pancreas is placed on the right side and the kidney on the left side (Fig. 8.5). Positioning of the pancreas is vital to its subsequent technical success. Appreciation of the final position of the pancreas is important for the orientation of both the venous and arterial anastomoses. The obvious final position for the pancreas is with its long axis at a 45° angle from the midline. The natural curve to the pancreas will result in a more vertical position for the body and tail. In its normal anatomical position, the portal vein passes behind the duodenum but in the transplant recipient, must pass downwards and away from the duodenum. To avoid kinking, the vein is kept to a minimum length but one that allows for easy anastomosis. The anastomosis is to the external iliac vein and at least 5 cm inferior to the point where the arterial anastomosis is subsequently performed.

One of the advantages and perhaps the only one for the use of the donor common iliac extension graft is a reduction in the size of the arteriotomy necessary for the arterial anastomosis. The donor common iliac artery is spatulated and anastomosed to the distal common iliac artery. If positioned correctly, the splenic artery anastomosis is lateral to the superior mesenteric artery anastomosis. The combined vascular

**Figure 8.5**
*Schematic representation of the pancreas transplant, with an aortic patch containing the coeliac trunk and superior mesenteric artery anastomosed to the common iliac artery and the portal vein to the external iliac vein. The segment of duodenum is anastomosed to the dome of the urinary bladder.*

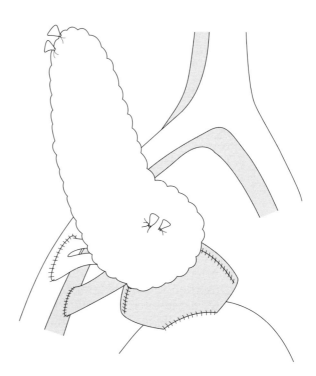

anastomosis time should be less than 35 min. A prolonged anastomotic time is associated with impaired graft function and an increased rate of thrombosis.[52] Keeping the pancreas cool during the anastomosis is technically awkward, made more difficult by the flat shape of the graft, but should be attempted.

Releasing the vascular clamps after completion of the pancreas anastomosis can be an exciting event. The anaesthetist should be well prepared with baseline measurements of blood gases, serum glucose and central venous pressure taken. Maximum safe intravascular filling of the recipient is obtained beforehand because unexpected bleeding can take place from inadequately ligated vessels, particularly in the region of the bowel mesentery anterior to the pancreas. Alternatively, hypotension may follow release of vasoactive substances from a poorly preserved pancreas. A well perfused pancreas will increase in size and will change from a pale appearance to a pink/orange colour. Prominent pulsation of the splenic artery and the ligated end of the superior mesenteric artery should be present. The duodenum also becomes pink and fills quickly with pancreatic juices. Unless the serum glucose is greater than 20 mmol $l^{-1}$, the insulin infusion can be discontinued. A constant low rate of dextrose infusion is continued. Blood sugar levels thereafter are repeated at half hourly intervals during the remainder of the transplant procedure. It is indeed satisfying for the surgeon to see the recipient insulin independent for the first time for more than 20 years.

Equally critical to the continuity of transplanted portal vein is the orientation of the duodenocystomy. The dome of the bladder is anastomosed side to side to the antimesenteric border of the duodenum in two layers of absorbable suture material. The length of the anastomosis is about 3 cm. An alternative technique using the GIA stapler for this anastomosis has not proved popular. The kidney is then transplanted in a conventional manner on the left side. Transplanting a kidney through a long midline incision, however, is more difficult than using a retroperitoneal approach. Care must be taken to avoid kinking of the ureter and the use of a ureteric stent is advisable. Drains are placed around the pancreas and the wound closed in layers.

**Postoperative management**

The recipient is extubated at the end of the surgical procedure and transferred to the renal transplant ward. Intensive care unit facilities are not necessary and management of the simultaneously transplanted kidney is no different from that of KTA. After SPK, primary renal function occurs in greater than 90% of transplants.

Primary renal function also facilitates the diagnosis of rejection and therefore forms an integral part of the successful management of the recipient of an SPK. Measurement of urine output and serum creatinine together with duplex ultrasound examination of the kidney are important markers for rejection after SPK.

Specific measures exist for managing the pancreas transplant. Hourly blood sugar levels for at least the first 24 h are necessary not only to monitor pancreas graft function, but also to protect the patient against hypoglycaemia. Thereafter, less frequent blood glucose levels are possible and provide a sensitive indicator of pancreas transplant catastrophe such as thrombosis, but not rejection. Delivery of a fixed rate of dextrose makes for easier management, particularly when the recipient is polyuric in the first days after transplantation. Parenteral nutrition is advisable until the patient is able to cope with oral intake. This may take a variable time and depends to an extent on the severity of the recipient's diabetic autonomic neuropathy. Generally, the recipients who vomited prior to transplantation have more trouble than those that did not.

Delayed endocrine pancreas graft function is almost a non-entity. Nevertheless, the Minneapolis group have reported a 69% incidence of delayed dysfunction, defined as requirement for exogenous insulin after day 5 in a technically successful pancreas transplant.[53] In contrast, the Leiden group has demonstrated immediate release of glucagon, insulin and pancreatic polypeptide from the transplanted pancreas. In 22 consecutive patients, the mean plasma glucose concentration was 8.3 mmol l$^{-1}$ 3 h after reperfusion.[54] The total cold ischaemia time was the only significant variable associated with a delay in fall in blood glucose and was associated with an increase in the swelling of the head of the pancreas and increased excretion of pancreatic polypeptide. It is probable that other vasoactive peptides are also released from the ischaemia-damaged pancreas and may be the reason for the occasional precipitous falls in blood pressure and metabolic acidosis encountered soon after reperfusion of the pancreas.

The more frequent complications of pancreas transplantation, which are discussed in detail later, are transplant venous thrombosis, collections and infection. The use of prophylactic heparin is controversial with intravenous infusion associated with local bleeding as well as haematuria. Subcutaneous heparin is a safer option and low-dose aspirin is advisable in the long term. Collections can occur around the pancreas for several reasons. In the initial days after transplantation, collections usually relate to pancreatitis with loss of fluid through the pancreas capsule into the peritoneal cavity. The collections often become loculated. A personal preference is to perform continuous peritoneal lavage with soft Jackson Pratt drains placed around the pancreas. Lavage is continued for 24–48 h with drains removed two days after transplantation, irrespective of the volume of fluid loss. Antibiotics are continued until such times as the drains are removed. The severity of the pancreatitis can be assessed by measurement of serum amylase, which is usually raised for the first 24–48 h, and serum calcium. It is not unusual for calcium replacement to be necessary for the first 48 h. Serum albumin may also fall precipitously, leading to peripheral oedema. Commonly, the recipient is 5–10 kg over dry weight at the end of the second day after transplantation.

Continuous collection of urine output is performed with measurement of total urinary amylase in a 24 h period.[55] Again as a reflection of the preservation injury to the pancreas and pancreatitis, the urinary amylase level falls to a nadir at 2–3 days after transplantation and then gradually increases reaching levels of 60 000–200 000 IU/24 h by the end of the second week after transplantation. As pancreatic function improves, so does the increase of bicarbonate loss into the urine. Intravenous bicarbonate replacement is usually necessary by the third day after transplantation and upwards of twelve bicarbonate capsules are necessary to prevent metabolic acidosis by the end of the second week after transplantation.

Reported median bed stay for the pancreas transplant recipient is about 20–25 days. It is exceptional for the patient to be discharged within 2 weeks of transplantation. The prolonged bed stay is a reflection of the frequency of complications after pancreas transplantation, as well as the management of factors specific to the diabetic patient such as postural hypotension and vomiting. Controlled trails of KTA in IDDM and SPK do not exist. However, a large USA multicentre analysis of diabetic patients transplanted between 1986 and 1989, aged 18–45 years, showed that KTA patients had a mean hospitalisation of 15 days compared to 23 days for SPK patients.[19] Interestingly, the same study demonstrated a significantly better kidney graft survival for SPK despite significantly worse HLA matching. Other studies have demonstrated higher re-admission rate after initial hospital discharge for the SPK patients.[22,56,57]

**Immuno-suppression**

The traditional immunosuppression protocol for pancreas transplantation in the United States includes induction therapy with antilymphocyte preparations together with triple therapy of cyclosporin, azathiaprine and prednisolone. The rationale for such therapy is based on the almost inevitable poor HLA matching of the donor and recipient. With such therapy, rejection is seen in about half the recipients at a median of about 30–40 days after transplantation.[58] In a randomised trial of OKT3 versus antilymphocyte globulin, the former proved more effective but three-quarters of recipients had major infections.[59]

In contrast, European centres have favoured the use of triple therapy with the use of antilymphocyte preparations reserved for treatment of rejection. This safer protocol is associated with earlier onset of rejection, usually in the second week after transplantation and with an incidence of more than 80%. The IPTR data have demonstrated no significant difference in graft survival of the pancreas or the kidney after SPK, with or without induction antilymphocyte therapy. Nevertheless, there is a significant difference in pancreas graft survival in favour of induction therapy for PTA and PAK. A misleading conclusion to make from these data would be that transplantation of the pancreas without a simultaneous kidney transplant is associated with more severe rejection. However, experimental data in dogs suggest otherwise with the advantage of induction antilymphocyte therapy being the ability to overcome the difficulty of diagnosing independent pancreas rejection.[60] Increasingly, units are avoiding the use of induction antilymphocyte therapy after SPK. It is possible that less acute rejection will be seen with the use of microemulsion formulations of cyclosporin that overcome, in part, the impaired cyclosporin absorption seen in diabetics. Higher cyclosporin levels in the early period after transplantation reduce rejection. Equally, initial multicentre experience with tacrolimus has shown it to be associated with a low rate of graft loss from rejection and a high rate of graft salvage when used for rescue or rejection therapy.[61] The initial concern of hyperglycaemia seen in liver transplant patients treated with tacrolimus has not been a major problem after SPK or PAK.

**Diagnosis of rejection**

Like any other solid organ allotransplant, the pancreas can be rejected hyperacutely, acutely or in a chronic manner. Hyperacute rejection can be diagnosed by the surgeon at the time of operation with the pancreas becoming grossly oedematous and then haemorrhagic within minutes.[62] In the first year after transplantation, the incidence of graft loss as a result of rejection is less than that for technical complications after SPK but the reverse after PTA or PAK. The difference is simply related to the paucity of specific and sensitive independent markers of pancreas rejection.

The diagnosis of acute rejection is problematic. There may be a low-grade fever and generally, an increase in size of the pancreas such that it becomes readily palpable and uncomfortable. The main differential diagnosis, particularly if the bladder is not defunctioned by a urinary catheter, is reflux pancreatitis. Short of a pancreas transplant biopsy, confirming the diagnosis of acute rejection is indeed difficult and after SPK, is made by implication by demonstrating rejection of the kidney from the same donor. The implied diagnosis is based on the assumption that the pancreas does not reject independently of the kidney.[63,64] Gruessner and Sutherland from Minneapolis, on the basis of considerable clinical experience and studies in pigs, believe that pancreas rejection can occur independent of the kidney. However, objective clinical data to support this, in particular by simultaneous biopsies of the pancreas and the kidney, are lacking.[65] In a small study in which biopsies of both organs were taken, rejection was seen in both organs in 75% and in the kidney only in the remainder.[66] A comprehensive longitudinal biopsy study in dogs undertaken by the Westmead demonstrated that independent pancreas rejection could occur after SPK but was in the order of 2% of simultaneous biopsies.[60] Furthermore, the study demonstrated histological evidence of rejection in the kidney to be the most sensitive and specific marker of pancreas rejection after SPK. Nevertheless, there is agreement that the severity of rejection in one or other organ is variable, with the severity in one not necessarily mirrored in the other, even for evidence of vascular rejection.[64]

Life for the transplant clinician looking after recipients of a PAK or PTA is not so easy. The markers of independent pancreas rejection are summarised in Table 8.3. Monitoring the principal function of the pancreas transplant, to normalise blood sugar levels, is complicated by the comparative resistance of islets to rejection and the considerable functional reserve provided by their large number. Hence, unless the pancreas is stressed with a large amount of glucose for example by measurement of the glucose disappearance rate after an intravenous glucose load, a diagnosis of rejection based on blood sugar levels is a late diagnosis of rejection.[67] The measurement of serum C-peptide and serum insulin is similarly a problem. Blunted first phase release of insulin in response to an intravenous glucose load is associated with acute rejection, but is not an investigation that would be done on a daily basis with same day results.[68]

On the other hand, the exocrine portion of the pancreas gland is affected early by rejection.[42] Not surprisingly, amylase enters the

**Table 8.3**  *Independent markers of pancreas rejection*

| Marker | Sensitive | Specific | Problems |
|---|---|---|---|
| Blood glucose | No | Yes | Late |
| Insulin release | Yes | Yes | Rarely measured on daily basis |
| C-peptide | No | Yes | Late |
| Serum amylase | No | No | Small to moderate increase only |
| Urinary amylase | No | Yes | Concentration also affected by fasting and diuresis |

circulation with acinar cell damage. The baseline level of serum amylase may double or triple, providing a comparatively early but nevertheless, soft marker of rejection. Equally, amylase can be measured in the urine provided the duodenum of the pancreas transplant is anastomosed to the bladder. Falls in urinary amylase occur earlier than significant rises in blood glucose levels but interpretation is made difficult unless the collection of urine is standardised, preferably by 24 h collection.[55] A 50% fall from baseline levels over several days is associated with biopsy proven rejection in about two-thirds of cases.[69,70] The concentration of amylase in the urine can be affected by diuresis or stimulation by gut hormones released after the intake of food. Nevertheless, it is perhaps the most useful marker of rejection in the absence of a simultaneously transplanted kidney. Serum amylase levels can also increase if urine containing amylase enters the peritoneal cavity. In such instances, the levels fall precipitously after insertion of a urinary catheter. More sensitive serum markers of damage to the exocrine portion of the pancreas is certainly an attractive option more so after PAK, PTA or enteric exocrine drainage of the pancreas transplant. Measurement of pancreas-specific protein, elastase, anodal trypsinogen and pancreatic secretory trypsin inhibitors have been measured in clinical situations and experimental models. Unfortunately, increased levels have been shown to be either non-specific or logistically difficult to measure on a daily basis.[64]

Imaging of the pancreas transplant for the diagnosis of rejection is equally problematic.[71,72] Unlike the kidney, the pancreas lacks a firm capsule, preventing monitoring on the basis of measurement of intra-vascular resistance by duplex ultrasonography. Ultrasound, however, confirms vascularity of the pancreas and demonstrates an increased size of the pancreas as well as areas of necrosis if the rejection process is advanced. Computed axial tomography offers little advantage over ultrasonography, and the same may be said for magnetic resonance imaging. Both investigations are nevertheless of value in demonstrating other graft-related pathology, particularly if compared to a previous study that can act as a baseline.

The gold standard for the diagnosis of rejection of the pancreas is the biopsy. Unexplained hypoamylasuria with falls of a greater than 50%, or less in the presence of graft signs and fever are probably the best indications for biopsy. Protocol biopsies in the initial months after transplantation are one way around the problem of non-specific and insensitive rejection markers.[21] Until the description of percutaneous biopsy of the pancreas using an automated biopsy gun and an 18 gauge trucut needle, a laparotomy was considered necessary to perform the biopsy.[66] To obtain a pancreatic biopsy by the percutaneous route, the pancreas must be palpable or at least adjacent to the anterior abdominal wall as demonstrated by an ultrasound examination. This is often not the case when a short portal vein is used for vascular anastomosis, and necessitates a transcystoscopic biopsy which can be performed with comparative safety, even though requiring the patient to visit the operating suite.[73] The needle is passed through the rigid cystoscope and into the duodenum and adjacent pancreatic head. Even if only the duodenum is biopsied, useful information can still be obtained.[74]

It is only in recent years that a histologic grading of pancreas acute allograft rejection has evolved and this has been made possible by the more frequent biopsy of the pancreas. Previously, histological specimens were dependent on incidental laparotomy for evaluation of a failing graft.[75] Longitudinal assessment was limited to studies in animals.[76] The cellular targets for rejection are endothelial cells and the acinar and ductal epithelial cells.[74,75,77] The presence of vasculitis and endothelialitis are the most specific findings in the diagnosis of rejection, whereas interstitial inflammation is less specific. The inflammatory cells are most prominent around ductal and vascular tissue. Fibrous tissue replaces the destroyed acinar tissue. With increasing severity of the rejection process, the polymorph infiltrate becomes more diffuse and includes destruction of islet cells.

The clinical diagnosis of chronic rejection of the pancreas is equally difficult. The functional reserve of the pancreas is such that the process is usually too late to reverse by the time hyperglycaemia has become apparent. Grafts lost after five years are from chronic rejection in 55% of instances, with overall graft lost at the rate of 5% per year thereafter.[78] Currently, the longest functioning pancreas graft is 16 years, a cadaveric pancreas transplanted after a living donor kidney. The hallmark of a chronic failing pancreas is a low C-peptide level in response to a glucose challenge. The histological features are the presence of dense septal fibrosis with acinar cell loss and fibrointimal vascular proliferation.

Recurrence of autoimmune diabetes is at least a theoretical, if not real cause for loss of pancreas graft function.[79] Certainly, if the donor is an identical twin and immunosuppressive therapy is not needed to prevent rejection, autoimmune disease may rapidly occur. The Stockholm group recently reported two patients with biopsy evidence of selective loss of beta cells after presenting with a slow decline in insulin secretion after a prolonged period of stable function. Both patients received cadaver grafts with poor HLA match.

## Complications

The reason for the significantly prolonged bed stay after pancreas transplantation compared to KTA is the frequency of complications.[20] These relate specifically to the pancreas, an organ that does not have a high blood flow, and the great majority of its parenchymal cells are associated with production of proteolytic enzymes for the digestion of food. The summary of the complications shown in Table 8.4 are either vascular in origin or relate to the exocrine function of the pancreas. The majority occur in the first few months after transplantation.

**Table 8.4**   *Complications of bladder drained pancreas transplantation*

|  | % |
| --- | --- |
| Mortality | 3–5 |
| Thrombosis | 2–15 |
| Duodenal leak | 5–15 |
| Reflux pancreatitis | 10–15 |
| Chronic haematuria | 5–35 |
| Recurrent urinary tract infection | 20–40 |

## Mortality

An experienced transplant unit might accept a mortality of 3–5% in the first year after transplantation. The commonest cause of death is overwhelming sepsis with cardiovascular causes kept to a minimum by careful screening prior to transplantation.[80] The risk of opportunistic infection increases with use of antilymphocyte preparations and tacrolimus. Striking a balance between this increased risk and immune graft loss is not always easy, but unlike heart and liver transplantation, it should be appreciated that the recipient will not die if the pancreas is lost.

## Thrombosis

Vascular thrombosis remains a major cause of graft loss after pancreas transplantation despite the use of the whole pancreas with duct drainage.[81–83] The presentation is usually in the first week after transplantation and is dramatic. The common scenario is of excellent pancreas graft function with acute onset of graft pain and loss of pancreas graft function. Venous thrombosis is more dramatic than arterial thrombosis in terms of increased size of the pancreas and patient discomfort. The aetiology is probably multifactorial and includes the variable blood supply to the pancreas, reperfusion injury and technical factors such as the alignment of the portal vein anastomosis. Additional insult to the pancreas from rejection may also further embarrass the blood flow to the pancreas and increase its susceptibility to thrombosis. Attempts to salvage the pancreas transplant are uniformly disappointing.

Arterial thrombosis has a different presentation with less florid local signs and may involve either the splenic artery, the superior mesenteric artery or both. Presentation will be dependent on the adequacy of the collateral circulation from one arterial system to the other, and the incidence is probably more common than appreciated. Transplant superior mesenteric thrombosis would increase the risk of producing a non-viable duodenal segment which may present initially with a grey appearance to the urine followed by duodenal segment leak of urine. Provided the splenic artery remains patent, the body and tail of the pancreas will remain viable and maintain normal or near normal glucose homeostasis. Exploration of the graft is inevitable if the transplant duodenum becomes non-viable and it may be possible to preserve the distal half of the pancreas, directly anastomosing it to the bladder. Alternatively, the body and tail of the pancreas may become non-viable, in which case presentation is usually late with a non-viable necrotic portion of the pancreas, perhaps with a pancreatic fistula into the peritoneal cavity. Usually, however, the necrotic portion of the pancreas develops into a localised collection which sooner or later will require formal drainage.

## Pancreatitis

Pancreatitis of variable extent occurs in the initial days after transplantation and results from handling of the pancreas during the donor and recipient procedures as well as reperfusion injury. It is usually self-limiting and rarely a problem. On the other hand, pancreatitis occurring weeks to months after pancreas transplantation is more likely related to reflux of urine, perhaps infected, into the pancreatic duct.[81,83] It is associated with a painful swollen pancreas graft, a low-grade fever and a raised serum amylase. The obvious differential diagnosis is acute rejection of the pancreas. Management involves exclusion of the diagnosis of rejection, perhaps by renal transplant biopsy, and urinary cathether drainage of the bladder. Symptoms usually subside over several days and it is recommended that the urinary catheter be kept in place for two weeks after the onset of symptoms, and appropriate antibiotics given if a urinary tract infection is also present. Most units also advocate resting the pancreas in the same way that one might treat native pancreatitis by limiting oral intake and providing parenteral nutrition.

## Haematuria and dysuria

As a group, the urological complications following pancreas transplantation are the most frequent, but fortunately, they do not have an adverse effect on long-term graft function. Again, their presence is a reflection of the unphysiological positioning of the pancreas transplant with the urinary tract mucosa not designed to cope with digestive enzymes. Theoretically, the enzymes should be in the inactive state, but evidence suggests otherwise, with possible activation by enzymes produced by the transplant duodenal mucosa and urea-splitting bacteria. Furthermore, a study of prospective SPK recipients demonstrated that 78% have bladder dysfunction, a third of which have high intravesical pressure.[84] The classic diabetic cystopathy involving a distended bladder was present in less than a fifth of patients. After SPK, recurrent urinary tract infections are common with incidences reported of up to 40%. They can be minimized by the use of prophylactic antibiotics, at least for the first six months after transplantation.

The effect of activated enzymes on the bladder mucosa can produce dysuria, particularly in the males' longer urethra.[85,86] The symptoms are easily controlled by placement of a urinary catheter for 2–4 weeks, allowing the bladder and urethral mucosa to heal. Inflammation of the urinary tract mucosa can also result in haematuria of a chronic nature. There is considerable variation in the reporting of the incidence of this problem which is probably a reflection of the definition of what is significant. Many units ignore intermittent haematuria which is present in perhaps as many as a third of successful recipients. Haematuria that results in clot retention and a need for transfusion is obviously of greater concern. These patients warrant cystoscopy to exclude the possibility of an anastomotic bleed or a transplant duodenal ulcer. Again, long-term urinary catheterisation is of benefit to many of these patients.

### Urine leak

The most troublesome of urinary tract complications is a leak of urine from around the anastomosis or the duodenal segment itself.[87] Commonly, the leak occurs from the staple line in what was the distal duodenum. Leaks elsewhere in the duodenum have been associated with cytomegalovirus infection. Often there is preceding chronic haematuria with the leaks occurring sometime in the first year of transplantation. Presentation is of lower abdominal pain in the suprapubic position and evidence of local peritonitis. Classically, the patient has an elevated serum amylase as a result of absorption from the peritoneal cavity, and symptoms and hyperamylasaemia are resolved by insertion of a urinary catheter. Often the leak is small or well contained by pelvic adhesions. Hence, demonstration of the leak by contrast studies is frequently unhelpful. The most useful study is an isotope-labelled cystogram with a late scan 2–4 h later.[88]

### Enteric conversion

The treatment of choice for the major urinary tract complications of duodenal leak, chronic haematuria and recurrent reflux pancreatitis is to convert the bladder-drained pancreas transplant into an enteric-drained pancreas transplant.[87,89] Some units report that as many as 30% of their patients have undergone so-called enteric conversion within three years of transplantation. The procedure can be performed with comparative safety, anastomosing an adjacent loop of small bowel to the duodenal segment. The success of the procedure begs a question of why not do this at time of initial transplantation. The simple answer is that the safety of the procedure is probably due to the fact that the patient is on baseline immunosuppression and has stable pancreas and renal graft function. Furthermore, the semi-elective procedure permits adequate bowel preparation.

**Glucose homeostasis**

Successful pancreas transplantation, by definition, means avoidance of the need for exogenous insulin. The need for even small amounts of insulin defines graft failure. For the recipients, this may be all that matters. For the diabetologists, success means the only form of treatment for IDDM patients that can produce normal haemoglobin $A^{1C}$ levels. However, it is unknown how perfect the glucose homeostasis needs to be to prevent further deterioration of neuropathy, retinopathy and recurrent nephropathy.

Many studies have shown that glucose haemostasis after SPK is not entirely normal.[90–92] Characteristically encountered least with systemic venous drainage are fasting hyperinsulinaemia, excessive insulin response to a glucose challenge when compared to a control group, and a delayed return to baseline levels (Fig. 8.6). In the long term, this may lead to islet exhaustion as is the case in Type II diabetics. In patients with impaired glucose tolerance, a reduced early phase insulin secretory response can be demonstrated. These patients usually also have reduced pancreatic exocrine secretion suggesting that the impaired response may follow perioperative influences such as ischaemia and the extent of rejection damage related to DR mismatches.

There are many reasons why pancreas transplant recipients may have an abnormal insulin response to a glucose challenge. First, most are

**Figure 8.6**
*Serum insulin in the response to an oral glucose tolerance test from 3 months to 4 years after pancreas transplantation with systemic venous drainage. The responses are compared to normal controls (mean ± 95% competence interval, hatched bars). From Nankivell BJ et al. Transplantation 1996; 61: 1705–11.*

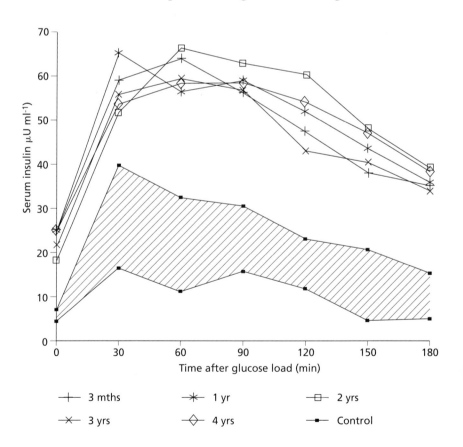

recipients of cyclosporin, tacrolimus or prednisolone – known diabeto-genic agents which increase peripheral resistance to insulin.[92] Secondly, the pancreas transplant is denervated which leads to the absence of suppression of insulin release by hyperinsulinaemia.[93] It remains to be determined which nerves are responsible for the insulin feedback but it is known that islets are innervated by sympathetic, parasympathetic and peptidergic nerves. Thirdly, experimental and clinical studies of portal venous drainage suggests that systemic delivery of insulin is the major reason for the hyperinsulinaemia observed after pancreas transplanta-tion.[46] Debate, however, continues as to which of these factors is the most important and whether or not hyperinsulinaemia is deleterious. The first two factors are unavoidable but the third, portal venous drainage, can at least be achieved. It remains to be seen whether the increased risk associated with pancreas portal vein anastomosis to a mesenteric vein is worth the advantage of lower fasting insulin levels.

**Effect on secondary complications of diabetes**

Despite the problems of increased risk of rejection, technical complica-tions specific to pancreas transplantation, and the abnormal insulin responses to a glucose challenge, improvement in quality of life after pancreas transplantation can be dramatic.[94,95] There is no longer the threat of hypoglycaemia and the shackles of the restrictive life style, and health risk from hyperglycaemia have been removed. For the patient, it is perhaps the single most important benefit of pancreas transplantation. As a group, the recipients of pancreas transplantation are exceptionally appreciative. They take their kidney for granted, but not the pancreas. Given the choice of a low morbidity KTA or a high morbidity SPK, the prospective recipients invariably opt for the latter, particularly after talking to other patients who have been successfully transplanted with a pancreas. Essentially, the prospective and actual recipients vote with their feet. Nevertheless, providing objective evidence of the advantages of SPK over KTA for insulin dependent diabetics is difficult and is limited to improved neuropathy and greater ability to function socially.

### Nephropathy

The principal reason for the Minneapolis group to consider SPK more than 30 years ago was to avoid recurrent diabetic nephropathy in the transplanted kidney.[10] Slowly but surely, evidence to support this hypothesis is accumulating.[96,97] Unfortunately, much of that evidence is cross-sectional in nature rather than a longitudinal biopsy study that includes a control group. There is little question that KTA for diabetics is associated with recurrent diabetic nephropathy and changes, both in function and histologically, can be demonstrated within two years of transplantation.[6,17,96] Not surprisingly, PTA cannot ameliorate estab-lished diabetic glomerular lesions in patients with their own kidneys.[16] Hence, PTA cannot be recommended for the treatment of the established lesions of diabetic nephropathy.

### Neuropathy

Studies of the effect of pancreas transplantation on autonomic and peripheral neuropathy provide the best objective evidence of the benefits of pancreas transplantation.[98–102] The first benefit experienced by the recipient, within months of pancreas transplantation, is the virtual disappearance of symptoms of postural hypotension. An echocardiography study which included a control group has demonstrated improved systolic and diastolic function of the heart which is reflected by less sudden death.[98] In a small group of patients, the Stockholm group have demonstrated improved nerve conduction up to eight years after SPK.[100] In comparison, KTA patients had an initial improvement in nerve conduction which might be expected with a reversal of the uraemia but no improvement thereafter. The Westmead group in a much larger longitudinal study demonstrated improvement in conduction velocity which was the primary reason for improved nerve conduction scores soon after transplantation (Fig. 8.7). More importantly, the group also demonstrated gradual sustained and late improvement in nerve action potential amplitudes which were consistent with axonal regeneration and partial reversal of diabetic neuropathy. Unfortunately, this improvement was only seen in patients with mild to moderate neuropathy at

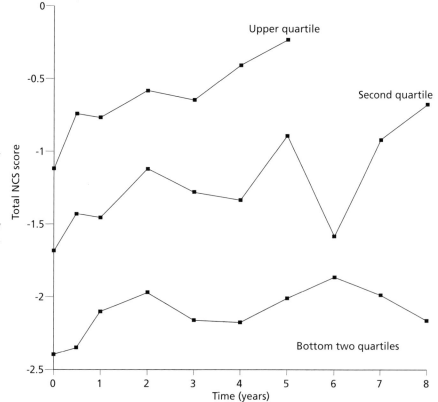

**Figure 8.7** *Total nerve conduction scored (NCS) according to time after SPK, stratified according to the severity of initial neuropathy. A zero score is normal, and increasing negative scores indicate greater neurological damage. The top line is the best quartile, the second line is moderate neurological damage designated by the second quartile, and the bottom line is the worst two quartiles combined. From Allen RDM et al. Transplantation 1997 (in press).*

time of transplantation and emphasises the need to offer pancreas transplantation early.

### Retinopathy

The effects of pancreas transplantation on retinopathy are difficult to quantitate for the reason that more than 75% of patients have had laser photocoagulation therapy prior to transplantation. One of the prerequisites for pancreas transplantation is stable retinopathy. Failure to observe this rule can increase the risk of haemorrhage and blindness during the not uncommon periods of anticoagulation and hypotension in the early post-transplant periods. Furthermore, visual acuity of pancreas transplant recipients can be affected by aggressive cataract formation associated with steroid therapy. The results of cataract surgery after transplantation are good and some of the reported improvement in visual acuity may relate to the resolution by surgery of cataracts that preceded transplantation.

### Macroangiopathy

A disappointing feature of pancreas transplantation has been the inability to prevent progressive macroangiopathy or large vessel disease. This is despite favourable effects of pancreas transplantation on the distribution and composition of plasma lipoproteins.[103] Evidence of progressive disease is based on the need for vascular intervention, amputation rates and increased carotid artery thickness.[104] A longitudinal study at Westmead has demonstrated progressive superficial femoral artery disease with 50% of legs at risk having significant progression of stenotic disease within five years of transplantation. Hence, it would seem that factors other than normalisation of glucose may be responsible. Hyperinsulinaemia is blamed but equally, the effect of chronic immunosuppressive therapy on glucose and free fatty acid metabolism could be involved.[105]

## Living-related pancreas transplantation

Before the widespread use of cyclosporin and in an attempt to increase the success rate of pancreas transplantation by reducing rejection, a living-related donor programme was commenced in Minneapolis in 1979.[10] Needless to say, prospective pancreas donor evaluation was done with care, ensuring the donors were at least 10 years older than the age of onset of diabetes in the recipient. In the subsequent five-year period to 1983, 36 of 89 pancreas transplants performed at that centre were from living-related donors. A variety of duct management techniques were used to cope with the donor pancreas segment. The best results were achieved in patients who previously had a kidney from the same donor. By 1994, 82 living-donor distal segment pancreas transplants had been performed in Minneapolis without donor operative mortality and preservation of the spleen in 95% of cases. Over a 16-year period to 1994, 31 sequential living donor segmental pancreas and kidney transplants had been performed with a one-year pancreas survival of 82%. It is therefore not surprising that the centre embarked on and was able to report the results of the first two successful simultaneous kidney and segmental pancreas transplants from living related donors.[106]

## Future prospects

Continuing concerns of hyperinsulinaemia and exocrine complications will dictate that greater numbers of portal venous drained pancreas transplants be performed, together with enteric drainage of the exocrine portion of the gland. However, the pancreas transplant surgeon, unless he or she has masochistic tendencies or a vested interest in vascularised pancreas transplantation, is most likely holding out for the procedure to be superseded by an alternative treatment option for insulin dependent diabetics. If genetic engineering of human cells to produce insulin cannot be achieved, the option of islet cell transplantation into the portal circulation is the most attractive option. Demand would require islet cell xenotransplantation, but the barriers to success remain daunting.[107,108] Until islet cell transplantation is achieved regularly and reproducibly, whole organ pancreas transplantation offers potential treatment for a group of patients who are otherwise notoriously difficult to manage.

### *Acknowledgement*

The author acknowledges the invaluable and expert assistance of Miss Melanie Reily in the preparation of this chapter.

## *References*

1. Nelson RG, Bennett PH, Beck GJ *et al*. Development and progression of renal disease in Pima Indians with non-insulin-dependent diabetes mellitus. N Engl J Med 1996; 335: 1636–41.
2. Reichard P, Nilsson B, Rosenqvist U. The effect of long-term intensified insulin treatment on the development of microvascular complications of diabetes mellitus. N Engl J Med 1993; 329: 304–9.
3. The Diabetes Control and Complications Trial Research Group. The effect of intensive treatment of diabetes on the development and progression of long term complications in insulin-dependent diabetes mellitus. N Engl J Med 1993; 329: 977–86.
4. Bojestig M, Arnqvist HJ, Hermansson G *et al*. Declining incidence of nephropathy in insulin-dependent diabetes mellitus. N Engl J Med 1994; 330: 5–18.
5. The Diabetes Control and Complications (DCCT) Research Group. Effect of intensive therapy on the development and progression of diabetic nephropathy in the Diabetes Control and Complications Trial. Kidney Int 1995; 47: 1708–20.
6. Najarian JS, Kaufman DB, Fryd DS *et al*. Long-term survival following kidney transplantation in 100 Type 1 diabetic patients. Transplantation 1989; 47: 106–13.
7. Ekberg H, Christensson A. Similar treatment success rate after renal transplantation in

diabetic and nondiabetic patients due to improved short and long-term diabetic patient survival. Transpl Int 1995; 9: 557–64.

8. Kelly WD, Lillehei RC, Merkel FK *et al.* Allotransplantation of the pancreas and duodenum along with the kidney in diabetic nephropathy. Surgery 1967; 61: 827–31.

9. Lillehei RC, Simmons RL, Najarian JS *et al.* Pancreatico-duodenal allotransplantation: experimental and clinical experience. Ann Surg 1970; 172: 405–36.

10. Sutherland DER, Gores PF, Farney AC *et al.* Evolution of kidney, pancreas, and islet transplantation for patients with diabetes at the University of Minnesota. Am J Surg 1993; 166: 456–91.

11. Dubernard JM, Monti LD, Faure JL *et al.* Report on 63 pancreas and kidney transplants in uremic diabetic patients. Transplant Proc 1986; 18: 1111–12.

12. Landgraf R, Landgraf-Leurs MMC, Burg D *et al.* Long-term follow-up of segmental pancreas transplantation in Type 1 diabetics. Transplant Proc 1986; 18: 1118.

13. Tyden G, Mellgren A, Brattstrom C *et al.* Stockholm experience with 32 combined renal and segmental pancreatic transplants. Transplant Proc 1986; 18: 1114.

14. Brekke IB, Dyrbekk D, Jakobsen A *et al.* Improved pancreas graft survival in combined pancreatic and renal transplantation. Transplant Proc 1986; 18: 1125.

15. Sollinger HW, Pirsch JD, D'Alessandro AM *et al.* Advantages of bladder drainage in pancreas transplantation: A personal view. Clin Transplant 1990; 4: 32–6.

16. Fioretto P, Mauer SM, Bilous RW *et al.* Effects of pancreas transplantation on glomerular structure in insulin-dependent diabetic patients with their own kidneys. Lancet 1993; 342: 1193–6.

17. Hariharan S, Smith RD, Viero R, First MR. Diabetic nephropathy after renal transplantation. Transplantation 1996; 62: 632–5.

18. Stratta RJ, Taylor RJ, Ozaki CF *et al.* A comparative analysis of results and morbidity in Type 1 diabetics undergoing pre-emptive versus post dialysis combined pancreas-kidney transplantation. Transplantation 1993; 55: 1097–1103.

19. Simultaneous kidney–pancreas transplantation versus kidney transplantation alone: patient survival, kidney graft survival, and post-transplant hospitalization. Am J Kidney Dis 1992; 20(Suppl. 2): 61–7.

20. Douzdjian V, Abecassis MM, Corry RJ *et al.* Simultaneous pancreas–kidney versus kidney-alone transplants in diabetics: increased risk of early cardiac death and acute rejection following pancreas transplants. Clin Transplant 1994; 8: 246–51.

21. Stratta RJ, Taylor RJ, Grune MT *et al.* Experience with protocol biopsies after solitary pancreas transplantation. Transplantation 1995; 60: 1431–7.

22. Stratta RJ, Taylor RJ, Ozaki CF *et al.* The analysis of benefit and risk of combined pancreatic and renal transplantation versus renal transplantation alone. Surg Gynecol Obstet 1993; 177: 163–71.

23. Manske CL, Wang Y, Rector T *et al.* Coronary revascularisation in insulin dependent diabetic patients with chronic renal failure. Lancet 1992; 340: 998–1002.

24. Bumgardner GL, Henry ML, Elkhammas E *et al.* Obesity as a risk factor after combined pancreas/kidney transplantation. Transplantation 1995; 60: 1426–30.

25. Stratta RJ, Taylor RJ, Wahl TO *et al.* Recipient selection and evaluation for vascularized pancreas transplantation. Transplantation 1993; 55: 1090–6.

26. Mizrahi SS, Jones JW, Bentley FR. Preparing for pancreas transplantation: Donor selection, retrieval technique, preservation, and back-table preparation. Transplant Rev 1996; 10: 1–12.

27. Squifflet JP. A quick technique for en bloc liver and pancreas procurement. Transpl Int 1996; 9: 520–1.

28. Kornblith PL, Boley SJ, Whitehouse BS. Anatomy of the splanchnic circulation. Surg Clin North Am 1992; 72: 1–6.

29. Mäkisalo H, Chaib E, Krokos N, Calne R. Hepatic arterial variations and liver related diseases of 100 consecutive donors. Transpl Int 1993; 6: 325–9.

30. Gruessner RW, Troppman C, Barroy B *et al.* Assessment of donor and recipient risk factors on pancreas transplant outcome. Transplant Proc 1994; 26: 437.

31. Nghiem DD, Corry RJ, Cottington EM. Function of simultaneous kidney and pancreas transplants from pediatric donors. Transplantation 1989; 47: 1075–9.

32. Dunn DL, Morel P, Schlumpf R *et al*. Evidence that combined procurement of pancreas and liver grafts does not affect transplant outcome. Transplantation 1991; 51: 150–7.

33. Imagawa DK, Olthoff KM, Yersiz H *et al*. Rapid en bloc technique for pancreas–liver procurement. Transplantation 1996; 61: 1605–9.

34. Shaffer D, Lewis WD, Jenkins RL, Monaco AP. Combined liver and whole pancreas procurement in donors with a replaced right hepatic artery. Surgery 1992; 175: 204–7.

35. Gores PF, Gillingham KJ, Dunn DL *et al*. Donor hyperglycaemia as a minor risk factor and immunologic variables as major risk factors for pancreas allograft loss in a multivariate analysis of a single institution's experience. Ann Surg 1992; 215: 217–23.

36. Masson F, Thicoipe M, Gin H *et al*. The endocrine pancreas in brain-dead donors. Transplantation 1993; 56: 363–7.

37. Wahlberg JA, Lover R, Landegaard L *et al*. 72-hour preservation of the canine pancreas. Transplantation 1987; 34: 5.

38. Sollinger HW, Vernon WB, D'Alessandro AM *et al*. Combined liver and pancreas procurement with Belzer-UW solution. Surgery 1989; 106: 685–91.

39. Nghiem DD, Cottington EM. Pancreatic flush injury in combined pancreas liver recovery. Transplant Int 1992; 5: 19–22.

40. Tyden G, Tibell A, Groth CG. Pancreaticoduodenal transplantation with enteric exocrine drainage: technical aspects. Clin Transplant 1991; 5: 36–9.

41. D'Alessandro AM, Sollinger HW, Stratta RJ *et al*. Comparison between duodenal button and duodenal segment in pancreas transplantation. Transplantation 1989; 47: 120–2.

42. Prieto M, Sutherland DER, Fernandez-Gruz L *et al*. Experimental and clinical experience with urine amylase monitoring for early diagnosis of rejection in pancreas transplantation. Transplantation 1987; 43: 73–9.

43. Barker RJ, Mayes JT, Schulak JA. Wound abscesses following retroperitoneal pancreas transplantation. Clin Transplant 1991; 5: 403–7.

44. Douzdjian V, Gugliuzza KK. The impact of midline versus transverse incisions on wound complications and outcome in simultaneous pancreas–kidney transplants: a retrospective analysis. Transpl Int 1996; 9: 62–7.

45. Muhlbacher F, Gnant MFX, Auinger M *et al*. Pancreatic venous drainage to the portal vein; a new method in human pancreas transplantation. Transplant Proc 1990; 22: 636–7.

46. Gaber OA, Shokouh-Amiri MH, Hathaway DK *et al*. Results of pancreas transplantation with portal venous and enteric drainage. Ann Surg 1995; 221: 613–24.

47. Corry RJ, Egidi MF, Shapiro R *et al*. Enteric drainage of pancreas transplants revisited. Transpl Proc 1995; 27: 3048–9.

48. Newell KA, Bruce DS, Cronin DC *et al*. Comparison of pancreas transplantation with portal venous and enteric exocrine drainage to the standard technique utilizing bladder drainage of exocrine secretions. Transplantation 1996; 62: 1353–6.

49. Yang HC, Gifford RRM, Dafoe DC *et al*. Arterial reconstruction of the pancreatic allograft for transplantation. Am J Surg 1991; 162: 262–4.

50. Nghiem DD. A technique for vascular reconstruction of pancreaticoduodenal allograft. A literature review and case report. Transpl Int 1995; 8: 411–13.

51. Fernandez-Cruz L, Astudillo E, Sanfey H *et al*. Combined whole pancreas and liver retrieval: comparison between Y-iliac graft and splenomesenteric anastomosis. Transplant Int 1992; 5: 54–6.

52. Nankivell BJ, Chapman JR, Bovington KJ *et al*. Clinical determinants of glucose homeostasis after pancreas transplantation. Transplantation 1996; 61: 1705–11.

53. Troppmann C, Gruessner AC, Papalois BE *et al*. Delayed endocrine pancreas graft function after simultaneous pancreas–kidney transplantation. Transplantation 1996; 61: 1323–30.

54. Tamsma JT, Schaapherder AFM, Van Bronswijk H *et al*. Islet cell hormone release immediately after human pancreatic transplantation. Transplantation 1993; 56: 1119–23.

55. Nankivell BJ, Allen RDM, Bell B *et al*. Factors affecting measurement of urinary amylase after bladder-drained pancreas transplantation. Clin Transplant 1991; 5: 392–7.
56. Cheung HAS, Sutherland DER, Gillingham KJ *et al*. Simultaneous pancreas kidney transplant versus kidney transplant alone in diabetic patients. Kidney Int 1992; 41: 924–9.
57. Schulak JA, Mayes JT, Hrick DE, Kidney transplantation in diabetic patients undergoing combined kidney–pancreas or kidney-only transplantation. Transplantation 1992; 53: 685–7.
58. Tesi RJ, Henry ML, Elkhammas EA *et al*. The frequency of rejection episodes after combined kidney–pancreas transplant – The impact of graft survival. Transplantation 1994; 58: 424–30.
59. Jones JW, Mizrahi SS, Bentley FR. Success and complications of pancreatic transplantation at one institution. Ann Surg 1996; 223: 757–64.
60. Hawthorne WJ, Allen RDM, Greenberg ML *et al*. Simultaneous pancreas and kidney transplant rejection: separate or synchronous events. Transplantation 1997; 63: 352–8.
61. Gruessner RW, Burke GW, Stratta R *et al*. A multicenter analysis of the first experience with FK506 for induction and rescue therapy after pancreas transplantation. Transplantation 1996; 61: 261–73.
62. Hawthorne WJ, Griffin AD, Lau H *et al*. Experimental hyperacute rejection in pancreas allotransplants. Transplantation 1996; 62: 324–9.
63. Gruessner RWG, Nakhleh R, Tzardis P *et al*. Differences in rejection grading after simultaneous pancreas and kidney transplantation in pigs. Transplantation 1994; 57: 1021–8.
64. Gruessner RWG, Sutherland DER. Clinical diagnosis in pancreatic allograft rejection. In Solez K, Racusen LC, Billingham ME (eds) Solid organ transplant rejection: mechanisms, pathology and diagnosis. New York: Marcel Dekker 1996, pp. 455–99.
65. Klassen DK, Hoehn-Saric EW, Weir MR *et al*. Isolated pancreas rejection in combined kidney pancreas transplantation. Transplantation 1996; 61: 974–7.
66. Allen RDM, Wilson TG, Grierson JM *et al*. Percutaneous biopsy of bladder drained pancreas transplants. Transplantation 1991; 51: 1213–16.
67. Elmer DS, Hathaway DK, Shokouh-Amiri H *et al*. The relationship of glucose disappearance rate ($k_G$) to acute pancreas allograft rejection. Transplantation 1994; 57: 1400–4.
68. Henry ML, Osei K, O'Dorisio TM *et al*. Concomitant reduction in urinary amylase and acute first-phase insulin release predict pancreatic allograft transplant rejection in type I diabetic recipients. Clin Transplant 1991; 5: 112–20.
69. Munn SR, Engen DE, Barr D *et al*. Differential diagnosis of hypoamylasuria in pancreas allograft recipients with urinary exocrine drainage. Transplantation 1990; 49: 359–62.
70. Benedetti E, Najarian JS, Gruessner AC *et al*. Correlation between cystoscopic biopsy results and hypoamylasuria in bladder-drained pancreas transplants. Surgery 1995; 118: 864–72.
71. Nghiem DD, Pancreatic allograft thrombosis: diagnostic and therapeutic importance of splenic venous flow velocity. Clin Transplant 1995; 9: 390–5.
72. Nelson NL, Largen PS, Stratta RJ *et al*. Pancreas allograft rejection: correlation of transduodenal core biopsy with Doppler resistive index. Radiology 1996; 200: 91–4.
73. Kuhr CS, Davis CL, Barr D *et al*. Use of ultrasound and cystoscopically guided pancreatic allograft biopsies and transabdominal renal allograft biopsies: safety and efficacy in kidney–pancreas transplant recipients. J Urol 1995; 153: 316–21.
74. Nakhleh RE. Pathology of pancreatic transplantation. In Solez K, Racusen LC, Billingham ME (eds) Solid organ transplant rejection: mechanisms, pathology and diagnosis. New York: Marcel Dekker, 1966, pp. 261–76.
75. Nakhleh RE, Sutherland DER. Pancreas rejection, significance of histopathologic findings with implications for classification of rejection. Am J Surg Pathol 1992; 16: 1098–107.
76. Allen RDM, Grierson JM, Ekberg H *et al*. Longitudinal histopathologic assessment of rejection after bladder-drained canine pancreas allograft transplantation. Am J Pathol 1991; 138: 303–12.
77. Drachenberg G, Klassen D, Bartlett S *et al*. Histologic grading of pancreas acute allograft rejection in percutaneous needle biopsies. Transplant Proc 1996; 28: 512–13.

78. Sutherland DER, Gruessner A. Long-term function (>5 years) of pancreas grafts from the international pancreas transplant registry database. Transplant Proc 1995; 27: 2977–80.

79. Tyden G, Reinholt FP, Sundkvist G, Bolinder J. Recurrence of autoimmune diabetes mellitus in recipients of cadaveric pancreatic grafts. N Engl J Med 1996; 335: 860–3.

80. Lumbreras C, Fernandez I, Velosa J et al. Infectious complications following pancreatic transplantation; incidence, microbiological and clinical characteristics, and outcome. Clin Infect Dis 1995; 20: 514–20.

81. Grewal HP, Garland L, Novak K et al. Risk factors for postimplantation pancreatitis and pancreatic thrombosis in pancreas transplant recipients. Transplantation 1993; 56: 609–12.

82. Fernandez-Cruz I, Sabater GR, Saenz A et al. Pancreas graft thrombosis: prompt diagnosis and immediate thrombectomy or re-transplantation. Clin Transplant 1993; 7: 230–4.

83. Douzdjian V, Abecassis MM, Cooper JL et al. Incidence, management and significance of surgical complications after pancreatic transplantation. Surgery 1993; 177: 451–6.

84. Sethi PS, Elkhammas EA, Pollifrone DL et al. Pre and post transplant urologic work-up in simultaneous kidney/pancreas transplant: preliminary results of an ongoing study. Transplant Proc 1995; 27: 3083–4.

85. Elkhammas EA, Henry ML, York JP et al. Pancreas transplantation and dysuria. J Urol 1994; 152: 881–3.

86. Ciancio G, Burke CW, Nery JR et al. Urethritis/dysuria after simultaneous pancreas–kidney transplantation. Clin Transplant 1996; 10: 67–70.

87. Sollinger HW, Messing EM, Eckhoff DE et al. Urological complications in 210 consecutive simultaneous pancreas–kidney transplants with bladder drainage. Ann Surg 1993; 218: 561–70.

88. Mouratidis B, Lomas F, Hurley B, Anastomotic leak of pancreatic transplants demonstrated by radionuclide cystography. Clin Nucl Med 1995; 20: 742–3.

89. Stephanian E, Gruessner RWG, Brayman KL et al. Conversion of exocrine secretions from bladder to enteric drainage in recipients of whole pancreaticoduodenal transplants. Ann Surg 1992; 216: 663–72.

90. Pfeffer F, Nauck MA, Benz S et al. Determinants of a normal (versus impaired) oral glucose tolerance after combined pancreas–kidney transplantation in IDDM patients. Diabetologia 1996; 39: 462–8.

91. Rooney DP, Robertson RP. Hepatic insulin resistance after pancreas transplantation in Type I diabetes. Diabetes 1996; 45: 134–8.

92. Hawthorne WJ, Griffin AD, Lau H et al. The effect of venous drainage on glucose homeostasis after experimental pancreas transplantation. Transplantation 1996; 62: 435–41.

93. Boden G, Chen X, DeSantis R et al. Evidence that suppression of insulin secretion by insulin itself is neurally mediated. Metabolism 1993; 42: 786–9.

94. Adang EMM, Engel GL, van Hooff JP, Kootstra G. Comparison before and after transplantation of pancreas–kidney and pancreas–kidney with loss of pancreas – A prospective controlled quality of life study. Transplantation 1996; 62: 754–8.

95. Milde FK, Hart LK, Zehr PS. Pancreatic transplantation. Impact on the quality of life of diabetic renal transplant recipients. Diabetes Care 1995; 18: 93–5.

96. Wilczek HE, Jaremko G, Tyden G, Groth CG. Evolution of diabetic nephropathy in kidney grafts. Transplantation 1995; 59: 51–7.

97. El-Gebely S, Hathaway DK, Elmer DS et al. An analysis of renal function in pancreas–kidney and diabetic kidney-alone recipients at two years following transplantation. Transplantation 1995; 59: 1410–15.

98. Gaber AO, El-Gebely S, Sugathan P et al. Early improvement in cardiac function occurs for pancreas–kidney but not diabetic kidney-alone transplant recipients. Transplantation 1995; 59: 1105–12.

99. Navarro X, Kennedy WR, Aeppli D, Sutherland DER. Neuropathy and mortality in diabetes: Influence of pancreas transplantation. Muscle Nerve 1996; 19: 1009–16.

100. Solders G, Tyden G, Tibell A et al. Improvement in nerve conduction 8 years after combined pancreatic and renal transplantation. Transplant Proc 1995; 27: 3091.

101. Laftavi MR, Chapuis F, Vial C et al. Diabetic polyneuropathy outcome after successful

pancreas transplantation: 1 to 9 year follow up. Transplant Proc 1995; 27: 1406–9.

102. Allen RD, Al Harbi IS, Morris J *et al*. Diabetic neuropathy after pancreas transplantation: determinants of recovery. Transplantation 1997; 63 (in press).

103. Foger B, Konigsrainer A, Ritsch A *et al*. Effects of pancreas transplantation on distribution and composition of plasma lipoproteins. Metabolism 1996; 45: 856–61.

104. Larsen JL, Lynch T, Al'Halawani M *et al*. Carotid intima-media thickness by ultrasound measurement in pancreas transplant candidates. Transplant Proc 1996; 27: 2996.

105. Luzi L, Groop LC, Perseghin G *et al*. Effect of pancreas transplantation on free fatty acid metabolism in uraemic IDDM patients. Diabetes 1996; 45: 354–60.

106. Gruessner RWG, Sutherland DER. Simultaneous kidney and segmental pancreas transplants from living related donors – the first two successful cases. Transplantation 1996; 61: 1265–8.

107. Kemp E. Xenotransplantation. J Int Med 1996; 239: 287–97.

108. Bach FH, Robson SC, Winkler H *et al*. Barriers to xenotransplantation. Nat Med 1995; 1: 869–73.

# 9 Pancreatic transplantation (islet cell)

*Reinhard G. Bretzel*

**Introduction**    Diabetes mellitus is the most common endocrine disease in Western countries. The estimated prevalence of insulin-dependent diabetes mellitus (IDDM) and non-insulin-dependent diabetes mellitus (NIDDM) world-wide was reported for 1994 as 11.5 million people and 98.9 million, respectively.[1] The authors expect more than a doubling of these prevalence rates by the year 2010 with 23.7 million people having IDDM and 215.6 million having NIDDM world-wide. At present, the incidence of diabetes mellitus in Europe is increasing, both for IDDM and NIDDM.[2,3] In Germany, the prevalence of IDDM patients younger than 40 years and of NIDDM patients is currently calculated to be 0.22% and 4.82%, respectively.[4,5] In the US, where the prevalence of diabetes is approximately 7% in adults, between 1987 and 1992 the total costs of diabetes more than quadrupled, from US\$ 20.4 billion to US\$ 91.8 billion, and the direct medical costs (US\$ 45.2 billion) alone represent 5.8% of the total personal health care expenditures in the US.[6]

People with diabetes are prone to many acute and chronic complications resulting in increased hospitalisations, disability and death. In particular, diabetic nephropathy, characterised by resistent proteinuria, hypertension and progressive loss of renal function, can develop with either IDDM or NIDDM. In the US, 30–40% of patients with IDDM and 10–40% of patients with NIDDM will develop nephropathy.[7] Once initiated, the course of diabetic nephropathy is one of progressive and relentless declining renal function, ending in chronic renal failure. It therefore comes as no surprise to any diabetologist and nephrologist to be told that diabetic nephropathy is now the commonest single cause of end-stage renal disease (ESRD). The most recent report of the United States Renal Data System[8] shows that, in 1992, 33.8% of all new patients accepted for renal replacement therapy were either IDDM or NIDDM patients,[8] and patients with diabetes and ESRD have a very low life expectancy, with a mean 5-year life expectancy of less than 20%.[9] However, a substantial number of patients with diabetic nephropathy die before reaching end-stage renal failure, since diabetic nephropathy confers an increased risk of macrovascular disease. A stratified random sample of almost 5000 diabetic patients aged 35–55 years participating in the WHO Multinational Study of Vascular Disease in Diabetes has been followed-up from 1975 to 1987. The recent report of the study clearly indicated that patients with both hypertension and proteinuria experienced a strikingly high mortality risk: 11-fold for men with IDDM and 18-fold for women with IDDM, and 5-fold for men with NIDDM and 8-fold for women with NIDDM.[10]

From clinical work it is accepted that poor glycaemic control is an important risk factor for the development of secondary complications.[11] It is, therefore, reasonable to propose that meticulous glycaemic control is important in prevention and delaying the progression of diabetic chronic complications. This has been best demonstrated by two prospective long-term studies.[12,13] These studies strongly suggest that tight control of blood glucose levels achieved by conventional intensive insulin treatment, self-blood glucose monitoring and patient education can significantly prevent the development and retard the progression of chronic complications of IDDM. However, the cost of this benefit was a threefold increase in the number of severe hypoglycaemic episodes, a significant increase of the body weight and dietary and other life-style restrictions affecting the quality of life.

By contrast, replacement of a patient's islets of Langerhans either by pancreas transplantation or by isolated islet transplantation is the only treatment of IDDM to achieve an insulin-independent, constant normoglycaemic state avoiding hypoglycaemic episodes.[14,15] The cost of this benefit is the need for immunosuppressive treatment of the recipient with all its potential risks. Thus, indications for pancreas or islet transplantation at present exist almost exclusively in patients with end-stage renal disease waiting on dialysis for a kidney graft or in diabetics with an established kidney graft; these patients are already obligated to receive immunosuppression. Pancreas transplants alone are primarily performed in highly selected non-uraemic patients with extreme problems of diabetes.[16] Recent studies have demonstrated that pancreas transplantation can delay the progression of diabetic secondary complications and probably prolong patient life expectancy.[17] Furthermore, there is no doubt that there is a dramatic improvement in quality of life.[18]

However, pancreas transplantation confers a certain risk and has its complications whereas islet transplantation is a rather minor procedure associated with only small, if any, risk.[17] Furthermore, islet transplantation offers the possibility to alter *in vitro* the islet immunogenicity and antigenicity, to induce an immunotolerance state or to encapsulate the islets so as to introduce only temporary immunosuppressive treatment of the recipient or to obviate the need for immunosuppression after islet allo- or xenotransplantation, the definite main attraction of islet transplantation.[17] The effectiveness of this concept was demonstrated in animal experiments and may be successfully transferred into the clinical situation.[19–21]

Unfortunately, islet isolation is still not as efficient as desired, and prevention of rejection of islet allografts appears to be even more difficult than prevention of pancreas allograft rejection.[22,23] However, insulin independence has been preserved with intraportal islet autotransplantation following total pancreatectomy for benign disease, and in this situation (no possibility of rejection) normoglycaemia can be maintained with a relatively small number of intrahepatic islets.[24-26] With the exception of one small preliminary trial with islet transplants alone, islet transplants in IDDM have been performed only simultaneously to, or after, kidney transplantations and this method is still a clinical investigational procedure. Nevertheless, the progress during the last three years has provided evidence that islet transplantation may, in principle, also establish insulin independence in IDDM patients, albeit prolonged insulin independence has been achieved in only a small number of cases.[27]

**Donor operation**

The criteria for selecting a pancreas donor for islet transplantation are similar to those for choosing a donor for whole pancreas organ transplantation, and exclusion criteria are listed in Table 9.1.

The technique of harvesting a pancreas is also the same as for whole organ grafting. Again, the pancreas must be treated extremely carefully in a no-touch way, and the spleen should be used for dissection and mobilisation of the gland. All vessels are ligated, electric cautery is avoided as much as possible and the capsule may not be disrupted. The pancreas is retrieved from the multiorgan donor, perfused with University of Wisconsin solution (UW-solution) after removal of heart, lung, liver and kidney. The organ is then shipped from donor centres to the isolation laboratory.

The impact of pre-organ donation factors on the outcome of islet isolation has been addressed elsewhere and recently studied in a small number of organ donors.[28] It appears that young (<21 years) donor age, low body mass index (<21), blood glucose levels above 10 mmol $l^{-1}$, and prolonged intensive care management are associated with significantly reduced or lower islet yields, whereas increased serum amylase levels are not associated with low islet yields.

**Table 9.1**  *Criteria for pancreatic islet donors*

| | |
|---|---|
| 1. Donor age (years) | 20–50 |
| 2. Donor weight (kg) | $\geqslant$ height (cm) − 100 |
| 3. Days on ICU | <7 |
| 4. Circulation | No hypotensive episodes with a subsequent increase of creatinine or transaminases >50% |
| 5. Blood glucose | <300 mg dl$^{-1}$ |
| 6. History | No alcohol or drug addiction |

ICU, intensive care unit.

Critical issues of human pancreas procurement are the warm ischaemia time, which should be as short as possible; an *in situ* vascular perfusion with cold UW-solution which appears superior to other solutions, e.g. Eurocollins; no overperfusion and no intrapancreatic venous hypertension; cold ischaemia time of no more than 12 h and, interestingly, no less than 2 h; and a well-preserved pancreatic capsule that allows subsequent intraductal collagenase distension.[29] At our islet isolation laboratory human pancreases are distended by inserting a catheter into the pancreatic duct and flushing with 5.0 mg ml$^{-1}$ collagenase dissolved in Hank's balanced salt solution (HBSS) at 24°C.

**Islet isolation and purification**

Islets are separated by an automated continuous digestion–filtration method as described by Ricordi *et al.*[30] (Fig. 9.1). In brief, the distended gland is placed in a stainless-steel digestion chamber (53 ml) connected to a tubing system and a peristaltic pump to fill the entire system with HBSS, passing a heat circuit to increase temperature progressively to a digestion temperature of 37–39°C for the human pancreas. Subsequently, the digestion chamber is set in vertical motion (300 oscillations min$^{-1}$) while the solution is recirculated (200 ml min$^{-1}$). During this first phase of digestion samples are taken to monitor the dissociation of the tissue. As soon as significant numbers of cleaved islets appear in the samples, the tubing system is opened and flushed with fresh HBSS also passing the heat circuit to maintain digestion temperature in the chamber. The suspension is then collected for further purification.

Purification of human islets is performed using a continuous gradient purification method. The linear continuous (500 mmol, 1070–1100 g/l) Ficoll–sodium diathrizoate (FSD) gradient is produced on a spinning Cobe 2991 centrifuge at 10°C using a commercially available gradient mixer according to the methods described by London *et al.*[31] The preformed gradient is top-layered during spinning with pancreatic digest dissolved in UW-solution. After centrifugation purified islet fractions are pooled for various quality controls.

**Assessment of human islet preparations and guidelines for islet quality control**

Several quality control measures need to be evaluated to ascertain whether an islet preparation merits transplantation into a patient. Parameters such as islet yield in terms of islet number and islet volume, islet purity, islet viability and islet sterility must be assessed. The most crucial point will be the transplantability, or what *in vitro* parameter best predicts the *in vivo* endocrine effect after islet transplantation.

### Islet number and volume

Based on calculations from historical and more recent work the average human pancreas, weighing 70 g, contains between 305 000 and

**Figure 9.1**
*Recirculation–*
*perfusion system for*
*digestion of*
*pancreatic tissue for*
*islet isolation. Phase 1:*
*digestion-perfusion;*
*phase 2: collection of*
*islet-rich suspension.*

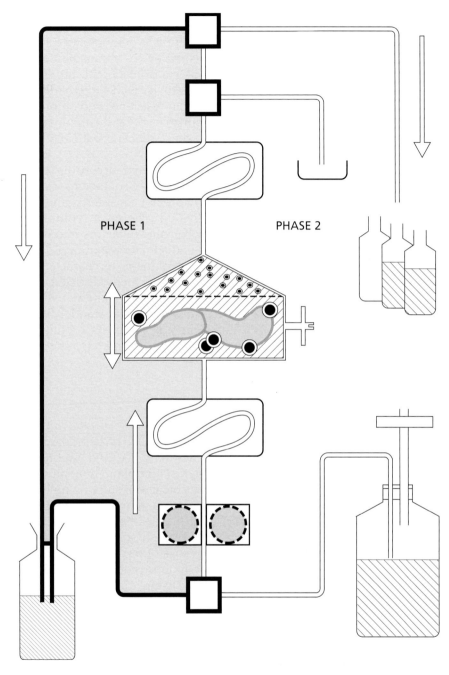

PHASE 1                    PHASE 2

1.5 million islets of 150 $\mu$m equivalent diameter (IEq), corresponding to between 0.5% and 4% of the total pancreatic volume. Where there is no insulin resistance (including diabetogenic immunosuppressive substances such as steroid and cyclosporin), a minimum of 265 000 human adult islets (3500/kg body weight of the recipient) may be enough to produce insulin independence with perfect metabolic control (fasting blood glucose, glycated haemoglobin, oral glucose test) after intraportal islet autotransplantation as demonstrated in patients after total pancreatectomy.[25] However, islets to be transplanted into type I diabetic patients will more often be confronted with an environment characterised by long-lasting glucose toxicity and microangiopathy (perhaps also in the portal system), insulin-resistance and autoimmune disease recurrence. It is, therefore, not surprising that the minimal number of islets required to render an adult type 1 diabetic patient insulin independent has been about 6000 IEq kg$^{-1}$.[32]

Stained islets are counted according to diameter classes using a calibrated grid in the eyepiece of the phase-contrast microscope. Particles smaller than 50 $\mu$m are not considered and islets larger than 350 $\mu$m are not further subdivided. The mean volume for each diameter class is assessed by using conversion factors into islets of 150 $\mu$m diameter. The total islet volume of the final preparation can also be estimated and may be a further useful parameter to characterise an islet preparation. The potential use of automated methods using computerised imaging analysers appears to be an attractive alternative to visual methods and may provide a more objective and standardised quantitative evaluation. Although this technology appears promising, it is expensive and too early in development to be proposed as a general standard.

## Islet purity

Transplanting highly purified islet preparations holds potential advantages of increased safety, reduced immunogenicity of the graft and probably improved islet implantation, although these issues have been questioned in light of new results obtained in a few diabetic patients using unpurified islet preparations.[33] However, reports of severe portal hypertension and three deaths resulting from intraportal autotransplantation of unpurified islet tissue should be a warning to use only highly purified (i.e. >80%) islet preparations for transplantation purposes.[34]

Large-scale, continuous-gradient centrifugation established on a Cobe 2991 cell processor using different or specifically designed gradient media is at present the preferred technique for rapid, effective and reproducible human islet purification.[31] When run in parallel, a test gradient for each individual pancreas may help to increase further the islet recovery and islet viability.

Although many approaches for determination of islet purity have been proposed (including insulin/amylase ratio and algebraic equations), each approach has inherent problems that result in assessment variabilities that are not easily controlled. Again, it is possible that the automatic methods using either specific stains or highly specific monoclonal antibodies will ultimately be used. For now, however, most investigators use the dithizone stain as an easy method to estimate the approximate degree of purity of the islets in any preparation.

## Islet viability and endocrine function

Islet viability is a critical factor that determines the outcome of transplantation. However, there is currently no entirely reliable method for standardising viability assessment. *In vitro* methods include light and electron microscopic morphology, fluorometric membrane integrity tests, colorimetric tests of mitochondrial function, and glucose-stimulated insulin release determined in static incubation or in continuous perifusion systems. Moreover, in studies of basic islet physiology and responses to pharmacological agents, insulin and protein synthesis and glucose utilisation have also been used to assess vital islet functions.

For rapid assessment of islet viability before islet transplantation, a fluorometric assay using inclusion and exclusion dyes that allows discrimination between intact and damaged cells is now widely used and recommended.[35] The combination of the inclusion and exclusion dyes acridine orange (AO) and propidium iodide (PI) have minimal background fluorescence, and when used in optimal concentrations (AO, 0.67 $\mu$mol l$^{-1}$; PI, 75 $\mu$mol l$^{-1}$), they stain living cells green and dead cells red. Using this fluorometric method, viable and non-viable whole islets may be differentiated, as may viable and non-viable components within an islet. The stability, cytotoxicity and reproducibility of the assay have been demonstrated on animal and human islets.

It is crucial that the isolated islets be shown not only to be viable but also able to respond appropriately to a glucose challenge. The standard in assessing *in vitro* islet endocrine function is the perifusion of islets with glucose, which provides a dynamic profile of the characteristics of glucose-mediated insulin release from prestored and newly synthesised insulin and of the ability of the islet endocrine cells to down-regulate insulin secretion after the glycaemic challenge is interrupted (return to baseline). Technical details have been described previously.[36]

Standards for reporting results of perifusion studies are critical for the accurate comparison of data. The absolute levels of insulin secretion during the prechallenge baseline period, the high glucose challenge and the last period of perifusion after return to low glucose concentration should be reported. The profile of insulin release is best reported as a plot that shows the release during the three consecutive periods.[37] Stimulation index estimated by determining the ratio between basal (last 15 min before high glucose and last 15 min after return to basal conditions) and stimulated insulin release (first 15 min and last 15 min of stimulation) identifies the secretory capacity but lacks details on basal insulin release, the quality of the biphasic response and return to basal secretion. However, *in vitro* insulin release does not necessarily predict *in vivo* transplant outcome, and the results of islet perifusion studies should therefore be interpreted with caution. Thus, cryopreserved rodent islets showed normal perifusion response but later failed to reverse diabetes, and vice versa, cryopreserved canine islets that failed to secrete insulin during perifusion induced normoglycaemia after autotransplantation. It has also been reported that a poor response from human islets during perifusion did not predict their *in vivo* function after transplantation.[38]

Therefore, the best index of viability is the ability of transplanted islets to withstand the rigours of engraftment in an ectopic site of a diabetic recipient until revascularisation is complete and to reverse diabetes in this recipient. *In vivo* endocrine function of human islets can be tested after transplantation (bioassay) of aliquots of the final islet preparation beneath the renal capsule of diabetic immunodeficient and athymic mouse or rat.[39]

## Islet sterility

Testing should start as usual with donor screening for viral antibodies (hepatitis A, B and C; human immunodeficiency viruses 1 and 2; cytomegalovirus). The demonstration that islets to be transplanted are free from bioburden risk is an important quality control test. This issue should be carefully considered because a period of tissue culture may amplify microbial contamination, and the induction of an immunosuppressed state in islet transplant recipients may render them susceptible to infections. It has been demonstrated that 42% of human donor pancreas had low level contaminants, usually of Gram-positive bacteria, and 15% had fungal contaminants.[40] During islet isolation, 97% of these contaminants are eliminated and only some new environmental contaminants are added, mostly fungal. However, holding the islets for 7 days and culturing the samples both at 24°C and at 37°C has prevented contaminated islet preparations from being transplanted into immunosuppressed recipients.[40] In contrast, other centres transplanting freshly isolated islets have reported septicaemia in two cases, whereas another centre observed no clinically apparent infection despite retrospectively demonstrable microbial contamination of the islet preparations.[41,42]

The various issues of the quality control programme suggested should serve as guidelines for investigators intending to initiate clinical islet

**Table 9.2** *Minimal requirements for islet preparation intended for clinical transplantation*

| | |
|---|---|
| ● Islet mass | >8000 IEq/kg body wt in type I diabetic recipient |
| | >3500 IEq/kg body wt in patients to be autotransplanted after pancreatectomy |
| ● Islet purity | >80% (percentage of the islet volume in the total cell volume) |
| ● Islet viability | >80% (assessed by a microfluorometric membrane integrity test) |
| ● Islet *in vitro* function | Documented biphasic response to a glucose challenge and return to baseline phenomenon |
| ● Islet culture | Exclusion of microbial contamination |

transplantation programmes. The main message should be that only an islet preparation with well-documented quantity, purity, viability, function and sterility (Table 9.2) before transplantation fulfils the criteria of transplantability and merits transplantation into a patient to mimic the complexity of the carbohydrate metabolism in normal subjects.

# Rejection of islet cells

Early studies with transplants of isolated adult islets have shown that islet allografts are highly susceptible to the recipient's immune mechanisms and will be destroyed within a few days after implantation. Some immunologically privileged properties have been ascribed to the portal venous bed or to the liver in mice and to the renal subcapsular space in rats. However, freshly isolated adult islet allografts are rejected rapidly if no measures are taken to prevent this event. Most of the classical techniques found to be successful for other organ allografts in rodents have been shown to suppress rejection of islet allografts to a much lesser degree. Furthermore, multiple factors such as heterogeneous combinations of donor–recipient pairs used, variability of donor source, the site of implantation/the number of islets transplanted and the lack of uniformity in the definition of rejection make it difficult to interpret and compare the results of the islet allograft experiments reported by various investigators. The rest of this chapter considers only those allograft experiments in which a sufficient number of islets were transplanted to an appropriate site with establishment of normoglycaemia, before rejection occurred.

## Induction of immunotolerance

First attempts with injection of donor antigens and antilymphocyte serum according to defined protocols resulted in a prolonged but not ultimate survival of islet allografts.[43] Difficulties appeared in using enhancement protocols with different sera. Very recently, rat islet allografts have been transplanted into the thymus of recipients treated with a single injection of antilymphocyte serum.[44] These islet allografts survived indefinitely. Interestingly, a state of donor-specific unresponsiveness was achieved by this procedure which permitted survival of a second donor-strain islet allograft transplanted to an extrathymic site. The authors speculated that maturation of precursors in a thymic microenvironment that is harbouring foreign alloantigen may induce the selective unresponsiveness. Tolerance to islet allografts was also induced in mice and rats by donor-specific bone marrow (intrathymic) inoculation.[45,46] In general, however, many experiments with the objective of inducing immunotolerance were performed under highly artificial conditions, and the specific protocols are not relevant to transplantation in humans. Therefore, another approach that has been demonstrated to prevent rejection in rodents is to manipulate the islet immunogenicity *in vitro* before transplantation.

### Immunoalteration

This concept starts with the hypothesis that antigen-presenting cells or passenger leukocytes within the graft are responsible for the induction of islet graft rejection exerted by the recipient's immunocompetent cells. The objective is to eliminate selectively donor immune cells or to suppress their antigen expression by various *in vitro* manipulations. It has been shown that prolonged *in vitro* culture at low temperature (22–24°C) or at 37°C, at high oxygen concentrations, by cryopreservation, by ultraviolet or gamma-irradiation and by pretreatment of islets with antibodies or substances directed to class-II antigens of the donor, significantly reduces islet allograft immunogenicity[47] (Table 9.3). These methods are very effective and may induce, with only a temporary immunosuppressive treatment of the recipient (e.g. a single dose of ALS on the day of operation) an indefinite prolongation of islet allograft survival across major histocompatibility barriers. Moreover, in our hands a combined cryopreservation–culture protocol induced a tremendous decrease in class II antigen expression in isolated adult rat pancreatic islets enabling long-term islet allograft survival in 80% of transplants across a major histocompatibility barrier without any immunosuppressive treatment of the recipient.

**Table 9.3** *Methods known for in vitro immunoalteration of isolated adult pancreatic islets. Adapted from Bretzel et al.[47]*

- Culture 22°C, 24°C, 37°C
- Hyperbaric/high oxygen culture
- Megaislets, pseudoislets
- UV-light
- Gamma-irradiation
- Cryopreservation
- Monoclonal antibodies against class-II antigen-bearing cells, dendritic cells or lymphocyte subpopulations
- Antineoplastic drugs
- Gangliosides

### Immunoisolation (micro- and macroencapsulation)

Immunoisolation of islets has been performed using an artificial membrane as a barrier to exclude cells or molecules able to mediate rejection while allowing flux of insulin and glucose. Millipore chambers and hollow fibres have been used with temporary but not long-term islet allograft and even limited xenograft survival.[48–50] More recently, our group provided evidence for the protection of islets inside the hollow fibre membrane from interleukin-1 toxicity.[51] Although the survival of isolated rat islets in hollow fibres lasts only a few weeks, there is one observation of much longer-lasting function of insulinoma cells or adult rat islets *in vivo*. More promising are the results using the technique of microencapsulation. In these cases, isolated islets are encapsulated in semipermeable hydrogels.[52] It has been clearly demonstrated that these microcapsules are permeable to glucose, arginine, theophylline and insulin, but they are nevertheless able to efficiently protect pancreatic beta cells against cytotoxic anti-islet antibodies and immunocompetent cells. A prolonged (more than 100 days) islet endocrine function has been observed *in vitro* as well as after allografting in spontaneously diabetic BB rats or in experimentally induced diabetic mice.[53] Unfortunately, the excellent *in vitro* function of encapsulated islets demonstrated by many groups has not been widely matched in transplantation experiments, with relatively few groups reporting long-term graft function. The major obstacle appears to be pericapsular fibrosis. Although recent advances in the purification of alginates provide a potential solution to this problem, much work is still required, particularly relating to the problems posed by spontaneously occurring long-term diabetic recipients. However, the ability to reduce greatly the size of the capsules and the advent of purified alginate preparations should allow considerable progress towards transplantation of encapsulated islets into type 1 diabetic patients.

## Prevention of diabetes recurrence

Islet grafts are susceptible to another immune-mediated pathway of destruction exerted by autoimmune mechanisms inherent in type I diabetes mellitus or in experimental models of spontaneously occurring diabetes mellitus in small animals (NOD mice; BB rats). Both experimental models and probably also the model of the immune-mediated low-dose streptozotocin diabetes mellitus provide an effective approach to study the mechanisms of recurrence of diabetes mellitus. This has been observed in non-immunosuppressed human recipients of pancreatic segment grafts from non-diabetic identical twin donors and also in the BB rat model when MHC-compatible islets had been grafted. Most of the studies show that the disease of the BB rats as well as diabetes recurrence after islet transplantation are restricted to the major histocompatibility complex (MHC) although two studies revealed conflicting results. Also in the natural model of autoimmune diabetes in non-obese diabetic mice (NOD) the pathogenic process seems to be MHC-restricted. Furthermore, isolated islets are more vulnerable to recurrent diabetes than vascularised pancreas grafts. The MHC-restriction of the disease would suggest that the problem of diabetes recurrence could be obviated by implanting an MHC-incompatible graft whose allograft immunogenicity had been controlled by pretreatment prior to allografting, since primed islet-autoreactive T cells would not recognise the islets. In fact, evidence to support this theory has been gathered by different measures in various studies using NOD mice and in the BB rat model. Considering recurrence of autoimmune diabetes, the survival of isolated islet grafts is highly dependent on the site of the islet implantation. Years ago it was shown that the kidney subcapsular space is superior to the liver, at least in rats. Our group recently confirmed that autoimmune damage has been avoided in all cases by adult rat pancreatic islet implantation into the renal subcapsular space of BB rats, where the islets survived indefinitely.[54] In principle, disease recurrence may also be prevented by any of the methods used for immunoisolation of islets by biomembrane constructs. But so far the results in spontaneous diabetes of small animals, in particular the NOD mouse, are not that encouraging and an additional recipient treatment (e.g. with monoclonal anti-CD4$^+$ antibodies) may be required. The interesting finding that in a model of natural diabetes, composite kidney–islet transplants function indefinitely suggests that the revascularising endothelium of the islets may play a role in resistance to autoimmune beta cell destruction.[55]

## Gene therapy to prevent islet graft rejection

Recent advances in molecular immunology have opened intriguing perspectives for improving the efficacy of islet transplantation by making use of gene therapeutic approaches.[56] Genetic modification of the islet cells may be a way of enhancing islet resistance to allogeneic, xenogeneic and autoimmune attacks by the host immune system. One approach may be to influence immune activation. T helper cells can respond to antigen presentation in different ways, such as ignorance, anergy, suppression or initiation of a destructive or non-destructive immune response. Th cells, and to some degree also cytotoxic lymphocytes (CTLs), can be divided in to those producing Th1 cytokines (such as interleukin-2 (IL-2) and interferon-$\gamma$ (IFN$\gamma$)), or Th2 cytokines (such as IL-4, IL-10, and transforming growth factor-$\beta$ (TGF-$\beta$)). At least in some rodent models (e.g. in autoimmune diabetes in NOD mice), destructive immune response is clearly correlated to the expression of Th1 cytokines, especially to IFN$\gamma$.[57] The current consensus seems to be that reduction of Th1 cytokine generation is the critical point for improving cell survival in conditions of autoimmune or allogeneic immune reactions, whether generation of Th2 cytokines may be activated or not. Th2 cell-response may be preliminary devised by nature for its antiparasite activity and additionally may be used as a last resort to inhibit exceeding Th1 activity. Despite much controversy in the details, it is accepted that T cells in the state of Th0 cells can be primed by the corresponding cytokines to become Th1 or Th2 cells, and after this differentiation usually do not revert to the opposite type. Therefore, a transitory transfection of cells to generate a local environment dominated by Th1 or Th2 cytokines may have permanent effects.[58] That gene transfer can be used to reduce the immunogenicity of islets was recently demonstrated by increased graft survival of cells genetically modified to express immunoregulatory molecules such as the adenovirus early region 3,[59] or viral IL-10 and TGF-$\beta$.[60–62]

Whereas transfection with cytokine DNAs is directed to modulate the initiation and amplification of the anti-islet immune response, transfection with DNA coding for Fas-ligand (FasL) is directed to paralyse anti-islet effector cells. Recently, programmed cell death (apoptosis) mediated via APO-1/Fas(CD95)–FasL interactions has been shown to play a pivotal role in maintaining immune-privileged sites where allogeneic or xenogeneic tissue grafts might enjoy prolonged survival probably avoiding life-long immunosuppressive treatment of the recipient.[56,63,64] FasL-expressing Sertoli cells prolonged discordant islet xenograft survival in mice, rats and monkeys.[65] Whether FasL abrogates preferentially CTLs, Th1 cells, or also APCs, awaits further analysis. In particular, it has not so far been documented that immunological privileged sites can be created simply by transducing FasL as postulated by Vaux.[56]

**Present clinical experience**

Significant advances have been made in the number and purity of islets that can be harvested from the human pancreas, thus encouraging several centres to resume clinical trials of islet cell transplantation in patients with IDDM.[30] Meanwhile, insulin independence has been achieved in several IDDM patients, at different institutions (Table 9.4).[66–71]

The aim of the author's human islet allograft programme started in 1992 at Giessen University Center, was twofold: first, to prevent early

**Table 9.4**   *Insulin independence after adult islet allotransplantation. Summary of cases to November 1995. *IEq: Islet equivalents (Δ 150 μm). Data source: ITR Giessen, 1996*

| | |
|---|---|
| • Number of cases (*n*) | 35 |
| • Institutions | Edmonton (2) |
| *n* = number of local | Giessen (3) |
| cases) | Miami (5) |
| | Miami–Pittsburgh (7) |
| | Milan (6) |
| | Milan–Nantes (2) |
| | Milan–Odense (1) |
| | Minneapolis (2) |
| | Paris (1) |
| | St. Louis (4) |
| | Verona-Padua (1) |
| | Zurich (1) |
| • Isolation method | Automated: 32; other: 3 |
| • IEq*/kg body wt | 6000 – 26 000 |
| • Purity | Unpurified: 3; Purified (40 to >90% islets): 32 |
| • Site of transplant | Liver: 33; Spleen: 1; Epiploic flap: 1 |
| • Recipient category | Islet after kidney: 11 Simultaneous islet–kidney: 9 Simultaneous islet–liver: 14 Islet transplant alone: 1 |
| • HLA | Random in nearly all cases |
| • Insulin treatment | Discontinued: <1 to 13 months post-transplant Resumed: 1 to >58 months post-transplant |

islet graft failure by optimised islet and recipient selection and improved transplant management and second, to identify better the reasons for potential graft failure by using characterised islets from a single donor. Experimental data suggest that strict metabolic control can lessen the number of islets required to reverse diabetes[72,73] and that maintaining a period of near-normoglycaemia after islet transplantation enhances the performance of an islet graft that would otherwise be expected to fail.[74] Therefore, we have introduced biostator-controlled or conventional intravenous insulin treatment and total parenteral nutrition in order to achieve tight blood glucose control both in the peripheral and in the portal circulation.[75] In addition, more technically and immunologically related features were part of the new protocol.[75]

### Islet after kidney (IAK) or simultaneous islet kidney (SIK) transplants

Between November 1992 and February 1996, islet allotransplantations were performed at our centre in 22 C-peptide negative IDDM patients of two different categories: previously or simultaneously kidney grafted patients (IAK, $n=14$; SIK $n=8$). Primary islet graft function (C-peptide secretion; CP) was established in all recipients. In all recipient groups, the islets were embolised into the liver after percutaneous–transhepatic catheter injection using local anaesthesia (Fig. 9.2). Ongoing islet graft function (basal CP $> 0.5$ ng ml$^{-1}$ after three months) was demonstrated in 7/14 IAK recipients and 7/8 SIK recipients, respectively.

**Figure 9.2** *X-ray imaging of a catheter transhepatically placed into the portal venous system in local anaesthesia for islet implantation.*

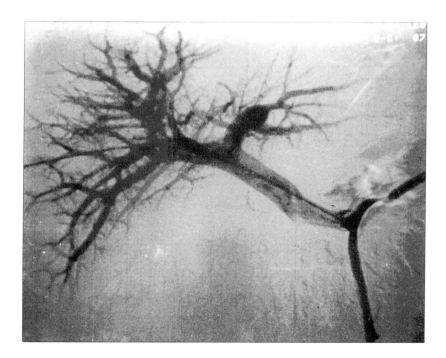

One patient of the IAK group, a 37-year-old woman, achieved insulin independence on day 400 after transplantation of islets derived from a single donor pancreas (Fig. 9.3). She is now insulin-independent for more than 2.5 years. Meanwhile, two further IAK recipients achieved insulin independence, eight to twelve months post transplant. To date, two of the SIK recipients have achieved insulin independence, 10 and 12 months after islet transplantation, respectively. Taken together, five islet allograft

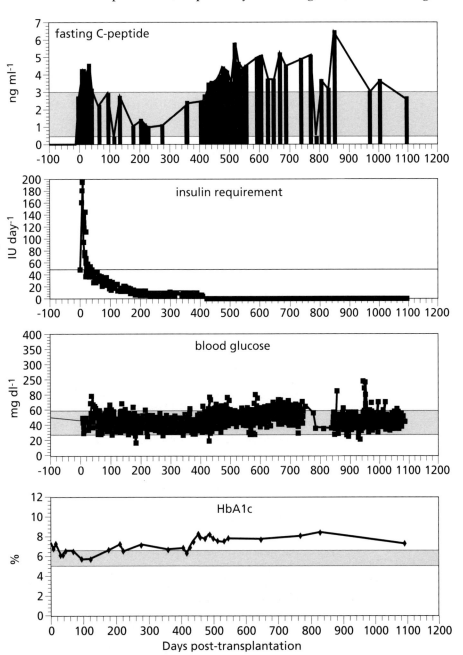

**Figure 9.3**  *Basal plasma C-peptide concentrations, daily insulin requirement, daily blood glucose profile and glycated haemoglobin A1c concentrations in an islet allograft type I diabetic recipient. Note insulin independence from 400 days after islet transplantation onwards. Shaded areas normal ranges.*

recipients have achieved insulin independence so far. In the remaining ten cases (IAK and SIK) with ongoing function (as defined by significant basal C-peptide release) a marked reduction of daily insulin requirement and reasonably good metabolic control was observed.

As far as overall complications are concerned, 7/22 of our islet transplanted patients experienced cytomegalovirus disease but were successfully treated with ganciclovir. One patient developed local herpes zoster infection and was also successfully treated. In two cases, subcapsular liver haemorrhage was observed but spontaneously resorbed. Portal hypertension was not observed in any case. No patient developed kidney graft failure even in case of islet graft loss.

The fact that the majority of islet transplant recipients remained insulin-dependent although many have near-normal or normal CP levels, may be explained in part by the insulin resistance observed in long-standing IDDM patients and by the treatment with potentially diabetogenic immunosuppressive drugs. To assess this, we have recently studied in a series of 15 allogeneic islet transplanted IDDM patients, transplanted either at the Milan Centre or at Giessen, the basal hepatic glucose production and the whole body glucose homeostasis and insulin action in comparison to a group of non-diabetic patients with chronic uveitis on the same immunosuppressive regimen.[76] We found that islet transplanted patients without optimal graft function have a higher basal hepatic glucose production (HGP) and a normal hepatic glucose production with a functioning graft.

However, even in case of functioning islet grafts, tissue glucose disposal was improved but still significantly different from normal controls. In a recent analysis on a single patient, near-normal insulin sensitivity index and C-peptide levels but continued insulin dependence have also been described after combined kidney–islet transplantation.[77] Furthermore, lack of success may also be ascribed to a significant loss of islets primarily not engrafted.

The definition of success should additionally include other indices of metabolic control. Islet transplants have resulted in C-peptide secretion and normalisation of HbA1c levels with no episodes of hypoglycaemia for periods of over four years. By contrast, this level of metabolic improvement, without the risk of hypoglycaemia is only achievable in less than 5% of patients with IDDM who receive intensive insulin treatment with multiple daily insulin injections and frequent measurements of capillary glucose in combination with diet and exercise, as reported in the Diabetes Control and Complications Trial Research Group.[12] An islet transplant that does not allow complete withdrawal of exogenous insulin, but results in continued C-peptide secretion, may be beneficial, too. In a prospective study, a three-month course of subcutaneous C-peptide administered to patients with IDDM ameliorated diabetic nephropathy and autonomic neuropathy.[78] These findings may become increasingly important when defining the indications for intensive insulin therapy, islet transplantation, and pancreas transplantation, respectively, in IDDM patients who have become incapacitated due to extremely labile diabetes (e.g. recurrent episodes of life-threatening severe hypoglycaemia).[79] Interestingly, successful pancreas transplants have been shown to improve the quality of life in previously diabetic recipients[80] and it is anticipated that a successful islet transplant would do the same. In addition, islet transplantation is associated with a lower incidence (nearly zero) of surgical morbidity. The challenge is to increase the success rate of islet transplants to that of pancreas transplants (currently 75% insulin independence rate at one year).[81]

According to the International Islet Transplant Registry (ITR), held at our institution in Giessen, from 1974 until 28 November, 1995, about 300 adult islet transplants had been performed at about 50 institutions world-wide in three different recipient categories. (1) Islet autografts to prevent diabetes in patients after pancreatectomy. These were patients with intractable pain from small duct chronic pancreatitis or failed drainage procedure, for whom total or near-total pancreatectomy appears to be the only treatment option. (2) Islet allografts to prevent diabetes in pancreatectomised recipients. In these cases islets have been implanted into simultaneously transplanted liver, following upper abdominal exenteration in patients suffering from primary or secondary hepatobiliary malignancies. (3) Islet allografts in IDDM recipients previously or simultaneously kidney-transplanted and already obligated for this reason to immunosuppression. Insulin independence after one year was achieved in 72% of the islet autograft pancreatectomised recipients and in 42% of islet allograft pancreatectomised recipients, respectively. However, insulin independence in IDDM patients was achieved in only 8% of cases. From this analysis of the Islet Transplant Registry (Fig. 9.4) and published remarkable results of islet autotransplantation[82] it becomes clear that (1) technical factors can be overcome;

**Figure 9.4**   *Insulin independence following islet transplantations in patients of different recipient categories. PIDM-Auto: autotransplantation in pancreatectomy-induced diabetes mellitus; PIDM-Allo: allotransplantations in pancreatectomy-induced diabetes mellitus; IDDM-Allo: allotransplantations in insulin-dependent-diabetes mellitus. Data source: ITR Giessen (1996).*

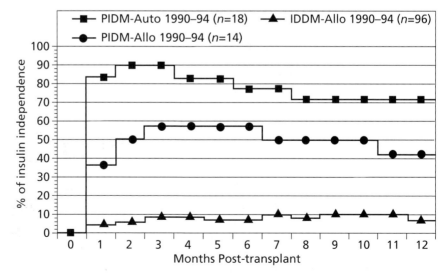

(2) the liver as an implantation site does not preclude maintenance of islet graft function as the experience with intraportal islet autografts in pancreatectomised dogs suggested;[83] (3) islets are apparently subjected both to allograft rejection[84] and to diabetes-specific factors including autoimmune destruction after clinical islet transplants[85,86] and even after whole pancreas gland transplantation under conventional immuno-suppression.[87]

The failure of islet allotransplantation consistently to establish insulin independence in IDDM patients may be attributed to another three primary obstacles: engraftment of an insufficient number of islets; toxic effects of current immunosuppressive drugs on islets, and lack of an appropriate rejection marker. It is becoming more and more appreciated that the relevant quantity of islets required to reverse diabetes is the amount of islet tissue effectively engrafted rather than the number of islets transplanted.[80] Rodent studies indicated that only about 25–50% of the islet mass originally transplanted engrafted and survived.[88] Early islet destruction and dysfunction is not mediated by classical T cell-mediated allograft rejection mechanisms which take 4–8 days to be manifested. Accumulating evidence suggests that early islet dysfunction/destruction are primarily mediated by macrophages or their by-products such as reactive oxygen intermediates, proinflammatory cytokines and nitric oxide. Islets are either destroyed, or their function is inhibited until classic T cell-mediated rejection ensues.[89–91] The low levels of enzymes which protect other cell types from free radical injury explain the specific susceptibility of islet beta-cells to early inflammatory mediators.[92,93] It appears that even when effective primary engraftment took place and rejection is prevented, islet function in immunosuppressed patients may be inadequate due to the diabetogenic side effects of currently used immunosuppression. The combination of cyclosporin, azathioprine and prednisone is associated with the development of abnormal glucose metabolism in up to 20% of non-diabetic kidney transplant recipients.[94] In order to maintain normoglycaemia, kidney transplant recipients on triple immunosuppressive therapy must increase insulin secretion 2.5 times.[95] This may not matter when there is a normal beta-cell mass as in patients with a whole pancreas transplant. However, a marginal mass of transplanted/engrafted islets cannot meet this demand. The diabetogenic effect of triple immunotherapy is largely ascribed to prednisone which is known to cause insulin resistance, and in part to cyclosporin which is known to inhibit insulin secretion.[96] The diabetogenic effect of prednisone and cyclosporin may be even synergistic and the incidence of post-transplant diabetes is significantly increased in patients receiving prednisone, cyclosporin and azathioprine in contrast to patients only on prednisone/azathioprine.[94]

## The future of islet transplantation

A revision of current concepts seems imperative if substantial progress is to be attained in clinical islet transplantation in IDDM patients in the not-too-distant future. At present, there are six centres, four in the United

**Table 9.5**   *Centres with > 10 islet transplantations in type 1 diabetic patients, 1990–95. Data source: ITR Giessen, 1996*

| Institution | No. of cases |
| --- | --- |
| • Minneapolis | 26 |
| • Giessen | 23 |
| • Pittsburgh | 22 |
| • Milan | 20 |
| • Miami | 14 |
| • St. Louis | 13 |

States and two in Europe, with experience of more than 10 islet transplants in IDDM patients performed between 1990 and 1995 (Table 9.5). These centres have used different protocols to allotransplant islets in diabetic patients either after or simultaneously with a kidney transplant. Their experiences are that at least three issues deserve particular attention: (1) more sensitive measures for monitoring islet cell grafts are needed; (2) means to control non-specific inflammatory damage have to be elaborated and (3) the use of immunomodulated islets may help to avoid the potential risk of adding other immunosuppressive drugs to the baseline immunosuppression of kidney-transplanted IDDM patients.

## Pancreas whole organ graft or islet graft?

The main attraction of islet transplantation is the potential to avoid chronic immunosuppression since islet transplantation in contrast to pancreas organ transplantation offers the possibility to alter *in vitro* the islet immunogenicity and antigenicity or to encapsulate the islets so as to introduce only temporary immunosuppressive treatment of the recipient, or even to obviate the need for immunosuppression after islet allo- or xenotransplantation.[17] Moreover, islet transplantation is a rather simple procedure associated with only minor risks, if any.[17] In this case, the indications for islet but not pancreas transplantation may be extended to islet transplants alone in non-uraemic IDDM patients (Fig. 9.5).

## Preliminary results in clinical islet transplants alone (ITA)

In 1995, for the first time world-wide, allogeneic islet transplants alone were performed at Giessen Islet Centre in five patients with hypoglycaemia unawareness and/or defect counterregulation. In this series of clinical islet transplants a temporary immunosuppressive protocol including anti-CD4 antibody treatment[97,98] together with cyclosporin was used. Islets were embolised into the liver after percutaneous-transhepatic catheter injection in local anaesthesia and peritransplant management was quite the same as in our SIK and IAK cases.

During the transient (four weeks) immunosuppressive treatment in these five non-uraemic IDDM patients without residual C-peptide secretion, re-establishment of C-peptide secretion was observed in all

**Figure 9.5**
*Pathogenesis and natural course of type I diabetes mellitus and transplantation. SPK: simultaneous-pancreas–kidney transplantation; PAK: pancreas-after-kidney transplantation; SIK: simultaneous-islet-kidney transplantation; IAK: islet-after-kidney transplantation; ITA: islet-transplant-alone. The latter offering the possibility to transplant patients before developing diabetic secondary complications and end-stage renal disease. [1]Death from acute complications; [2]Death from secondary vascular complications (myocardial infarction and stroke).*

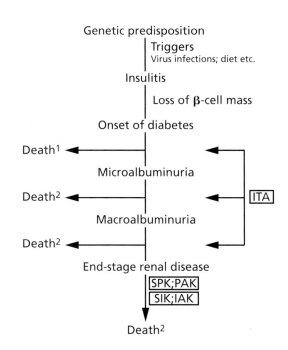

cases. One patient achieved insulin independence for two weeks and two patients could significantly reduce their daily insulin dosage to four units per day. In two patients islet graft loss was observed despite immunosuppressive treatment whereas in the other three patients islet graft function was lost after withdrawal of immunosuppressive drugs after four weeks.

As far as the clinical outcome is concerned, we observed in three of these patients re-tested with hyperinsulinaemic–hypoglycaemic clamp techniques and cognitive function tests, a restitution of hypoglycaemia awareness, an improved adrenaline counterregulation, and an adequate suppression during insulin-induced hypoglycaemia of endogenous insulin secreted by the grafted islets but no restitution of glucagon counterregulation, probably due to an inhibitory effect of the hepatic site of implantation on glucagon secretion of the islet graft.[99,100]

The mediator between islets engrafted and amelioration of hypoglycaemia awareness/counter regulation may be C-peptide provided by the transplant, since it has been most recently demonstrated that C-peptide improves autonomic nerve function in IDDM patients by an intravenous infusion over 3 h.[101] However, further studies in islet transplant recipients are needed to evaluate this hypothesis. In contrast to hypoglycaemia-prevention studies,[102] the secretory response of adrenaline largely recovers even in long-standing IDDM patients suggesting a beneficial effect of C-peptide. Additionally, autonomic warning symptoms improve, which both make it less likely that severe hypoglycaemia occurs even if insulin independence is not achieved. We therefore propose from a clinician's standpoint, that intraportal islet transplantation should be considered as a treatment in selected IDDM patients with recurrent episodes of severe hypoglycaemia refractory to intensive patient education, frequent self-monitoring of blood glucose levels and safe treatment goals. The final message of this first clinical experiment on islet transplants alone in non-uraemic IDDM patients may be that it is possible to achieve C-peptide secretion, and even insulin independence by using temporary immunosuppressive treatment.

### Islet xenotransplantation

Provided the problems with islet graft rejection are solved and islet transplantation becomes widely applied to the treatment of diabetes, the supply of human pancreases will not suffice. Since porcine insulin substitutes for human insulin, pig islets offer an attractive alternative. Transplanted islets presumably become vascularised by host vessels. Thus, hyperacute rejection as seen with vascularising xenograft may not occur after pig-to-human islet transplantation. Also, it is highly likely that the pig islets will be able to perform their physiological function when residing in humans.

There are important questions about whether these islets should come from fetal, neonatal or adult pigs. There are also difficult questions about what steps must be taken to control the discordant xenograft rejection process that will occur, with the main strategies being immunobarrier devices, immunosuppressive drugs and manoeuvres that might induce tolerance.

In March 1995, some 50 investigators from ten different countries gathered for the First International Workshop on Pig-To-Man Islet Transplantation, held at the Nobel Forum at the Karolinska Institute in Stockholm, Sweden. The first day of the workshop was devoted to production and quality control of porcine islets; the second day was spent discussing the problems of xenorejection as it applies to xenografts in general and xenoislets in particular. The workshop ended with evidence that islet xenotransplantation in diabetic patients has a much more realistic future.[103]

To conclude, islet transplantation will probably supersede pancreas transplantation as the method of endocrine replacement therapy and may be extended to non-uraemic IDDM patients including diabetic children. This group of patients is the ultimate target group for the islet transplant concept.

## References

1. Zimmet P, McCarthy D. The NIDDM epidemic: global estimates and projections – a look into the crystal ball. IDF Bull 1995; 40: 8–16.
2. Bingley PJ, Gale EAM. Rising incidence of IDDM in Europe. Diabetes Care 1989; 12: 289–95.
3. Pozza G, Garancini P, Gallus G. Prevalence and incidence of NIDDM. In: Williams R, Papoz L, Fuller J (eds) Diabetes in Europe. London: John Libbey, 1994, pp. 21–38.
4. Hauner H, von Ferber L, Köster I. Prävalenz und ambulante Versorgung insulinbehandelter Diabetiker im Alter unter 40 Jahren. Eine

Analyse von Krankenkassendaten der AOK Dortmund. Diab Stoffw 1996; 5: 101–6.

5. Hauner H, von Ferber L, Köster I. Schätzung der Diabeteshäufigkeit in der Bundesrepublik Deutschland anhand von Krankenkassendaten. Dtsch Med Wochenschr 1992; 117: 645–50.

6. American Diabetes Association. Direct and indirect costs of diabetes in the United States in 1992. Alexandria, VA, American Diabetes Association, 1993.

7. Tuttle KR, Stein JH, De Fronzo RA. The natural history of diabetic nephropathy. Semin Nephrol 1990; 10: 185–93.

8. US Renal Data System. USRDS 1994 Annual Data Report. Incidence and causes of treated renal disease. Am J Kid Dis 1994; 24 (suppl 2): S48–S56.

9. The National Institutes of Health, The National Institute of Diabetes and Digestive and Kidney Diseases, Division of Kidney, Urologic and Hematologic Disease: United States Renal Data System, 1993, Annual Data Report. March 1993, pp. 55–67.

10. Wang SL, Head J, Stevens L, Fuller JH, World Health Organisation Multinational Study Group: Excess mortality and its relation to hypertension and proteinuria in diabetic patients. The World Health Organisation Multinational Study of Vascular Disease in Diabetes. Diabetes Care 1996; 19: 305–12.

11. Hansen KF, Dahl-Jorgensen K, Lauritzen T, Feld-Rasmussen, Bircman-Hansen O, Deckert T. Diabetic control and microvascular complications: the near normoglycemic experience. Diabetologia 1986; 29: 677–84.

12. The Diabetes Control and Complications Trial Research Group. The effect of intensive treatment of diabetes on the development and progression of long-term complications in insulin-dependent diabetes mellitus. N Engl J Med 1993; 329: 977–86.

13. Reichart P, Nilsson BY, Rosenquist U. The effect of long-term intensified insulin treatment on the development of microvascular complications of diabetes mellitus. N Engl J Med 1993; 329: 304–9.

14. Sutherland DER. Pancreatic transplantation. An update. Diab Rev 1993; 1: 152–65.

15. Bretzel RG, Browatzki CC, Schultz A et al. Clinical islet transplantation – report of the Islet Transplant Registry and the Giessen center experience. Diab Stoffw 1993; 2: 378–90.

16. Sutherland DER, Kendall DM, Moudry KC et al. Pancreas transplantation in nonuremic, type I diabetic recipients. Surgery 1988; 104: 453–63.

17. American Diabetes Association (ADA). Pancreas transplantation for patients with diabetes mellitus. Diabetes Care 1992; 15: 1668–72.

18. Zehrer CL, Gross CR. Quality of life of pancreas transplant recipients. Diabetologia 1991; 34 suppl 1: S145–9.

19. Federlin KF, Bretzel RG. The effect of islet transplantation on complications in experimental diabetes of the rat. World J Surg 1984; 8: 169–78.

20. Lacy PE. Status of islet cell transplantation. Diab Rev 1993; 1: 76–92.

21. Hering BJ, Browatzki CC, Schultz A et al. Clinical islet transplantation – registry report, accomplishments in the past and future research needs. Cell Transplant 1993; 2: 269–82.

22. Ricordi C, Hering BJ, London NJM et al. Islet isolation assessment. In: Ricordi C (ed) Pancreatic islet cell transplantation. Austin: Landes, 1992, pp. 132–42.

23. Ricordi C, Tzakis AG, Carroll PB et al. Human islet isolation and allotransplantation in 22 consecutive cases. Transplantation 1992; 53: 407–14.

24. Farney AC, Najarian JS, Nakhleh RE et al. Autotransplantation of dispersed pancreatic islet tissue combined with total or near-total pancreatectomy for treatment of chronic pancreatitis. Surgery 1991; 110: 427–39.

25. Pyzdrowski KL, Kendall DM, Halter JB, Nakleh RE, Sutherland DE, Robertson RP. Preserved insulin secretion and insulin independence in recipients of islet autografts. N Engl J Med 1992; 327: 220–6.

26. Farney AC, Najarian JS, Nakhleh RE et al. Long-term function of islet autotransplants. Transplant Proc 1992; 24: 969–71.

27. Federlin KF, Bretzel RG, Hering BJ. Islet transplantation: state-of-the-art. Diab News 1994; 15: 6–8.

28. Brandhorst D, Hering BJ, Brandhorst H, Federlin K, Bretzel RG. Influence of donor data and organ procurement on human islet isolation. Transplant Proc 1994; 26: 592–3.

29. Ricordi C, Mazzaferro V, Casavilla A *et al.* Pancreas procurement from multiorgan donors for islet isolation. Diab Nutr Metab 1992; 5 suppl 1: 39.

30. Ricordi C, Lacy PE, Finke E, Olack B, Scharp DW: Automated method for isolation of human pancreatic islets. Diabetes 1988; 37: 413–20.

31. London NJ, Robertson GSM, Chadwick D *et al.* Purification of human pancreatic islets by large-scale continuous density gradient centrifugation. Horm Metab Res 1993; 25: 61.

32. Bretzel RG, Hering BJ, Brandhorst D *et al.* Insulin independence in type 1 diabetes achieved by intraportal transplantation of purified pancreatic islets. Diabetologia 1994; 37 suppl 1: A38.

33. Gray DW. The role of exocrine tissue in pancreatic islet transplantation. Transplant Int 1989; 2: 41–5.

34. Memsic L, Busuttil RW, Traverso LW. Bleeding esophageal varices and portal vein thrombosis after pancreatic mixed-cell autotransplantation. Surgery 1984; 95: 238–42.

35. London NJM, Contractor H, Lake SP *et al.* A microfluorometric viability assay for isolated human and rat islets of Langerhans. Diab Res 1989; 12: 141–9.

36. Bretzel RG, Alejandro R, Hering, BJ *et al.* Clinical islet transplantation: guidelines for islet quality control. Transplant Proc 1994; 26: 388–92.

37. Warnock GL, Ellis D, Rajotte RV *et al.* Studies of the isolation and viability of human islets of Langerhans. Transplantation 1988; 45: 957–63.

38. Socci C, Davalli AM, Vignali A *et al.* Evidence of *in vivo* human islet graft function despite a weak response to *in vitro* function. Transplant Proc 1992; 24: 3056–7.

39. Lake SP, Chamberlain J, Bassett PD *et al.* Successful reversal of diabetes in nude rats by transplantation of isolated adult human islets of Langerhans. Diabetes 1989; 38: 244–8.

40. Scharp DW, Lacy PE, McLear M *et al.* The bioburden of 590 consecutive human pancreata for islet transplant research. Transplant Proc 1992; 24: 974–5.

41. Warnock GL, Lakey JRT, Taylor GD *et al.* Microbial studies of a tissue bank of cryopreserved human islet cells. Transplant Proc 1994; 26: 827.

42. Casanova D, Xenos E, Lloveras JJ *et al.* Comparison of human islet isolation from the stored and nonstored pancreas with two different protocols using UW solution. Transplant Proc 1994; 26: 588.

43. Vialettes B, Sutherland DER, Payne WA *et al.* Synergistic effect of donor specific soluble membrane antigen injection and antilymphocyte globulin administration on the survival of islet allografts in rats. Transplantation 1978; 25: 336.

44. Posselt AM, Barker CF, Tomaszewski JE *et al.* Induction of donor-specific unresponsiveness by intrathymic islet transplantation. Science 1990; 249: 1293–5.

45. Markees TG, De Fazio SR, Gozzo JJ. Prolongation of impure murine islet allografts with antilymphocyte serum and donor-specific bone marrow. Transplantation 1992; 53: 521–7.

46. Posselt AM, Odorico JS, Barker CF *et al.* Promotion of pancreatic islet allograft survival by intrathymic transplantation of bone marrow. Diabetes 1992; 41: 771–5.

47. Bretzel RG, Hering BJ, Federlin K. Islet cell transplantation in diabetes mellitus – from bench to bedside. Exp Clin Endocrinol Diabetes 1995; 103 suppl 2: 143–159.

48. Strautz RL. Studies of hereditary-obese mice (ob/ob) after implantation of pancreatic islets in Millipore filter capsules. Diabetologia 1970; 6: 306.

49. Chick WL, Perris JJ, Lauris V *et al.* Artificial pancreas using living beta cells: effect on glucose homeostasis in diabetic rats. Science 1977; 197: 780.

50. Tze WJ, Wong FC, Chen LM *et al.* Implantable artificial endocrine pancreas unit used to restore normoglycemia in the diabetic rat. Nature 1976; 264: 466.

51. Zekorn T, Siebers U, Bretzel RG *et al.* Protection of islets of Langerhans from interleukin-1 toxicity by artificial membranes. Transplantation 1990; 50: 391–4.

52. Lim F, Sun AN. Microencapsulated islets as bioartificial endocrine pancreas. Science 1980; 210: 908.

53. Zekorn T, Siebers U, Horcher A *et al*. Barium-alginate beads for immunoisolated transplantation of islet of Langerhans. Transplant Proc 1992; 24: 937–9.

54. Woehrle M, Pullmann J, Bretzel RG *et al*. Prevention of recurrent autoimmune diabetes in the BB rat by islet transplantation under the renal capsule. Transplantation 1992; 53: 1099–102.

55. Bartlett ST, Hadley GA, Dirden B *et al*. Composite kidney–islet transplantation prevents recurrent autoimmune beta-cell destruction. Surgery 1993; 114: 211–17.

56. Vaux DL. Ways around rejection. Nature 1995; 377: 576–7.

57. Muir A, Peck A, Clare-Salzer M *et al*. Insulin immunization in nonobese diabetic mice induces a protective insulitis characterized by diminished intraislet interferon (transcription). J Clin Invest 1995; 95: 628–34.

58. Swain SL. Generation and *in vivo* persistence of polarized Th1 and Th2 memory cells. Immunity 1994; 1: 543–52.

59. Efrat S, Fejer G, Brownlee M, Horwitz HS. Prolonged survival of pancreatic islet allografts mediated by adenovirus immunoregulatory transgenes. Proc Natl Acad Sci USA 1995; 92: 6947–51.

60. Golsorkhi AA, Min JK, Shaked A, Barker C, Naji A. Prolongation of islet allograft survival by vector-mediated gene transfer of TGF-beta and IL-10. Abstract 2361. XVI. Int. Congress of the Transplantation Society, Barcelona 1996.

61. Deng S, Ketchum RJ, Kucher T, Shaked A, Naji A, Brayman KL. Adenoviral transfection of canine islet xenografts with immunosuppressive cytokine genes abrogates primary non-function and prolongs graft survival. Abstract 2511. XVI. Int Congress of the Transplantation Society, Barcelona, 1996.

62. Deng, S, Yang ZD, Ketchum RJ, Shaked A, Naji A, Brayman KL. Analysis of human islet function, *in vitro* and *in vivo*, following adenoviral infection and cytokine gene transfer. Abstract 2513. XVI. Int Congress of the Transplantation Society, Barcelona, 1996.

63. Bellgrau D, Gold D, Selawry H, Moore J, Franzusoff A, Duke RC. A role for CD95 ligand in preventing graft rejection. Nature 1995; 377: 630–2.

64. Griffith TS, Brunner T, Fletcher SM, Green DR, Ferguson TA. Fas ligand-induced apoptosis as a mechanism of immune privilege. Science 1995; 270: 1189–92.

65. Gerling I, Wang X, Alloush L, Selawry H. Sertoli cells prolong discordant xenograft survival in mice, rats and monkeys. Autoimmunity 1995; 21: 83.

66. Scharp DW, Lacy PE, Santiago JV *et al*. Insulin-independence after islet transplantation into type 1 diabetic patients. Diabetes 1990; 39: 515–18.

67. Socci C, Falqui L, Davalli AM *et al*. Fresh human islet transplantation to replace pancreatic endocrine function in type I diabetic patients. Acta Diabetol 1991; 28: 151–7.

68. Warnock G, Kneteman NM, Ryan EA, Rabinovitch A, Rajotte RV: Long-term follow-up after transplantation of insulin-producing pancreatic islets into patients with type I (insulin-dependent) diabetes mellitus. Diabetologia 1992; 35: 89–95.

69. Alejandro R, Burke G, Shapiro ET *et al*. Long-term survival of intraportal islet allografts in type I diabetes mellitus. In: C. Ricordi (ed.) Pancreatic islet cell transplantation. Austin: R. G. Landes, 1992, pp. 410–13.

70. Gores PF, Najarian JS, Stephanian E, Lloveras JJ, Kelly SL, Sutherland DE: Insulin independence in type I diabetes after transplantation of unpurified islets from single donor with 15-deoxyspergualin. Lancet 1993; 341: 19–21.

71. Bretzel RG, Hering BJ, Brandhorst D *et al*. Insulin independence in type 1 diabetes achieved by intraportal transplantation of purified pancreatic islets. Diabetologia 1994; 37 suppl 1: A38.

72. Hayek A, Lopez AD, Beattie GM. Decrease in the number of neonatal islets required for successful transplantation by strict metabolic control of diabetic rats. Transplantation 1988; 45: 940–2.

73. Rajab AA, Ahren B, Bengmark S. Islet transplantation to the renal subcapsular space in streptozotocin-diabetic rats: short-term effects on glucose-stimulated insulin secretion. Diab Res Clin Pract 1989; 7: 197–204.

74. Juang JH, Bonner-Weir S, Wu YJ, Weir GC. Beneficial influence of glycemic control upon

the growth and function of transplanted islets. Diabetes 1994; 43: 1334–9.

75. Hering BJ, Bretzel RG, Hopt UT *et al*. New protocol toward prevention of early human islet allograft failure. Transplant Proc 1994; 26: 570–1.

76. Luzi L, Hering BJ, Socci C *et al*. Metabolic effects of successful intraportal islet transplantation in IDDM. J Clin Invest 1996; 97: 2611–18.

77. Atkison PR, Zucker P, Hramiak I *et al*. Continued insulin dependence despite normal range insulin sensitivity and insulin connecting peptide levels in a kidney/islet transplant patient. Diabetes Care 1996; 19: 236–40.

78. Wahren J. Experimental and clinical studies with C-peptide in type 1 diabetes. Presented at the Satellite Symposium to the 15th International Diabetes Federation Congress: Advances in diabetes therapy: From insulin to gluco-active peptides and beyond. Kobe, Japan, 3–4 Nov, 1994.

79. Cryer PE. Banting lecture. Hypoglycemia: the limiting factor in the management of IDDM. Diabetes 1994; 43: 1378–89.

80. Sutherland DER. Pancreatic transplantation: an update. Diab Rev 1993; 1: 152–65.

81. Gruessner A, Sutherland DER. Pancreas transplant results in the United Network for Organ Sharing (UNOS) United States of America (USA) Registry compared with non-USA data in the International Registry. In: Terasaki and Zecka (eds) Clinical transplants 1994, Los Angeles: UCLA Tissue Typing Laboratory, 1994, pp. 47–68.

82. Wahoff DC, Papalois BE, Najarian JS *et al*. Autologous islet transplantation to prevent diabetes after pancreatic resection. Ann Surg 1995; 222: 562–75.

83. Alejandro R, Cutfield RG, Shienvold FL *et al*. Natural history of intrahepatic canine islet cell autografts. J Clin Invest 1986; 78: 1339–48.

84. Ricordi C, Tzakis A, Carroll P. Human islet allotransplantation in 18 diabetic patients. Transplant Proc 1992; 24: 961.

85. Jaeger C, Hering BJ, Dyrberg T, Federlin K, Bretzel RG. Islet cell antibodies and glutamic acid decarboxylase antibodies in patients with insulin-dependent diabetes mellitus undergoing kidney and islet-after-kidney transplantation. Transplantation 1996; 62: 424–6.

86. Stegall MD, Lafferty KJ, Kam I, Gill RG. Evidence of recurrent autoimmunity in human allogeneic islet transplantation. Transplantation 1996; 61: 1272–4.

87. Tyden G, Reinholt FP, Sundkvist G, Bolinder J. Recurrence of autoimmune diabetes mellitus in recipients of cadaveric pancreatic grafts. N Engl J Med 1996; 335: 860–3.

88. Davalli AM, Ogava Y, Ricordi C, Scharp DW, Bonner-Weir S, Weir GC. A selective decrease in the beta-cell mass of human islets transplanted into diabetic nude mice. Transplantation 1995; 59: 817–20.

89. Kaufman DB, Platt JL, Rabe FL, Dunn DL, Bach FH, Sutherland DER. Differential roles of Mac-1+ cells, and CD4+ and CD8+ T-lymphocytes in primary nonfunction and classic rejection of islet allografts. J Exp Med 1990; 172: 291–302.

90. Nagata M, Mullen Y, Matsuo S, Hereira M, Clare-Salzler M. Destruction of islet isografts by severe nonspecific inflammation. Transplant Proc 1990; 22: 855–6.

91. Nussler AK, Carroll PB, Di Silvio M *et al*. Hepatic nitric oxide generation as a putative mechanism for failure of intrahepatic islet cell grafts. Transplant Proc 1992; 24: 2997.

92. Bonner-Weir S, Baxter LA, Schuppin GT, Smith FE. A second pathway for regeneration of adult exocrine and endocrine pancreas. A possible recapitulation of embryonic development. Diabetes 1993; 52: 1715–20.

93. Malaisse WJ, Malaisse-Lagae F, Sener A, Pipeleers DG. Determinants of the selective toxicity of aloxan to the pancreatic b-cell. Proc Natl Acad Sci USA 1982; 79: 927–30.

94. Boudreaux JP, McHugh L, Canafax DM, Ascher N. The impact of cyclosporine and combination immunosuppression on the incidence of posttransplant diabetes in renal allograft recipients. Transplantation 1987; 44: 376–81.

95. Christiansen E, Andersen HB, Rasmussen K *et al*. Pancreatic beta-cell function and glucose metabolism in human segmental pancreas and kidney transplantation. Am J Physiol 1993; 264: E441–9.

96. Andersson A, Borg H, Halberg A, Hellerström C, Sandler S, Schnell A. Long-term effects of cyclosporine A on cultured mouse pancreatic islets. Diabetologia 1984; 27: 66–9.

97. Emmrich J, Seyfarth M, Fleig WE, Emmrich F. Treatment of inflammatory bowel disease with anti-CD4 monoclonal antibody. Lancet 1991; 338: 570–1.

98. Reinke P, Volk HD, Miller H *et al.* Anti-CD4 therapy of acute rejection in long term renal allograft recipients [letter]. Lancet 1991; 338: 702–3.

99. Gupta V, Rooney D, Kendall D, Sutherland D, Wahoff D, Robertson R. Defective glucagon responses from intrahepatic transplanted islets during hypoglycemia is transplanta-tion-site determined. Diabetes 1996; 45 suppl 2: 60A (abstr.)

100. Teuscher A, Seaquist E, Kendall D, Robertson R. Alpha cell function in human recipients of pancreatic islet autografts. Cell Transplant 1994; 3: 228 (abstr.).

101. Johansson BL, Bork K, Fernqvist-Forbes E, Odergren T, Remahl S, Wahren J. C-peptide improves autonomic nerve function in IDDM patients. Diabetologia 1996; 39: 687–95.

102. Fanelli C, Pampanelli S, Epifano L *et al.* Long-term recovery from unawareness, deficient counterregulation and lack of cognitive dys-function during hypoglycaemia, following institution of rational, intensive insulin therapy in IDDM. Diabetologia 1994; 37: 1265–76.

103. Groth CG, Moeller E, Hellerström C, Tibell A, Wennberg L. Proceedings of the First International Workshop on Pig-to-Man Islet Transplantation. Xenotransplantation 1995; 2: 107–240.

# 10 Small bowel transplantation

*Stephen G. Pollard*

**Introduction**

For many years intestinal transplantation had been regarded as the 'Forbidden Fruit' of transplant surgeons. This followed an early experience with a group of eight patients who were transplanted in various centres during the 1960s as an emergency treatment of massive intestinal infarction. They all died from intractable rejection, graft thrombosis or sepsis. Therefore with a greater understanding of nutritional requirements and the introduction of hypertonic total parenteral nutrition solutions in 1969, bowel transplantation fell into disrepute and was not revisited for some twenty years.

With advances in immunosuppression, coupled with improved surgical techniques and a greater understanding of the pathophysiology of the transplanted bowel, isolated reports of successful cases started to appear in the literature in the late 1980s.[1–3] Intestinal transplantation is now finally emerging as a viable treatment option for patients with intestinal failure who are unlikely to survive long-term on parenteral nutrition.

In 1995 an International Registry for all cases of intestinal transplantation was set up in London, Ontario, under the supervision of Dr David Grant, whose group had reported the first successful combined liver/small bowel transplant in 1988. By the time of the first report from the group,[4] which had collected data up to June 1995, 182 transplants had been performed in 172 patients from 25 centres.

**Indications and incidence**

The various recognised indications for intestinal transplantation are shown in Table 10.1 for children and Table 10.2 for adults. In the paediatric group, some cases suffer from a physiological failure of the bowel, whereas the remainder together with the adult group suffer from loss of intestine for various reasons to a point where nutrition cannot be maintained via the enteral route.

Each year in the UK approximately 100 patients (i.e. 2 per million) can be expected to commence long-term total parenteral nutrition (TPN) and of these perhaps half would be suitable for consideration of small bowel

**Table 10.1** *Indications for small bowel transplantation: paediatric*

Necrotising enterocolitis
Volvulus neonatorum
Gastroschisis
Extensive atresia
Pseudo-obstruction
Hirschprung's disease
Microvillus inclusion disease

**Table 10.2** *Indications for small bowel transplantation: adult*

Superior mesenteric artery thrombosis
Superior mesenteric vein thrombosis
Radiation enteritis
Small bowel volvulus
Crohn's disease
Extensive gastrointestinal polyposis
Tumours, e.g. mesenteric desmoid

transplantation; exclusions being on the basis of age, other medical contraindications such as active sepsis or malignancy, or eventual return to enteral diet following adaptation.[5] Currently patients are more likely to survive on total parenteral nutrition than with a transplant; data from the Cleveland clinic gives one-year survival rates of 75–95% (according to the underlying disease), which on the face of it compares very favourably with the results for intestinal transplantation. It must be remembered, however, that if one considers transplantation as an option only for those patients who are dying from the complications of total parenteral nutrition then it is much more viable as a treatment option; at present intestinal transplantation should be viewed as a treatment for patients who are unlikely to survive on total parenteral nutrition.

## Investigative techniques

### Recipient assessment

Long-term TPN can lead to irreversible structural changes in the liver, and an important part of the assessment of a potential recipient is to assess their liver function with biochemical liver function tests, particularly looking at synthetic function such as clotting indices, serum albumin and bilirubin. Doppler studies of the hepatic vessels should be performed to exclude portal hypertension and portal vein thrombosis, and liver biopsy to look for the irreversible structural changes of fibrosis and cirrhosis as a consequence of long-term TPN. Cirrhotic patients will require a combined liver/intestine transplant. It is important to define how much bowel remains. This allows some prediction as to whether with maximal adaptation the patient might resume independent enteral nutrition, and this information is important when planning the anastomoses if a transplant is to be performed.

Cardiovascular assessment and pulmonary function tests are similar to those required for liver transplantation with chest X-ray and electrocardiogram, supplemented if need be by pulmonary function tests, echocardiography, dynamic isotope imaging and coronary angiography. Isolated small bowel transplantation is a less exacting procedure than combined liver/bowel transplantation and requires less cardiorespiratory reserve. The assessment must also include a careful evaluation of the patency of the great veins of the head and neck and the femoral veins and vena cava which may have thrombosed from repeated venous access for TPN. Baseline renal function should be measured by glomerular filtration rate (GFR), since tacrolimus is nephrotoxic in the high doses used as is amphotericin which is often required for treatment of fungal sepsis postoperatively.

It is also advisable for any potential candidates to undergo careful psychological assessment prior to embarking on the operation in order to reduce the risk of non-compliance with immunosuppression and of failure to rehabilitate following what may be prolonged hospitalisation.

## Donor selection

The majority of intestinal transplants have used cadaveric donors, although isolated successful cases have been performed using an intestinal segment from a living related donor. Great care must be exercised in selecting potential cadaveric bowel donors. There must be no history of malignancy outside the central nervous system (CNS), liver disease, bowel disease or substance abuse and no systemic or abdominal sepsis.

Donor and recipient should be ABO identical and size matched – ideally the donor should be smaller than recipient since the abdominal cavity of the recipient is likely to be contracted and one expects some swelling of the graft following preservation and reperfusion.

The donor should have normal liver function tests and electrolytes, negative serology for Hepatitis A, B, C, HIV and be cytomegalovirus (CMV) matched to the recipient with no excessive inotrope requirement and no significant hypotensive episodes. Currently there is no functional assessment of the intestine which is helpful prior to retrieval. The need for a negative white cell cross-match is currently unknown.

For assessment of a potential living related donor, first the claimed relationship must be confirmed by tissue typing with or without DNA studies, and ABO compatibility confirmed. In addition to the biochemical and serological tests outlined above, the potential donor must be assessed for their general fitness to undergo extensive small bowel resection, and a mesenteric arteriogram performed to define a usable segment of intestine for grafting. In the first UK case of live related intestinal transplantation, which was performed successfully by the author in Leeds in 1995, a 180 cm segment of distal ileum was taken on an ileocolic artery and vein pedicle and transplanted from mother to daughter, leaving the mother with 270 cm of small bowel, and her ileocaecal valve.

## Management options

### Non-transplant options

The early attempts at small bowel transplantation in the 1960s were doomed to fail, not just because of an inability to control the immunological events in the graft but also from performing the operation as an emergency procedure in septic, malnourished and catabolic individuals shortly after massive bowel resection. The advent of total parenteral nutrition has allowed the introduction of the dimension of time to allow careful evaluation and stabilisation of candidates for intestinal grafting in addition to removing the need for such a transplant in many.

Failure of total parenteral nutrition is commonly due to catheter-related sepsis and catheter occlusion, access difficulties following multiple venous thromboses and impaired liver function. Liver impairment is multifactorial, including lack of enteral stimulation, bacterial overgrowth, disruption of the enterohepatic circulation, reduced bile flow, imbalance of amino acids, lipids and trace elements and iron overload. Other problems seen due to long-term TPN include altered bone metabolism and severe psychological problems with inability to eat, particularly in children if sham feeding is not performed.

Bowel transplantation is a treatment option for a proportion of these patients who have short gut syndrome and are failing on total parenteral nutrition. However, although opinion is slowly changing, a bowel transplant is still widely regarded as the last resort for the patient in whom all else has failed. It is currently essential to explore other alternatives in patients who are failing on total parenteral nutrition to ascertain whether partial or complete independence with enteral nutrition may be restored before considering transplantation. These alternative measures which might obviate the need for a transplant in the short gut patient will now be considered.

First and foremost, these patients must be allowed a period of adaptation following resection, during which time the function of the residual small bowel will improve, and any remaining colon will develop some nutrient absorptive functions. Adaptation is due to bowel dilatation and lengthening, with villus hyperplasia and an effective increase in the absorptive surface area. The mechanism of this adaptation is multifactorial, but it is stimulated by a raised nutrient load being presented to the remaining bowel and/or the increase in pancreatic and biliary secretion which this causes, and by increased levels of enteroglucagon and possibly gastrin, prostaglandin $E_2$ and epidermal growth factor. There is some evidence that this adaptation can be enhanced by growth hormone.[6] Somatostatin has the reverse effect, inhibiting adaptation, possibly by inhibiting secretion of enteroglucagon and pancreatic juice. This should be borne in mind when considering its use in short gut syndrome.

During this adaptation period it is essential to stabilise the patient on TPN and to eradicate any septic foci; not only will active sepsis be a contraindication to transplantation, but also liver dysfunction is much more likely to occur with TPN if there is superadded infection. Catheter sepsis is a particular problem; infection of the venous feeding line can be reduced or prevented by use of a dedicated line and meticulous attention to sterility when connecting the feed to the access port. Treated with care such lines can last for many years.

Other sequelae of short gut include gastric hypersecretion from raised levels of gastrin and reduced levels of gastric inhibitory hormones such as GIP (gastric inhibitory peptide), VIP (vasoactive intestinal peptide) and serotonin which are produced by the small bowel. Loss of the bile salt pool from impaired reabsorption leads to cholelithiasis and steatorrhoea. Steatorrhoea leads to excessive fats entering the colon, which binds calcium in preference to oxalate which is then absorbed. This can lead to urinary oxalate calculi.

There are a number of manoeuvres which can be considered to optimise usage of the remaining bowel. The output from a proximal stoma can be redirected into a mucus fistula leading into a distal loop of defunctioned bowel. Special catheters with retaining balloons on both ends have been designed for this purpose and in addition to increasing absorption, this will discourage atrophy of the defunctioned segment.

Some operative procedures have been designed to slow transit and improve absorption; these include the interposition of a segment of colon into the remaining small bowel, the creation of reversed (antiperistaltic) small bowel segments to delay transit, and the construction of an artificial ileocaecal valve to both increase transit time and reduce colonisation of the small bowel. One of the adaptive responses to massive resection is dilatation of the remaining bowel and this can be counterproductive from ineffective peristalsis/stasis, and bacterial overgrowth. Operations to taper or plicate this dilated bowel are generally unsuccessful in the long term however, as the problem is likely to recur. The fashioning of recirculating loops to allow repeated exposure of luminal nutrients to the mucosa should also be discouraged since they promote colonisation and function poorly. An innovative operation described by Bianchi[7] aims to increase bowel length at the cost of this ineffective dilatation by dividing the bowel lengthways along both its mesenteric and antimesenteric borders, with each of the resulting sheets supplied by half the mesenteric vessels. The sheets are rolled into tubes and joined together, effectively doubling the length of this segment. This creation of two tubes from one can be performed as a single manoeuvre with the use of a linear stapling device. Other imaginative techniques such as growing small bowel mucosa on other surfaces such as the colonic serosa and the abdominal wall for eventual incorporation into the gastrointestinal (GI) tract, and retrograde electrical pacing to slow transit, although attractive theoretically, have yet to be applied successfully clinically.

It is generally considered that in adults with a terminal stoma, about 100 cm of small bowel is the minimum that can allow independence on an enteral diet. This can be reduced to as little as 30 cm of small bowel if the colon and ileocaecal valve remain; the prognosis is better if ileum rather than jejunum is retained because of the tight junctions which allow osmotic differences to develop between the lumen and the extracellular fluid. As little as 10–20 cm of bowel in the neonate may be sufficient to allow eventual weaning from TPN.

During the period of adaptation it is important to monitor liver and renal function and replace trace elements. $H_2$ antagonists should be given as these patients have high levels of gastrin and are prone to peptic ulceration. The addition of glutamine as an enterocyte fuel can improve the function of the remaining small bowel and short chain fatty acids fulfil a similar role as a preferred fuel for colonocytes. Arginine enrichment of the diet appears to improve integrity of the bowel wall and despite dependence on parenteral nutrition it is important to feed the patient orally, both to minimise liver damage and to improve the integrity and reduce atrophy and abnormal colonisation of the remaining gut. It is also important to feed orally to avoid the difficult problem in children who have never been fed who fail to learn how to eat following successful bowel replacement.

There will emerge a group of patients, however, in whom enteral nutrition cannot be restored despite all the above measures and in whom the complications of total parenteral nutrition make this unlikely to succeed as a long-term option. In these cases bowel transplantation should be considered.

## Transplant options

Once the decision has been made to consider a patient for intestinal transplantation, it is necessary to determine the most appropriate type of graft. Early enthusiasm for combined transplantation of liver and intestine was based on the observation that both experimentally and clinically the transplanted liver is able to impart a degree of donor specific immunosuppression to other organs simultaneously grafted from the same donor. The morbidity of combined transplants is higher, however, and with the advent of newer and more powerful immunosuppressive agents, particularly tacrolimus, simultaneous transplantation of the liver is only required in cases where the liver has failed, for example from TPN-induced cholestasis progressing to cirrhosis. Early enthusiasm for composite grafts including the colon and ileocaecal valve has now waned because of clear evidence of an inferior outcome in such cases, as will be discussed later.

**Technical aspects**

## Isolated bowel transplantation

### Cadaveric donor procedure

The abdomen is opened through a long midline or cruciate incision. The root of the small bowel mesentery is mobilised from the posterior abdominal wall and the front of the aorta to the origin of the superior mesenteric artery. The right colon and transverse colon are mobilised and the mesocolon divided where it meets the mesentery, ligating the contained middle and right colic arteries arising from the right side of the superior mesenteric artery. The superior mesenteric artery is identified and mobilised from the uncinate lobe of the pancreas, and cleared down to its origin from the aorta having Kocherised the duodenum and head of the pancreas. The superior mesenteric vein is similarly identified where it crosses the third part of the duodenum and mobilised towards the liver. This necessitates dividing the pancreas and duodenum with a stapling device in front of the portal vein followed by meticulous ligation and division of all the branches entering it from the pancreas. A reasonable length of splenic vein is preserved to be used as a vent following reperfusion in the recipient. A series of fine sutures picking up just the adventitia of the anterior wall of the portal vein are inserted and used for orientation, since it is easy to inadvertently twist the vessel (Fig. 10.1). The graft is perfused with University of Wisconsin

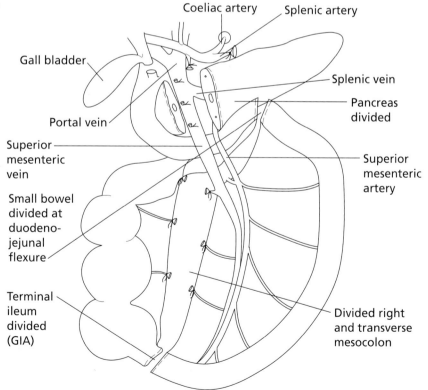

**Figure 10.1**  *Completed dissection for small bowel retrieval.*

Coeliac artery

Splenic artery

Gall bladder

Splenic vein

Pancreas divided

Portal vein

Superior mesenteric vein

Superior mesenteric artery

Small bowel divided at duodeno-jejunal flexure

Terminal ileum divided (GIA)

Divided right and transverse mesocolon

(UW) preservation solution through a cannula in the aorta having applied an aortic cross-clamp at the level of the oesophageal hiatus. The jejunum just beyond the duodenojejunal flexure, and the terminal ileum are then divided with linear staplers and the graft placed in a bath of UW solution at 4°C. The lumen of the distal bowel is not occluded earlier in order to allow the small bowel to continue to empty its contents during the dissection. The portal vein is divided just above the level of the duodenum ensuring that sufficient portal vein remains with the liver for grafting this organ. The origin of the superior mesenteric artery together with a surrounding Carrel patch of aorta is removed with the graft.

In general the liver will also be harvested for another recipient, but removal of the pancreas and duodenal segment for whole organ pancreas transplantation cannot be performed since the neck of the pancreas is divided to gain access to the superior mesenteric vein and portal vein.

### Live related donor procedure

If the graft is being procured from a living donor, the superior mesenteric artery is identified in the mesentery and mobilised with the adjacent vein at a point predetermined by a preoperative angiogram beyond the origin of the right colic artery. The mesentery is then divided up to the bowel wall to create a vascularised segment of 150–200 cm of ileum. It is important to measure the entire length of small intestine in the donor at the outset and to ensure that both an adequate length of small bowel (at least 250 cm) and the ileocaecal valve remain.

### Recipient procedure

The bowel is placed orthotopically in the peritoneal cavity. In paediatric cases with motility disorders the existing bowel is resected at the time of operation, but in patients with previous massive resection there can be logistic problems in housing the graft in the abdominal cavity which has often collapsed and become obliterated by adhesions.

The infrarenal aorta is mobilised and controlled with slings, as is the portal vein or the inferior vena cava, depending on the preferred method of venous drainage (see below). If the graft has been procured from a living donor, the rather short vascular pedicle will not reach the portal vein and must be anastomosed to the vena cava (Fig. 10.2). The graft is revascularised by anastomosis of the superior mesenteric artery on its patch of aorta end-to-side to the aorta, having applied a side biting clamp to the recipient vessel. The portal vein of the graft is anastomosed end-to-side to the inferior vena cava or to the portal vein (Fig. 10.3), leaving the splenic vein stump on the donor portal vein open. The graft is revascularised by releasing the clamp on the recipient aorta, and the first 200–300 ml of blood allowed to escape from the splenic vein orifice which is then ligated with release of the clamp

**Figure 10.2**  *Isolated small bowel transplant implantation with systemic venous drainage.*

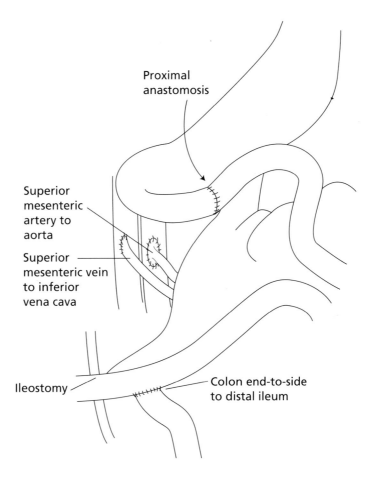

**Figure 10.2**  *Isolated small bowel transplant implantation with systemic venous drainage.*

Proximal anastomosis

Superior mesenteric artery to aorta

Superior mesenteric vein to inferior vena cava

Ileostomy

Colon end-to-side to distal ileum

controlling the vena cava/portal vein. This is to prevent the cold hyperkalaemic, acidotic blood from the reperfused graft entering the recipient circulation since it may precipitate a cardiac arrest. Intestinal continuity is restored by anastomosis of the proximal recipient bowel (usually the distal duodenum) to the proximal end of the graft using standard techniques over a nasojejunal tube. It is important to identify the proximal end of the graft with a suture in the donor to ensure that it is placed isoperistaltically. The distal end of the graft is exteriorised as a spouted ileostomy, and the end of the distal recipient bowel, if present, is anastomosed to the side of the graft a few inches proximal to the stoma. Immediate restoration of continuity allows restoration of normal gut flora and the early reintroduction of enteral feeding. A stoma is needed for observation, to access for biopsy, and to sample the intestinal contents and is sited at the distal end – a proximally sited stoma tends to atrophy and give biopsies which may be non-representative. The use of a distal end-to-side anastomosis makes closure of the stoma a straightforward procedure, which can be performed extraperitoneally.

**Figure 10.3** *Isolated small bowel transplant implantation with portal venous drainage.*

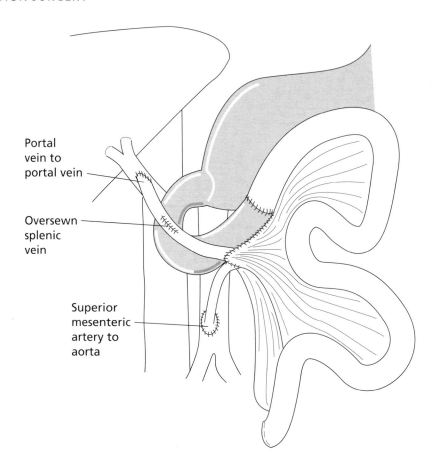

Portal vein to portal vein

Oversewn splenic vein

Superior mesenteric artery to aorta

## Combined liver/small bowel transplantation

### *Donor procedure*

Unlike the isolated small bowel graft, with this composite graft the portal vein is kept in continuity. The mobilisation of the bowel proceeds as above, and the liver is mobilised as described elsewhere with division of the common bile duct. The coeliac artery is dissected right down to the aorta with ligation of the splenic and left gastric vessels. In addition there are frequently two small phrenic arteries arising from the coeliac artery just beyond its origin and these are also ligated. The portal vein is skeletonised as it passes through the pancreas and a reasonable length of splenic vein is dissected. Following cross-clamping of the aorta, arterial perfusion of the liver and the bowel is effected by a cannula in the lower aorta, via the coeliac and superior mesenteric arteries. Portal perfusion of the liver is initially by drainage from the small intestine. Once the liver is removed portal perfusion is completed by a cannula placed in the portal vein via the splenic vein orifice. Excessive perfusion of the bowel with preservation solution will lead to excessive bowel swelling and should be avoided. The graft is removed by division of the inferior vena cava

**Figure 10.4** *Liver/ small bowel graft.*

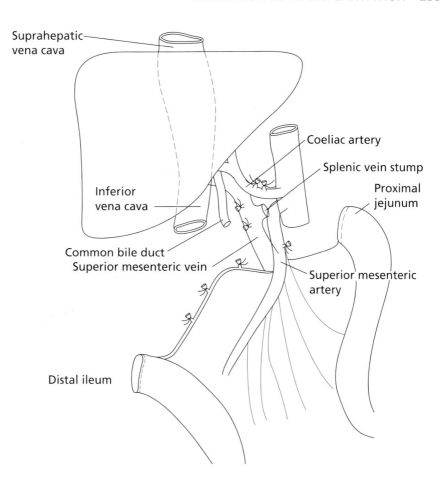

above and below the liver and excision of either a large patch of aorta bearing both coeliac and superior mesenteric orifices, or of a segment of aorta (Fig. 10.4). The proximal jejunum and terminal ileum are divided as stated above.

### Recipient procedure

In cases of combined small bowel/liver transplantation, but not isolated small bowel transplantation, it is necessary to allow venous decompression of the remaining recipient viscera – generally the stomach, duodenum, pancreas, spleen and colon; for this reason an external portasystemic shunt is employed in addition to venovenous bypass from the femoral vein to the internal jugular vein to prevent undue haemodynamic disturbance when the inferior vena cava is divided. The portal vein is divided close to the liver and cannulated to allow this portal bypass. The recipient's liver is removed, with ligation and division of the hepatic artery and common bile duct, and clamping and division of the vena cava above and below the liver. The graft is placed orthotopically and following anastomosis of the inferior vena cava above the liver, the arterial supply to the entire graft is established by anastomosis of the Carrel patch/aortic segment bearing the orifices of the coeliac and superior mesenteric arteries to the recipient's infrarenal aorta. Arterial reperfusion is commenced, initially allowing the venous blood to drain out of the liver from the infrahepatic inferior vena caval anastomosis which is then completed with removal of the suprahepatic caval clamp. The native portal vein, which had been draining into a portasystemic shunt circuit is now anastomosed to the side of the portal vein of the transplant, using a side-biting clamp on the recipient vessel. The biliary anastomosis is fashioned to the end of the recipient bile duct or to the proximal end of the bowel graft and intestinal continuity is restored by anastomosis of the proximal bowel to the end of the graft, or to its side if the end has been used to establish biliary drainage. The distal end of the graft is brought out as an ileostomy with side-to-end anastomosis to the distal recipient bowel just proximal to the stoma (Fig. 10.5).

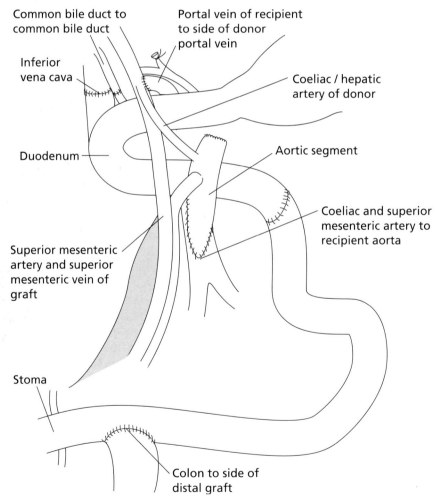

**Figure 10.5**
*Completed implantation of liver/small bowel graft.*

Debate has arisen as to whether it is necessary to institute portal rather than systemic venous drainage of the graft in cases of isolated bowel transplantation.

Clearly to drain the graft into the portal vein is more physiological than to drain it into the systemic venous system, but technically this can be difficult and hazardous and there is some debate as to how important it is. Creation of an experimental Eck fistula, diverting the entire portal vein drainage into the vena cava can lead to liver atrophy and clinically, portosystemic shunts to relieve portal hypertension can lead to hepatic encephalopathy. This argument was initially cited in favour of portal venous drainage of the isolated bowel graft. The situation following isolated intestinal transplantation, however, differs in two major respects. First, to drain the graft into the vena cava is not comparable to an experimental Eck fistula, since these patients will still deliver blood into their portal vein from their remaining viscera such as the stomach, pancreas, spleen and colon. Indeed there is evidence that insulin is one of the more important 'hepatotrophic' factors in the portal blood. Secondly, the encephalopathy which follows shunting for portal hypertension occurs in patients with parenchymal liver disease. Indeed these patients will often become encephalopathic without a surgical shunt as a consequence of their liver disease. As stated earlier, significant liver dysfunction is a contraindication to isolated bowel transplantation – such patients should be considered for a combined liver–bowel graft, and although it has been shown that the circulating levels of ammonia and free amino acids are less with portal than systemic drainage, the clinical importance of this is currently undefined and overall systemic venous drainage seems perfectly acceptable.

**Patho-physiology of bowel transplantation**

Transplantation of the intestine leads to a number of physiological and pathological sequelae, the consequences of which will be discussed in the context of what has been learned from both clinical and experimental bowel transplantation.

The act of transplanting the bowel involves division of its neurological and lymphatic connections, preservation and reperfusion injury, and, following transplantation, a two-way immunological engagement between the host and the graft.[8]

Much has been learned about these pathophysiological effects from the use of inbred rodent species. Transplantation between inbred animals of the same strain allows the study of the physical effects of the transplant (e.g. denervation, lymphatic interruption) without any super-added immunological factors being involved. The use of appropriately selected inbred rodent species has allowed the study of the graft-versus-host response in the absence of rejection, by employing transplantation of grafts from homozygous parental strains into their first generation hybrid offspring ($F_1$). Although the $F_1$ host will not recognise the graft as foreign, the immunocytes in the graft will respond to those antigens which the host inherited from the other parent. This has allowed the response of the graft to the foreign host antigens to be studied in the absence of any immune response of the host to the graft. Similarly, rejection responses can be studied in isolation in this same model without interference by any graft-versus-host response by transplantation of the bowel from the $F_1$ hybrid into the homozygous parental strain.[9]

## Sequelae of transplantation

### Effect of denervation

The net sympathetic effector pathways act as a brake on crypt activity and denervation acutely will lead to enhanced secretion of sodium and water into the gut lumen. The contractile properties of the totally denervated intestine appear unaltered in the long term. Acutely there is a loss of intrinsic inhibition leading to a transient phase of hyperacute peristalsis and large stomal fluid losses.[10,11]

### Effect of lymphatic interruption

The act of transplanting the intestine will require the division with or without ligation of the draining lymphatics and immediately after transplantation absorbed fats will drain freely into the peritoneal cavity although this is generally unimportant since these patients are still on TPN. Within 2 weeks of transplantation there is evidence of lymphatic channels reforming and within a month there is some restoration of lymph drainage from the gut, with drainage into the recipient's cisterna chyli. Long-term lymphatic function probably approaches normal.[12,13]

### Effect on mucosal barrier mechanisms

A number of factors tend to cause a breakdown of the mucosal barrier and encourage bacterial translocation across the bowel wall following bowel transplantation.[14]

The ischaemia of preservation and more importantly the injury due to reperfusion from the generation of superoxide radicals, leads to breakdown of the integrity of the mucosa with focal denudation of the epithelium lining the graft. This will usually recover within about 10 days. In addition, flushing the lumen of the graft during retrieval will remove the mucus which forms an important physiological barrier to bacteria by preventing their adhesion to the epithelium.

During acute rejection, the assault on the graft will culminate in epithelial ulceration, and bacterial translocation will be further encouraged by the loss of peristalsis which may accompany the rejection encouraging stasis and bacterial proliferation.

In addition, secretion of IgA by the graft is transiently halted, but will recover with secretion by host B cells once the donor lymphocytes in the graft have been replaced by recipient derived cells.

## Graft rejection

With rejection, morbidity and mortality is related to sepsis from bacterial translocation across the bowel wall once its integrity is lost. This is unlike the situation in heart, liver and kidney transplantation where the graft is not colonised and loss of graft function *per se* causes the problems from rejection.

The unmodified response to bowel transplantation is a sequential attack first on the graft-derived lymphatic tissue, followed by the epithelial and vascular elements of the transplants.[14,15] After 2 days the graft lymph nodes enlarge from infiltration by host lymphocytes – possibly also with an element of lymphatic obstruction. Host lymphocytes will then appear in the Peyer's patches of the graft and after about 4 days start to appear in the lamina propria of the graft, and around the blood vessels. This is followed by blunting and oedema of the villi with some loss of the brush border enzymes and after about 6–7 days there is a mixed inflammatory infiltration of the submucosa of the graft with sloughing of the mucosa. If the acute rejection response is modified by immunosuppression, the graft remains susceptible both to further episodes of acute rejection, and to chronic rejection in which there is villous atrophy and fibrosis, with only a sparse, scattered infiltration of the lamina propria and submucosa by lymphocytes and macrophages resulting in little crypt necrosis or ulceration. Vessels in the submucosa of the graft show features of endarteritis obliterans.

## Graft-versus-host disease

The small intestine normally contains abundant lymphoid tissue. These lymphocytes are found in organised groups in the Peyer's patches and within lymph nodes and are also diffusely distributed through the lamina propria and epithelium. The T cell component of the graft is sufficient to repopulate the host. These lymphocytes have the capacity to migrate out of the graft and infiltrate various sites such as the skin, the liver, and residual host intestine. In these sites they respond to foreign (i.e. recipient) antigens and release various lymphokines such as tumour necrosis factor and Gamma interferon and this can lead to the clinical picture of graft-versus-host disease (GVHD). Experimentally it occurs after 10–14 days and is generally self-limiting, being held in check by rejection responses to the graft lymphocytes. Once the donor lymphocytes have been cleared, the GVHD cannot recur as there is no capacity for regeneration of the donor lymphocytes. The GVHD is in itself immunosuppressive by the assault on host lymphocytes. Clinically various manoeuvres have been used to reduce the immunogenicity of the graft and to reduce the intensity of any graft versus host response. These include, graft lymphadenectomy, and lymphocyte depletion by methods such as irradiation and *ex vivo* perfusion with antilymphocyte preparations, as well as more obvious strategies such as the use of shorter grafts and better HLA matching.

However, in clinical small bowel transplantation with immunosuppressed recipients, the rejection response outweighs any GVHD and GVHD has proven to be rather less of a clinical problem than had been predicted. It may manifest as a transient skin rash, and it is not uncommon to find circulating lymphocytes with the specificity of the donor and no apparent symptoms or signs. Indeed this state of microchimerism with two cell populations co-existing harmoniously may be of importance in the establishment of a state of operational tolerance to the graft.[8]

## Postoperative management

### General measures: feeding

Postoperatively patients will require management on the intensive therapy unit (ITU) and ventilation for a variable period of time, because of a tendency for pulmonary oedema to occur, in addition to the ventilatory problems which can arise from raised intra-abdominal pressure secondary to swelling of the graft. After approximately two weeks it is usually possible to institute oral feeding with an isotonic dipeptide solution enriched with medium-chain triglycerides and glutamine, and changing to a gluten- and lactose-free diet within 2–4 weeks, and eventually weaning to a normal diet. The majority of patients with isolated bowel grafts are independent of TPN within a month, although patients with combined liver/bowel grafts tend to take longer. During rejection episodes the oral feed is withheld and TPN resumed. Ganciclovir prophylaxis should be given for 14 days in all cases of CMV mismatch (i.e. donor serologically positive, recipient negative) and in any cases where the CMV titre in the recipient circulation rises. Patients generally remain on $H_2$ blockers, and receive misoprostol (Cytotec) both to protect the stomach mucosa from steroid induced damage, and to protect the kidney from tacrolimus-induced nephrotoxicity, although the evidence for this protective ability is somewhat weak. If all is well, the stoma can be closed after 3–6 months.

### Immunosuppression

There remains debate as to whether lymphocyte depletion of the graft is clinically advantageous. Experimentally these manoeuvres will reduce the intensity of GVHD, but this has not proven to be a major clinical problem and may even be advantageous in counteracting rejection responses. In addition there have been concerns that lymphocyte depletion might increase the risk of lymphoma in the recipient. In general, it is currently considered unnecessary to deplete the graft of its lymphoid elements, although it is still practised by some units.

Although there have been successes with cyclosporin-based regimens of immunosuppression it is generally considered necessary to use the more potent agent tacrolimus, which is combined with azathioprine or mycophenolate mofetil (MMF) and corticosteroids. Initially these drugs are given intravenously, the tacrolimus being administered in near-nephrotoxic doses in conjunction with prostacyclin which is believed to reduce its nephrotoxicity, aiming for a steady state level of around $30 \, \text{ng ml}^{-1}$. Once gut function is recovering, oral tacrolimus is introduced, overlapping with the i.v. preparation which is gradually withdrawn. Careful monitoring of blood levels allows conversion to oral dosing without the risk of subtherapeutic levels, aiming for a 12 h trough level of $10–20 \, \text{ng ml}^{-1}$. Most patients are fully converted to oral tacrolimus within a month of transplantation. Azathioprine is commenced at $2 \, \text{mg kg}^{-1} \, \text{day}^{-1}$ or MMF at $2 \, \text{g day}^{-1}$ and reduced if there are signs of bone marrow toxicity. Many centres withdraw azathioprine after the first month. Following a peroperative 1000 mg bolus of methyl prednisolone, corticosteroids are given at $200 \, \text{mg day}^{-1}$ and rapidly reduced to 20 mg within 2 weeks and thence gradually to a maintenance dose of around $0.15 \, \text{mg kg}^{-1} \, \text{day}^{-1}$. Once gut function has recovered, the drugs are given orally; the majority of patients can be weaned to tacrolimus monotherapy within 3–6 months.

Episodes of acute rejection require temporary intensification of the immunosuppression, either with a short course of high dose intravenous corticosteroids (e.g. 500 or $1000 \, \text{mg day}^{-1}$ for 3–5 days) or with a 1–2 week course of a monoclonal or polyclonal antilymphocyte preparation such as OKT3 or ATG.

### Graft monitoring

#### Clinical observation

The changes associated with rejection are increased stomal losses, bleeding from the lumen, oedema and cyanosis of the stoma, followed by ulceration. The patient develops abdominal pain, ileus and fever progressing to septic shock from bacterial translocation.

#### Immunological assessment

Rejection is to be expected in around 80% of recipients, and is generally reversed with high-dose steroids or antilymphocyte preparations such as OKT3 or ATG together with optimisation of the tacrolimus dose. Biopsies taken from inside the stoma with a gastroscopy biopsy forceps are examined histologically. The findings are of oedema and lymphocytic infiltration of the lamina propria with an inflammatory infiltration of the crypts; in severe cases there is epithelial ulceration and crypt destruction with formation of an inflammatory pseudomembrane.

Microchimerism, the finding of circulating lymphocytes of donor specificity may be important in tolerance and must not be confused with GVHD, a clinical condition manifested by skin rash and multiorgan failure, and diagnosed by the identification of donor lymphocytes in biopsies taken from skin lesions.

#### Functional tests

A number of tests can be used to quantify the functional integrity of the graft.

1. $^{51}$Cr-labelled EDTA absorption.[17] The EDTA is not normally absorbed and if >5% of an orally administered dose is absorbed (and appears in the urine) this indicates abnormal permeability, as occurs in rejection.
2. $^{14}$C-labelled mannitol. Given orally, normally >10% is absorbed, appearing in the urine. Less than this indicates impaired absorption.
3. Oral glucose or D-xylose tolerance test.
4. Schilling test to measure absorption of vitamin B$_{12}$, a function of the terminal ileum.
5. Faecal fat excretion. This is usually abnormal with raised faecal fat levels even in the presence of apparently excellent graft function.
6. The absorption of orally administered tacrolimus (with measurement of blood levels 1, 2 and 3 h post-dose) can be a useful measure of absorptive function and confirm that it is safe to convert from intravenous administration.

### Microbiology

It is essential to frequently sample the rectal and stomal effluent, and nasojejunal aspirate. Rather than sterilise the bowel with antibiotics, the aim is to encourage the development of benign flora which can be treated swiftly if they undergo translocation. It is also important to survey for serological evidence of CMV infection or reactivation. Symptomatic CMV infection has proven to be a major problem in bowel transplantation presumably because of the large amounts of immunosuppression which have to be given. Fungal prophylaxis with fluconazole and pneumocystis prophylaxis with cotrimoxazole or pentamidine inhalations are generally given for 3–6 months after the transplant during the period of maximal immunosuppression.

### Radiological imaging

Doppler studies can be used to document flow in the mesenteric vessels of the graft with arteriography if concern arises.

Barium or water-soluble contrast studies allow assessment of peristalsis and integrity of the enteric anastomoses. Rejection is manifested by mucosal oedema, and, in severe cases with loss of epithelium, the bowel may appear as a series of featureless tubes.

Radiolabelled white cell scanning is a means of assessing the graft for infiltration by lymphocytes, as occurs in rejection. Rejection can be a patchy process, and stomal biopsies alone may be non-representative.

## Postoperative complications

### Technical problems

1. Mesenteric artery or vein thrombosis which invariably leads to infarction of the graft and requires swift action with laparotomy and graft excision.

**2.** Anastomotic leakage must be treated aggressively at laparotomy – conservative management puts the patients at risk of overwhelming sepsis. Non-anastomotic strictures may be features of chronic graft rejection.

### Motility disorders

Motility disorders occur both in the graft and in the native gut. The initial response to denervation is hypermotility with excessive secretion. This tends to be self-limiting but can be treated with agents such as loperamide or somatostatin if problematic or persistent. The development of an ileus should arouse suspicion that the graft is suffering rejection. Poor emptying of the native stomach has been a problem after bowel transplantation. This seems to be due to atony of the gastric musculature combined with failure of the pylorus to relax but the underlying cause is unclear. It might reflect a loss of retrograde pacing from the proximal jejunum. It may respond to treatment with metoclopramide, cisapride or clonidine. In the long term it tends to be self-limiting, but it can be very troublesome during the early weeks.

### Immunological

These have been more fully discussed above.

**1.** Acute rejection with mucosal ulceration and bacterial translocation.
**2.** Chronic rejection with fibrosis and loss of absorptive/peristaltic ability.
**3.** Graft-versus-host disease which tends to be mild and self-limiting clinically, but can lead to liver dysfunction, fever, skin rash etc.

### Infection

This represents a major cause of morbidity and mortality.

**1.** Bacterial sepsis: this is either from translocation, leakage, catheter sepsis or other sources such as the urinary tract or chest.
**2.** Viral: cytomegalovirus infections causing hepatic dysfunction, bone marrow suppression and pneumonitis are more severe if due to a primary infection (infection from blood products or from a seropositive donor) than if due to reactivation of the dormant virus in the recipient. Epstein–Barr virus reactivation or transmission from the graft can lead to a viral type illness, or to post-transplant lymphoproliferative disease (PTLD) which merges as a continuum with B cell lymphoma. This may be due to chronic viral infection combined with selective suppression of T cells and is a particular problem in patients receiving large doses of anti-T cell agents such as the monoclonal antibody OKT3. Oral and oesophageal lesions from herpes simplex respond swiftly to acyclovir or ganciclovir therapy and prophylaxis is probably not merited.
**3.** Fungal/yeast: oropharyngeal candidiasis can lead to lesions in the mouth and oesophagus, with colonisation of the graft following aggressive antibiotic treatment. Topical treatment with nystatin or

amphotericin lozenges can be replaced by systemic treatment with fluconazole. This will cover *Candida albicans* but is less effective against other strains such as *Candida tropicalis*, and amphotericin may be needed. The potential nephrotoxicity of this drug may be reduced if the lysosomal preparation is used. This drug is also used to treat aspergillosis which can lead to a severe pneumonia or to overwhelming sepsis and death from multisystem failure.

4. Protozoa: *Pneumocystis carinii* can lead to a severe chest infection in the immunocompromised host, presenting with hypoxia and visible infiltrates on a chest radiograph although the initial changes can be subtle. The diagnosis is confirmed with bronchoscopy and broncho-alveolar lavage or transbronchial biopsy; the characteristic pathogens are demonstrated with silver staining. Treatment is with oxygen with or without ventilatory support, high dose co-trimoxazole and reduc-tion/withdrawal of immunosuppression.

## Results and recom-mendations

The initial results reported from the modern era of bowel transplantation are strikingly good when compared with the equivalent results for heart and kidney transplantation when these procedures were at their genesis.

The largest single centre experience has been reported from Pittsburgh and this forms approximately one-third of the world experience. The international small bowel transplant registry data were made available in 1995 and derives figures from a pooled experience of 182 cases operated on in 25 centres worldwide.[5] More than half the cases are paediatric and more than half of the patients were hospitalised at the time of their transplant. The majority were for short gut syndrome complicated by central line difficulties (sepsis and loss of access sites) and/or liver dysfunction. Of the 182 cases, 38% received isolated intestine transplants, 46% were bowel + liver, and the remaining 16% were composite multivisceral grafts including at least one additional organ.

The majority (72%) of patients received an immunosuppressive regimen based on tacrolimus with the remainder treated by cyclo-sporin-based therapy.

Results are better for patients treated with tacrolimus than with cyclosporin, both in the isolated small bowel and composite graft recipients. In tacrolimus-treated patients, the one-year actuarial graft survival for isolated bowel transplants is 60%, falling to around 33% by three years. The patient survival in this group is higher – 80% at one year, and 50% at three years since loss of the graft is not inevitably fatal, and excision of the graft allows withdrawal of immunosuppression. This, of course, is not the case for combined liver/bowel transplants where both patient and graft survival is around 60% at one year and 40% at three years. There is concern regarding this graft attrition rate after the first year.

Overall, 84 (49%) of the recipients have died, chiefly from multiorgan failure or sepsis. It is of concern that 55% of these died with a functioning graft and it seems likely that if immunosuppression had been withdrawn sooner and the graft removed there might have been less deaths from septic complications.

Of the 86 survivors, nine (10%) have had the intestinal graft removed, 67 (78%) have stopped TPN and the remaining 10 (12%) require partial TPN.

In a select subgroup derived from the Pittsburgh series, where only CMV-negative donors without inclusion of the colon are studied, results are significantly better with 70% actuarial 4-year survival.

## Conclusions and the way ahead

The advent of powerful immunosuppressive agents, in particular tacrolimus, has allowed transplantation of the isolated bowel graft without inevitable failure from rejection. Despite this, rejection is still a major problem and in addition to advances in immunosuppressive drugs, biological methods to induce microchimerism by simultaneous infusion of bone marrow from the donor are currently being evaluated in Pittsburgh. Although the composite liver/bowel graft has the attraction of donor-specific protection of the bowel by the liver, this is outweighed by the disadvantage that, unlike the isolated bowel graft, the status quo cannot be restored in cases of graft failure and immunosuppression cannot be withdrawn. Failure of the transplanted bowel is often complicated by sepsis from bacterial translocation and in such cases it would be desirable to withdraw all immunosuppression but this cannot be done if the recipient still bears a transplanted liver. For this reason, bowel transplantation is preferable to the combined procedure if the liver is healthy. GVHD has not proven to be the problem that had been predicted experimentally and is generally self-limiting and may even be advantageous in some cases. There does not appear to be any detrimental effect long term from having an intestine which is denervated with the normal lymphatic channels interrupted. With the evolution of techniques of rapid tissue typing it should become possible to improve HLA matching of donors and recipients. It is hoped that immunosuppression will continue to improve and become more selective for rejection responses, thus reducing the risk of opportunistic infection and lymphoma. The use of anti-Epstein–Barr virus (EBV) immunoglobulin and less non-specific T cell depletion may reduce the incidence of EBV driven B cell lymphoma which has been shown to be due to host-derived virus.[18] The selective use of CMV-negative donors and excluding colon from the graft would be predicted to improve results by reducing the risk of sepsis.

Although the long-term results such as the yearly attrition rate from chronic rejection and the lymphoma incidence remain unknown and hence areas of concern, it seems likely that we will see bowel transplantation being introduced more widely as a therapeutic modality in many of the larger transplant units around the world. The continued reporting of cases to the International Registry, supervised by Dr David Grant in London, Ontario, is essential while data are being derived from a large number of centres around the world. It seems most appropriate that small bowel transplant programmes only develop in units with a pre-existing liver transplant programme. This has already been the case in the UK where clinical bowel transplant programmes are cautiously underway in three units (Leeds, Cambridge and Birmingham) by the same teams of surgeons who have developed liver transplantation in these centres.

## References

1. Cohen Z, Silverman RE, Wassef *et al*. Small intestinal transplantation using cyclosporin. Transplantation 1986; 42: 613–21.
2. Grant D, Wall W, Mimeault R *et al*. Successful small bowel/liver transplantation. Lancet 1990; 335: 181–4.
3. Revillon Y, Jan D, Goulet O *et al*. Small bowel transplantation in seven children: preservation technique. Transplant Proc 1991; 23: 2350–3.
4. Grant D. Current results of intestinal transplantation. Lancet 1996; 347: 1801.
5. Lennard-Jones, JE. Indications and need for long term parenteral nutrition: implications for intestinal transplantation. Transplant Proc 1990; 22: 2427–9.
6. Byrne, TA, Persinger RL, Young LS, Ziegler TR, Wilmore DW. A new treatment for patients with short-bowel syndrome. Ann Surg 1995; 222: 243–55.
7. Bianchi A. Intestinal loop lengthening – a technique for increasing small intestinal length. J Paediatr Surg 1980; 15: 145–51.
8. Iwaki Y, Starzl TE, Yagihasi A *et al*. Replacement of donor lymphoid tissue in small bowel transplants. Lancet 1991; 337: 818–19.
9. Diflo T, Maki T, Balogh K, Monaco AP. Graft-versus-host disease in fully allogeneic small bowel transplantation in the rat. Transplantation 1989; 47: 7–11.
10. Ballinger WFII, Christy MG, Ashby WB. Auto-transplantation of the small intestine: the effect of denervation. Surgery 1962; 52: 151–64.
11. Cooke HJ. Neurobiology of the intestinal mucosa. Gastroenterology 1986; 90: 1057–81.
12. Goott B, Lillehei RC, Miller FA. Mesenteric lymphatic regeneration after autografts of small bowel in dogs. Surgery 1960; 48: 571–5.
13. Olivier C, Rettori R, Camilleri JP. Interruption of the lymphatic vessels and its consequences in total homotransplantation of the small intestine and right side of the colon in man. Lymphology 1972; 5: 24–31.
14. Collins BH, Bollinger RR. The mucosal barrier. In: Grant DR, Wood RFM (eds) Small bowel transplantation. London: Edward Arnold, 1994, pp. 53–69.
15. Holmes JT, Klein MS, Winawer SJ *et al*. Morphologic studies of rejection in canine jejunal grafts. Gastroenterology 1971; 61: 693–706.
16. Rosemurgy AS, Schraut WH. Small bowel allografts: sequence of histologic changes in acute and chronic rejection. Am J Surg 1986; 151: 470–5.
17. Grant D, Hurlbut D, Zhong R *et al*. Intestinal permeability and bacterial translocation following small bowel transplantation in the rat. Transplantation 1991; 52: 221–4.
18. Tibbles L, Gawley WF, McAlister VC *et al*. CD21 and CD24 monoclonal antibodies for the treatment of Epstein–Barr virus induced lymphoproliferative syndrome in a patient with a multi-visceral transplant. Clin Invest Med 1991; 14: A140.

# 11 Heart, lung and heart–lung transplantation

*Jonathan Forty*

Data on cardiopulmonary transplants are collected annually by the International Society for Heart and Lung Transplantation and although not every centre in the world contributes to these figures, nonetheless they give a good indication of activity and outcome. A total of 34 326 procedures has been recorded in the 14 years of the Registry. Early steady growth in activity has plateaued with around 4000 transplants registered in 1995 of which 75% were cardiac operations and 25% were pulmonary.[1]

Heart transplantation is the most common thoracic transplant and is performed for end-stage cardiac failure or intractable cardiac pathology. Pulmonary replacement can be performed as a single lung transplant when the remaining native lung will not compromise the recipient or as a bilateral (sequential) transplant when it is necessary to remove all native lung tissue. True, en-bloc double lung transplant with a tracheal anastomosis has fallen into disuse. When both heart and lungs are involved in the pathological process an en-bloc heart and lung transplant is performed with central anastomoses.

## Heart transplantation

### Indications for heart transplantation

In adults heart grafting is performed for end-stage failure in assorted cardiomyopathies, the most common aetiology being ischaemic (coronary) heart disease. Rarely, transplantation may be necessitated by untreatable angina or the complications of ischaemic heart disease (e.g. intractable ventricular tachycardia) which cannot be managed by conventional cardiac surgery even though ventricular function is preserved. Other unusual indications include inoperable valve disease, congenital defects, drug toxicity and re-transplantation. The frequency of indications is shown in Fig. 11.1.

The heart is usually placed in its correct anatomical site with both systemic and pulmonary circulations supported by the graft with the native heart removed (orthotopic). A much smaller number of hetero-

**Figure 11.1** *The common indications for adult cardiac transplantation* (from the ISHLT Registry).

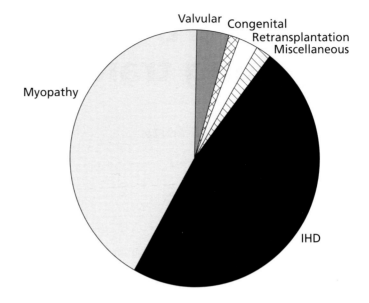

topic transplants has been performed in which the systemic venous connection is superior cava to cava, the left atrial connection is direct, the donor aorta is anastomosed end-to-side onto the recipient ascending aorta and the pulmonary arterial connection is with a Dacron interposition graft. The usual reasons for adopting this approach are acute cardiac failure where a sufficiently large donor heart is not available or for patients with excessively elevated pulmonary vascular resistance (see discussion below). In these circumstances the preserved native heart continues to give some support to the graft and the circulation.

Paediatric heart transplantation (age 0–16 years) is a more recent field, though now well established with many designated centres throughout

**Figure 11.2** *The common indications for paediatric cardiac transplantation* (from the ISHLT Registry).

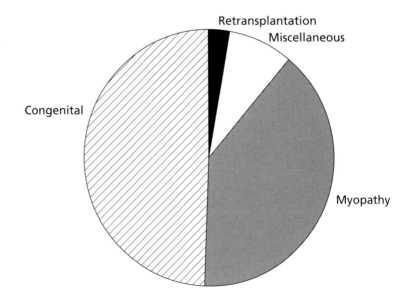

the world. The indications for transplantation differ from those seen in the adult population with congenital defects replacing ischaemic heart disease as the most common pathology. Acute cardiomyopathies are also more common in this age group (Fig. 11.2).

Heart and lung transplantation combined is undertaken for primary cardiac pathology when the cardiac lesion has produced irreversible pulmonary hypertension to a degree that prevents cardiac replacement alone since this would result in acute failure of the graft right ventricle as it attempts to eject into the abnormal pulmonary vasculature. Examples include pulmonary hypertension resulting from chronic left heart failure or exposure to systemic pressures through a congenital defect with a left-to-right shunt (reversal of the shunt as pulmonary hypertension develops, produces the cyanosis of Eisenmenger's syndrome).

## Heart recipient assessment and selection

Patients with end-stage cardiac failure are admitted for a three-day assessment programme. They undergo a medical assessment with particular emphasis on cardiac function, other organ failure and the identification of previously undetected pathologies. They also undergo psychological and social evaluation to ensure they will be able to cope with the new problems associated with successful transplantation and that they have adequate social support to manage their own care subsequent to transplantation. The assessment period should be seen as a two-way process where patients are given the opportunity to learn the realities of transplantation and perhaps meet successful recipients. At the end of the assessment a recommendation for future treatment can be given to the patient. If this is transplantation, then the surgeon explains the risks and benefits of the operation so that the patient can make an informed decision to allow inclusion on the transplant waiting list.

The heart assessment programme is designed to ascertain that all conventional (medical and surgical) options have been exhausted, that the patient is sufficiently disabled to need transplantation on symptomatic or prognostic grounds and that there are no contraindications to transplantation. The timing of listing for transplant is critical. Since life expectancy with a graft is limited (typically eight to ten years) and in the context of limited donor availability retransplantation is uncommon, premature transplantation can curtail prognostic benefit. Equally, excessive delay in patients with prognostic markers (see below) can result in the development of contraindications to transplantation (general debility, nutritional failure and irreversible multiorgan damage) or, of course, death whilst waiting.

The assessment tests are summarised in Table 11.1. Some tests help to exclude pathology which could be managed by conventional means (e.g. coronary grafting); coronary angiography, thallium scanning and dobutamine stress echocardiography are therefore performed only if indicated. Others are designed to identify prognostic indices (summarised in Table 11.2). These include the pulmonary capillary wedge pressure

**Table 11.1**  *Assessment tests for potential cardiac transplant recipients*

| | |
|---|---|
| **All patients** | Full blood count, platelets, coag screen |
| | Blood group and antibody screen |
| | Urea, electrolytes, creatinine and liver function tests |
| | Uric acid |
| | Hepatitis B/C and HIV |
| | Fasting glucose and lipids |
| | Chromium EDTA GFR |
| | Chest radiograph (PA and lateral) |
| | 12 lead ECG and 24 hour tape |
| | Echocardiogram |
| | Right heart catheter |
| |    mean PAP |
| |    mean PCWP |
| |    cardiac index |
| |    calculated pulmonary gradient and PVR |
| |    manipulation of PVR |
| | Spirometry |
| | Swabs of nose, throat, axilla, perineum |
| | MSU and sputum to microbiology |
| **If conventional surgery considered** | Coronary angiography |
| | Thallium scan |
| | Dobutamine stress echo |
| **After acceptance** | CMV, Herpes, EBV, Legionella |
| | Viral screen |
| | Tissue typing and lymphocyte cross-match |
| | Auto-antibody screen |

**Table 11.2**  *Prognostic indicators in heart failure (see text for abbreviations)*

NYHA class III or IV
Left ventricular ejection fraction $<20\%$
Increased PCWP
Non-sustained VT
Failed sudden death
Use of anti-arrhythmic agents
Elevated serum catecholamines
Low serum sodium
Raised blood urea
Maximum oxygen consumption $<14\,\mathrm{ml\,kg^{-1}\,min^{-1}}$

(obtained at right heart catheterisation) which reflects the rising left atrial pressure resulting from a progressively failing left ventricle. A maximal oxygen consumption under exercise conditions ($MVO_2$) less than $14\,\mathrm{ml\,kg^{-1}\,min^{-1}}$ is thought to indicate poor prognosis. A history of cardiac arrhythmias or easily induced ventricular tachycardia at electrophysiological study is also valuable as a prognostic marker. Further tests assess any impairment in other systems in an attempt to identify contra-indications to transplantation. Relative and absolute contraindications are summarised in Table 11.3.

Measurement of pulmonary vascular resistance (PVR) at right heart catheterisation with a pulmonary artery flotation catheter is essential. Patients with a fixed elevated PVR cannot be managed with heart transplantation alone but if the patient is otherwise unblemished the patient might be considered for en-bloc heart and lung transplantation. A PVR of greater than 6 Wood units is considered to preclude heart transplantation. Patients with a PVR at the upper end of the range can be transplanted but a larger donor must be used (see comments on matching donor to recipient below). At the time of right heart catheter-isation attempts are made to manipulate an elevated PVR. Techniques used range from supplemental oxygen, through simple vasodilators such as sodium nitroprusside or gliceryl trinitrate to direct infusion of prostacyclins into the pulmonary artery. If a raised PVR can be brought down with manipulation the patient can be listed but will need to be admitted a little earlier prior to transplant so that a pulmonary artery flotation catheter can be inserted and manipulation can be performed prior to and during the operation and in the immediate postoperative period. Chronic control of PVR can also be achieved with prostaglandin therapy.[2]

Most patients assessed have a degree of renal impairment. This can result from underperfusion and high venous pressures, drug therapy

**Table 11.3.**  *Contraindications to cardiac transplantation (see text for abbreviations)*

| | |
|---|---|
| **Absolute** | Multiorgan failure |
| | On-going sepsis |
| | Current malignancy |
| | Active peptic ulceration |
| | PVR >6 Wood units |
| | Reversible causes of heart failure or inadequate therapy |
| |    reversible ischaemia |
| |    inadequate control of AF |
| |    continued alcohol use |
| |    untreated endocrine disorder |
| |    poor salt and water control |
| |    ineffective use of vasodilators or antiarrythmics |
| **Relative** | Diabetes |
| | Peripheral and cerebral vascular disease |
| | Obesity and raised PVR |
| | Osteoporosis |
| | Chronic pulmonary disease |
| | Cardiac cachexia |

(diuretics and ACE inhibitors) or intrinsic renal disease including renal artery stenosis. Renal function is assessed by glomerular filtration and renal biopsy if indicated. A small number of patients are accepted for combined heart and kidney replacement.

It is now recognised that it is possible to support patients in heart failure with mechanical ventricular assist devices for months if necessary. Provided potential recipients remain sepsis-free with single organ failure they can be assessed for transplantation in the knowledge that the outcome for such 'bridge to transplant' patients is comparable to that for unsupported patients. However, those who have undergone some catastrophic cardiac event and are ventilator dependent with incipient multiorgan failure do less well. Here there is only a small window of opportunity for grafting and such referrals should be treated with caution. Acute retransplantation for graft failure is also associated with poor outcome[3] and many centres have a policy not to undertake such transplants.

## Heart donor criteria and selection

The general considerations and criteria for organ donation are described in Chapter 2. Management of the donor during the perioperative period is a multidisciplinary process as the requirement is met for optimal function of different organs.

Specific considerations for heart donation are shown in Table 11.4. The mechanisms of coning and brain-stem death have a significant impact on the heart and circulatory system. Many donors when referred are on significant doses of ATP-depleting inotropes and receive large volumes of crystalloid in an attempt to fill a vasodilated circulation and maintain the perfusion pressure to other organs. Neither is good for the heart. The judicious use of vasoconstrictors under these circumstances (arginine vasopressin can be especially effective)[4] will often permit weaning of inotropes prior to heart removal without compromise to other organs. The early arrival of a donor team who can insert and use a pulmonary artery flotation catheter to optimise the haemodynamics can be invaluable.[5] The final assessment of ventricular function is a visual one performed by the surgeon aided by knowledge of the systemic arterial

**Table 11.4** *Organ donation for cardiac transplantation*

| Requirements | Age up to 60 years |
| --- | --- |
| | No previous proven or treated ischaemia |
| | No prolonged cardiac arrest |
| | Minimal inotropic support |
| | Vasopressin as a substitute for ATP-depleting inotropes |
| Will consider | Chest trauma |
| | Single vessel coronary disease |
| | Primary cerebral malignancy |

and venous pressures supplemented by a line in the left atrium or the data from a pulmonary catheter.

Donors are considered up to the age of 60 years in our unit though many centres are more restrictive. Many older donors will have intrinsic cardiac disease but some do not and in a donor-restricted practice consideration of such hearts is valid. Predonation assessment of coronary disease is impractical so again a judgement is made by the donor surgeon on visual inspection of the coronary arteries.

### Heart recipient–donor matching (see also Chapter 4)

As a result of the poor prognosis of heart failure, waiting lists for cardiac transplantation never contain large numbers of patients. Consequently, even on a national basis, matching of donor to recipient can be performed only to crude criteria.

When a donor organ is offered to a transplant centre the first match is by ABO blood group. Patients with a positive lymphocyte cross-match must be prospectively matched with donor blood. The next consideration is size. Recipients with a low pulmonary vascular resistance can accept the heart of a donor some 20% smaller and some reports describe using hearts considerably smaller.[6] Larger hearts can occasionally cause difficulty due to restricted space in the chest though this consideration really applies only to paediatric recipients; examination of chest radiographs can be helpful in these circumstances. If the PVR is elevated, a proportionately larger donor is needed. In general, weight is equated with size but some attention can also be applied to height. It will be obvious that since the typical donor is younger and tends to be smaller than the typical recipient, patients who are larger or have a raised PVR will wait longer for transplantation and will have a poorer survival on the waiting list.

In the context of small donor and recipient pools, matching for tissue type is impractical though retrospective studies have shown mismatches to be more likely to reject.[7] Although cytomegalovirus (CMV) mismatch has clinical implications in the postoperative period, it is not feasible to match for this variable as a routine.

### Heart retrieval and preservation

The thoracic organs are approached through a median sternotomy. In a multiorgan retrieval, this will often have been performed by the liver retrieval team to assist with access to the upper abdominal organs. When liver mobilisation is complete, the heart retrieval team can join the operating table and open the pericardium. The heart can now be inspected and carefully palpated to ensure that there is no obvious coronary artery disease and observed for normal contractility. The patient is fully heparinised.

The pericardium is held up with stay sutures and a sling is placed around the ascending aorta. The superior (SVC) and inferior vena cavae

(IVC) are mobilised and two ligatures are placed around the SVC but left untied. A perfusion cannula for the administration of cardioplegic solution is placed in the ascending aorta. When the perfusion apparatus for the other organs has been established the heart can now be removed. The ligatures around the superior vena cava are tied and it is divided. The inferior vena cava is clamped above the diaphragm. The aorta is now cross-clamped and the heart cardiopleged with an infusion of St Thomas' crystalloid cardioplegia with simultaneous topical cooling to produce electromechanical arrest in diastole. During infusion the heart can be retracted and the left superior pulmonary vein incised to vent the heart and prevent ventricular distension.

Simultaneously, the abdominal organs are perfused and cooled. When all the cardioplegia has been given, the heart can be completely excised. The inferior vena cava is divided taking care not to damage the coronary sinus which is nearby. The ascending aorta is divided just below the cross-clamp and the left and right pulmonary arteries and the left and right pulmonary veins are now divided flush with the pericardium to complete the excision.

The heart is now examined to ensure that the ligature on the SVC is secured, that there is no unsuspected patent foramen ovale and that heart valves are macroscopically normal. The heart is then placed in cold St Thomas' cardioplegic solution and wrapped in a sterile polythene bag. This bag is wrapped in turn in a further series of two bags, each containing cold physiological solution. The resulting package can be packed with ice and transferred in a cold box to the recipient hospital.

The retrieval of a heart and lung bloc for combined transplant is described in the section on the lung donor operation.

A variety of different solutions have been used for cardiac preservation and transport in an attempt to lengthen ischaemic times (and hence range of donation) and minimise ischaemic or reperfusion injury. University of Wisconsin solution has theoretical advantages[8] but no solution has been demonstrated to be significantly superior to St Thomas' cardioplegic solution in clinical application.

### Heart implantation

The patient is anaesthetised with full monitoring. Left internal jugular cannulation is performed to preserve the right side for access for future endomyocardial biopsies for rejection surveillance. A median sternotomy is performed. The patient is fully heparinised and placed on cardiopulmonary bypass with an inflow cannula in the ascending aorta and cannulae draining the venous circulation placed into the inferior and superior vena cavae through the right atrium. These are snared to facilitate removal of the heart. If separate caval anastomoses are to be performed, the superior vena caval cannulation is through the side of the cava rather than through the native atrium itself.

Cardiopulmonary bypass is now commenced with systemic cooling to 28°C and the aorta is cross-clamped. The heart is excised by serially incising the free wall of the right atrium down towards the coronary sinus and round to the root of the left atrium. The interatrial septum is now opened. The aorta is transected above the aortic valve and coronary ostia and the pulmonary artery divided at the same level. All that remains is to excise the left atrium. The incision is continued from the septum along the coronary sinus and across the free wall of the left atrium posteriorly. Care is taken not to carry this excision down into the left pulmonary veins. Fig. 11.3 shows the pericardial cavity awaiting the graft and the right atrial anastomosis.

**Figure 11.3** *The pericardial cavity awaiting the graft and the right atrial anastomosis.*

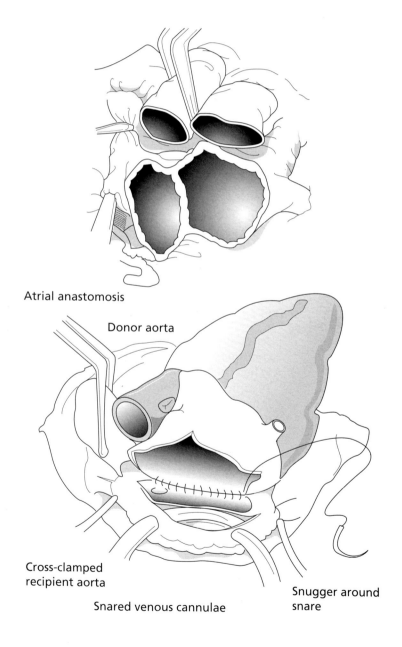

Atrial anastomosis

Donor aorta

Cross-clamped
recipient aorta

Snared venous cannulae

Snugger around
snare

The donor heart is now prepared by trimming the pulmonary artery back to the main bifurcation and separating this from the ascending aorta. The left atrium is opened by joining the pulmonary veins but the right atrium is left intact at this stage.

At this point it may be appropriate to recardioplege the donor heart with blood cardioplegia (recipient blood). Implantation proceeds with the left atrial anastomosis performed with a continuous 3/0 Prolene suture along the free margin of the left atrium and then along the interatrial septum. The heart is kept covered with a cold swab during this period or a cold infusion may be run over its surface. The pulmonary artery anastomosis is performed next with a 4/0 Prolene suture taking care that there is no kinking of either donor or recipient pulmonary artery. The right atrial anastomosis follows after opening the right atrium from the inferior cava up towards the right atrial appendage, taking care not to damage the sino-atrial node. A 3/0 Prolene suture is used to complete the anastomosis commencing at the septum and then working along the free margin of the atrium. An alternative at this point is not to open the atrium but to perform direct caval anastomoses with 4/0 Prolene sutures. The recent fashion to perform separate 'bicaval anastomoses' for systemic venous connection in place of a right atrial anastomosis carries the benefits of lower incidence of tricuspid regurgitation (this can cause significant morbidity in a small number of recipients) and of atrial dysrhythmias.[9] The technique is not without its complications however, with anastomotic stenoses being reported.

The implantation is now completed by anastomosing the aorta with a continuous 4/0 Prolene suture. The patient is rewarmed and after careful de-airing the aortic cross-clamp is removed to reperfuse the organ. DC cardioversion may be needed to establish sinus rhythm but often the heart spontaneously defibrillates.

Ventricular and atrial pacing wires are applied and can be used for sequential atrioventricular pacing. An isoprenaline infusion is also commenced. Sinus rhythm at a rate of 100–110 beats $min^{-1}$ is desirable. When the patient is warm and the organ has been reperfused for about 20 minutes cardiopulmonary bypass can be weaned with care. It is important to ensure that the right ventricle does not overdistend during this period particularly if the recipient PVR is elevated. Two chest drains are placed into the pericardium and routine closure follows.

Patients are usually extubated within 8 h and can return to the ward from the intensive care unit within 12 h.

## Heart–lung implantation

Access is via a median sternotomy. Cannulation for bypass is with an aortic inflow cannula and separate snared caval cannulae. The heart is removed as described above and the oblique sinus is then opened so the entire left atrium can subsequently be removed with the lungs. The pericardium is incised anterior to each hilum and the pulmonary veins are separated from the posterior pericardium with electrocautery taking

**Figure 11.4** *The tracheal anastomosis in heart-and-lung transplantation.*

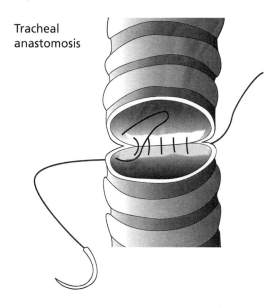

Tracheal anastomosis

care not to damage the oesophagus and aorta which are adjacent. The interatrial septum is preserved as the right-sided pulmonary veins are mobilised. The left and right lungs are now removed sequentially. The pleura is opened on each side and the inferior pulmonary ligaments are divided up to the level of the inferior pulmonary veins. This dissection continues posterior to the hilum on each side. The pulmonary artery is divided on each side and left and right bronchi are stapled prior to completing excision of the lungs. During mobilisation of each hilum great awareness of the phrenic nerves is required. The carina and remnants of the bronchi are now excised from behind the ascending aorta with meticulous haemostasis.

The donor trachea is trimmed just above the carina and the organs are inserted into the chest, passing the lungs through the pericardial window on each side. The tracheal anastomosis is performed with continuous 3/0 Prolene (Fig. 11.4). Right atrial and aortic anastomoses are completed as described for heart transplantation. De-airing, rewarming and reperfusion follow before cardiopulmonary bypass is weaned. Pleural and pericardial drains are placed and the sternotomy is closed. After stabilisation in the intensive care unit the patient can be extubated and returned to the ward.

### Peri- and postoperative care for heart transplants

Patients are admitted from the waiting list for heart transplantation at short notice and are rapidly re-assessed to detect intercurrent infections, new organ failure and unacceptable deterioration. Anaesthesia commences as soon as the donor organ has been safely removed and is in transit. The recipient will not have been starved so 'crash induction' techniques are used.

Inotropic support for the transplanted heart is needed only occasionally though dopamine administered at a renal dose is routinely used. An isoprenaline infusion is commenced during reperfusion to achieve a heart rate of around 110 beats min$^{-1}$ and reduce end diastolic volume. Isoprenaline is also helpful as a pulmonary vasodilator; right ventricular failure as the patient is weaned from cardiopulmonary bypass is not uncommon especially if the PVR is elevated. If sinus rhythm and a suitable rate cannot be achieved then atrioventricular sequential pacing is employed. This may need to be continued for days or even weeks until native sinus rhythm at an acceptable rate is established. Maintenance of these conditions is essential to preserve renal function and help clear oedema in the postoperative period. On occasion permanent pacing is needed.

Immunosuppression is commenced prior to the operation with azathioprine (4 mg kg$^{-1}$ orally) and cyclosporin A (CsA) (4–6 mg kg$^{-1}$) if renal function is not impaired (a peak in the serum CsA level whilst on cardiopulmonary bypass is sufficient to produce acute renal failure in already compromised kidneys). If CsA is withheld it is commenced in the early postoperative period once there is an adequate urine output and serum creatinine begins to fall. CsA is given twice daily by the intravenous route and subsequently orally to achieve morning serum trough levels of 400 ng l$^{-1}$ (this is reduced to 200 ng l$^{-1}$ at 6 weeks). If poor renal function precludes administration of CsA then antithymocyte globulin (ATG) is given, a daily flow cytometry count indicating the level of T-cell destruction. Although we use cytolytic therapy only in these circumstances, some centres still use it as adjunctive immunosuppression routinely. Methyl prednisolone (500 mg) is administered at the time of reperfusion of the graft and subsequently 8 hourly for the first 24 h. Oral steroids are then commenced with a reducing dose commencing at 1 mg kg$^{-1}$ day$^{-1}$ until a maintenance dose of 0.2 mg kg$^{-1}$ day$^{-1}$ is achieved. In the absence of rejection this can be reduced still further at six months. Azathioprine is maintained at a dose of 1.5–3.0 mg kg$^{-1}$ provided the white cell count does not become depressed.

In paediatric recipients this regimen is modified with the routine use of ATG cytolytic therapy for seven days. Methyl prednisolone (15 mg kg$^{-1}$) is given at reperfusion and as three subsequent doses (3 mg kg$^{-1}$) 8 hourly. Oral steroids are then only given to those children over five years of age and these are weaned after six weeks.

Antibiotic prophylaxis is given at induction (flucloxacillin for Gram positive cover is adequate). This is continued for 48 h and then stopped. Further antibiotics are only given if indicated by positive cultures. Acyclovir is used as prophylaxis against herpetic infection and oral nystatin against candidiasis. If there is a CMV mismatch, CMV immunoglobulin is given until seroconversion occurs. *Pneumocystis carinii* prophylaxis is with co-trimoxazole given at weekends.

Immunosuppressive and antimicrobial treatments often require modification as the agents used produce unwanted side effects; the marrow suppression of azathioprine, ganciclovir and antifungal agents and the

**Table 11.5**  *Grading of cardiac allograft rejection*

| acute rejection | 0 | none |
|---|---|---|
| | 1 | mild – focal infiltrate |
| | 3 | moderate – multifocal aggressive infiltrates with myocyte damage |
| | 4 | severe – infiltrate, oedema, vasculitis, necrosis, haemorrhage |

nephrotoxic effects of CsA for example. Daily monitoring of haematological and biochemical levels are therefore important.

Routine endocardial biopsies are performed to detect rejection. Biopsies are taken at weekly intervals for six weeks, fortnightly up to 12 weeks, monthly up to six months, every three months to a year and then annually unless additional biopsies are clinically indicated. A bioptome is introduced under X-ray screening from the right internal jugular vein into the right ventricle where endomyocardial samples are taken and examined histologically. In addition coronary angiography to detect occlusive disease is performed annually from two years onwards.

Rejection grading is summarised in Table 11.5.[10] Grade 1 does not require treatment. Grades 3 and 4 are treated. Grade 2 rejection, represented by very focal lymphocyte infiltration is often included in Grade 1 and requires treatment only if there are additional clinical concerns. Treatment is by augmentation of steroid therapy (three days of intravenous methyl prednisolone (500 mg) and subsequent augmentation of oral steroids).

## Outcomes and complications of heart transplantation

The actuarial survival of recipients of orthotopic heart transplants in the modern era (postintroduction of CsA) is shown in Fig. 11.5 for adults. These are aggregate world-wide data and survival in the Freeman Hospital series is also shown to demonstrate what can be achieved in an established unit. All curves have an early shoulder which reflects operative mortality and early donor organ dysfunction, infection and rejection as immunosuppression is established. Paediatric survival data is shown in Fig. 11.6. In general the outcome for paediatric transplants is similar to that for adult transplants though the younger the child the worse the survival.[1]

Perioperative mortality reflects a number of factors. Acute donor organ dysfunction may result from ATP depletion after inotrope usage in the donor, from poor preservation or reperfusion injury. Renal failure or other multisystem failure may develop in the sick recipient. Sepsis may intervene as immunosuppression is established.

Hyperacute rejection is an antibody-mediated phenomenon and results in rapid graft failure within hours of reperfusion. Plasmapheresis and mechanical support may help but survival is rare. Acute rejection can be seen from a few days after transplant. It may present as acute graft

**Figure 11.5** *The actuarial survival of recipients of orthotopic heart transplants in the modern era (postintroduction of CsA).* Freeman and ISHLT Registry data.

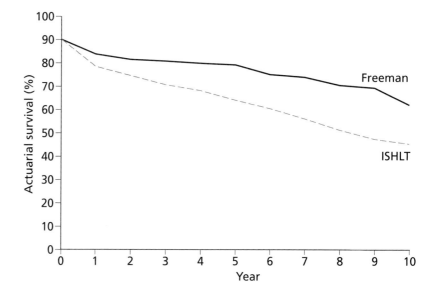

**Figure 11.6** *Actuarial survival after paediatric heart transplantation.* ISHLT Registry data.

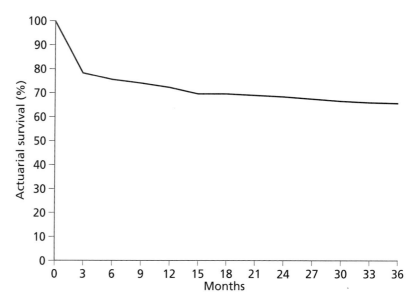

failure or more insidiously with fever, leukocytosis, oedema and tiredness. Suspected rejection is investigated with cardiac biopsy and treated as described above. Patients treated for rejection are re-biopsied after a week; continuing rejection may necessitate cytolytic therapy with ATG, monoclonal therapy or a change in immunosuppressive agent, to tacrolimus for example.

Long-term immunosuppression predisposes recipients to malignancies of all cell types. Lymphoproliferative disorders are the most common form. It is believed that this condition results from uncontrolled Epstein–Barr virus (EBV) driven proliferation of B cells in the context of T-cell depression. Patients particularly at risk are EBV negative pretransplant and receive greater than average immunosuppression.[11] Management is therefore directed to reducing immunosuppression as much as possible and administering the antiviral agent acyclovir. If this is unsuccessful, chemotherapy is used although patients requiring this have a poor prognosis.

Chronic rejection seems to manifest itself in the transplanted heart as occlusive disease in the coronary arteries.[12] As such, diagnosis is made at angiography rather than on endomyocardial biopsy. Unlike coronary atheroma this phenomenon is neither focal nor proximal and is therefore not suitable for conventional revascularisation procedures. There seems to be an association between multiple episodes of early aggressive rejection and the development of coronary occlusion. Sudden death several years after transplant is a common source of mortality in patients who are known to have occlusive disease.

Numerous quality-of-life studies have shown improvement in symptom status and life satisfaction though return to work rates are low.[13] Those patients with continuing symptoms still cope well with little functional restriction.[14] Whether heart transplantation is a cost-effective approach to end-stage cardiac failure is more difficult to ascertain. It is difficult to cost all follow-up and subsequent treatment costs and costs for a non-transplanted group of patients will be less as survival is curtailed. However, using a cost per quality adjusted life year model, indicators of effectiveness are favourable.[15]

Survival data for en-bloc heart and lung transplantation for cardiac indications are more difficult to ascertain since most reported series do not disaggregate survival data from transplants performed for pulmonary pathologies. However, survival for cardiac indications is probably similar to that for orthotopic heart transplantation. The complications, in contrast, are more in line with those seen in lung transplantation (see below) although it is important to recognise that cardiac rejection can be seen in these grafts in the absence of lung rejection.

## Lung transplantation

### Indications for lung transplantation

Bilateral (sequential) lung transplantation (BSLT) is performed where it is necessary to remove all native lung tissue. For example, with the chronic lung sepsis of cystic fibrosis (the most common indication for BSLT) or bronchiectasis single lung replacement would fail with infection spilling over from the native lung into the graft. Similarly, extensive destruction of both lungs in emphysema may encourage bilateral replacement to avoid air-trapping in a remaining native lung, which may result in mediastinal shift and compromise to the contralateral graft. Superadded sepsis in emphysematous lungs is also an indication for bilateral transplant.

Single lung transplantation (SLT) is an attractive approach to the treatment of lung failure. The operation can often be performed without the acute injury to lung tissue and other attendant risks of cardiopulmonary bypass. There is an economy in use of scarce donor organs with two lung recipients benefiting from each donor and, in the event of acute or chronic injury to the graft, some viable native lung tissue will remain. Fibrotic lung conditions with normal pulmonary vasculature, a relatively immobile mediastinum and no native overinflation are most suited to this modality of pulmonary replacement. However, SLT is used with varying enthusiasm between centres for selected patients with emphysema (with or without $\alpha_1$-antitrypsin deficiency), life-threatening asthma and sarcoidosis.

A controversial area is transplantation for primary pulmonary hypertension. Here, in the absence of structural injury to the heart, BSLT may suffice though many centres still advocate en-bloc heart and lung transplantation. Some centres are performing SLT alone in these circumstances. Survival for all three modalities of treatment for primary pulmonary hypertension is similar.

Transplantation of both lungs en-bloc with the heart for pulmonary pathology is becoming less popular although this was the early means of lung replacement. Some centres still use this approach in circumstances where total lung tissue replacement is required (the same indications as for BSLT). Although at first sight this may seem wasteful of scarce donor hearts since BSLT will suffice, the (normal) recipient heart is harvested and used as a living organ donation for a heart transplant candidate (the 'domino' operation).[16]

The indications for each modality of lung replacement are summarised in Fig. 11.7 together with an indication of the popularity of each approach in world-wide practice.

## Lung recipient assessment and selection

The general aspects of assessment for lung transplantation are identical to those for heart assessment. Again, after inpatient assessment, a recommendation is made to the patient by the surgeon after ensuring that all conventional treatment is exhausted and timing for listing is appropriate.

The lung assessment tests are summarised in Table 11.6. The six-minute walk test measures the distance a patient is able to walk in a given time and the degree of arterial desaturation that results during the exertion. Not only does this give a measure of symptomatic restriction but it also has prognostic value. Values of less than 300 m are seen in patients in end-stage pulmonary failure.

Computerised tomography (CT) is used to study the texture of lung parenchyma and identify areas of maximal lung destruction or bullous disease with anatomical precision. This, along with the results of ventilation-perfusion scanning assists with the decision of whether to perform BSLT or SLT in those conditions where either might be considered and, if SLT is selected, which side should be transplanted (or whether either side will suffice). It is desirable to explant a lung if there is evidence of chronic sepsis within it or if a bullus that is likely to

**Figure 11.7**  *Usage of each modality of pulmonary replacement by pathology.*

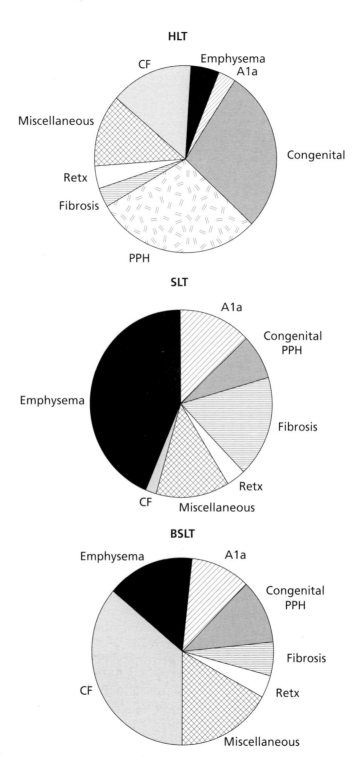

**Table 11.6** *Assessment tests for potential lung transplant recipients*

| | |
|---|---|
| **All patients** | Full blood count, platelets, coag screen |
| | Blood group and antibody screen |
| | Urea, electrolytes, creatinine and liver function tests |
| | Uric acid |
| | Hepatitis B/C and HIV |
| | Fasting glucose and lipids |
| | Chromium EDTA GFR |
| | Chest radiograph (PA and lateral) |
| | 12 lead ECG |
| | Echocardiogram |
| | Gated heart scan if indicated |
| | Coronary angiogram if indicated |
| | Sputum for aspergillus |
| | Aspergillus precipitins |
| | Pulmonary function tests |
| | 6-minute walk test |
| | Ventilation/perfusion scan (single lung recipients) |
| | Alpha-1 level and phenotype (for emphysema patients) |
| | Isotope liver scan (alpha-1 deficiency and cystic fibrosis) |
| | Swabs of nose, throat, axilla, perineum |
| | MSU and sputum to microbiology |
| **After acceptance** | CMV, Herpes, EBV, Legionella |
| | Viral screen |
| | Tissue typing and lymphocyte cross-match |
| | Autoantibody screen |

rupture is present. For SLT it is usual to replace the lung with poorer perfusion. These investigations also help to identify those emphysematous patients who might be suitable for lung-reduction surgery to improve their ventilatory mechanics with symptomatic relief as an alternative to transplantation (see below).

Detailed microbiological screening is an essential part of the assessment with attention also paid to cultures performed over the preceding months and years at the referring centre. An awareness of microbiological history identifies patients likely to be colonised with multiply resistant organisms (especially pseudomonads in the cystic population) and helps direct antibiotic prophylaxis in the perioperative period. Again, in the cystic patients with chronic sepsis and malabsorption, a nutritional assessment is vital since if all muscle bulk is lost insufficient respiratory power will remain to allow the patient to be weaned from the ventilator with a painful thoracotomy wound in the postoperative period. Wound healing is also impaired.

Cardiopulmonary bypass is used routinely for BSLT and on occasion for SLT so coincidental cardiac disease must be identified. Older patients and those with relevant risk profiles undergo cardiac catheterisation

**Table 11.7** *Contraindications to lung transplantation*

| Absolute | Multiorgan failure |
| --- | --- |
| | On-going sepsis |
| | Current malignancy |
| | Active peptic ulceration |
| | Inadequate therapy for pulmonary disease |
| Relative | Diabetes |
| | Peripheral and cerebral vascular disease |
| | Obesity |
| | Osteoporosis |
| | Ischaemic heart disease |
| | Nutritional failure (esp in cystic fibrosis) |

with coronary angiography. Right heart catheterisation is undertaken in patients considered for lung transplantation for pulmonary hypertension. This can be supplemented by pulmonary angiography if pulmonary thromboendarterectomy might be considered as an alternative to grafting.

The remainder of the assessment is designed to identify contraindications to organ replacement. Unlike patients with cardiac failure most candidates for lung replacement have intact renal function. Relative and absolute contraindications for lung transplantation are summarised in Table 11.7.

On occasion patients who have acute pulmonary failure (ARDS, drug overdose or after childbirth) and are ventilator-dependent are referred for transplant consideration. Transplantation is rarely successful under these circumstances as sepsis and other multiorgan failure are common. However, if attempted, it is worth considering single lung replacement since the potential for recovery in the native lung is present in many cases of acute respiratory disease.

## Lung donor criteria and selection

Specific considerations for lung donation are shown in Table 11.8. The circumstances of organ donation lead to potential lung injury in a number of ways. Trauma is not uncommon. Although a haemothorax and fractured ribs may indicate parenchymal damage this is not always so and the contralateral lung may in any case be uninjured.[17] Aspiration of gastric contents at the time of injury or cardiac arrest is not uncommon. Injudicious fluid replacement can produce pulmonary oedema. Transfusion of a large volume of blood products also predisposes to lung injury (sometimes becoming apparent only after implantation) and fat embolus from long bone fractures with catastrophic result has been reported.[17] In all these circumstances infection is more likely and will compound the injury.

**Table 11.8** *Organ donation for pulmonary transplantation*

| | |
|---|---|
| **Requirements** | Age up to 60 years |
| | Good gas exchange |
| | ($P_{AO_2}$ > 50 kPa on 100% $O_2$ with 5 mmHg PEEP) |
| | No evidence of aspiration or embolism |
| | No evidence of pneumonia (CXR and Gram stain) |
| **Will consider** | Chest trauma |
| | Primary cerebral malignancy |
| | Asthma |
| | Smoker |

Examination of the chest radiograph is essential. Aspirates taken from the endotracheal tube should be stained and microscoped in the donor hospital. Mixed Gram-negative and -positive organisms and numerous polymorphs in the aspirate may indicate potentially unacceptable infection. Previous culture results should be requested and considered. Use of broad spectrum antibiotics in the absence of specific organism sensitivities should also be treated with caution. Flexible bronchoscopy can be useful to facilitate full expansion of the lungs and obtain good specimens of pulmonary secretions.

Lung function is assessed by gas exchange. A useful measure is the $P_{AO_2}$ with the donor ventilated on 100% oxygen and with 5 mmHg of positive end-expiratory pressure to optimise ventilation. A value of less than 50 kPa is an indicator of significant lung injury.

Final assessment of the lungs is performed by the donor surgeon who can see bullae and traumatised lung and feel areas of consolidation. Oedematous lungs feel heavy and spongy.

## Lung recipient–donor matching

As with heart donors, matching of donor and recipient for lung transplantation is a crude process with no prospective match for tissue type.

There is a larger pool of lung recipients available to a transplant centre at a given time than there is for hearts. This allows more attention to be paid to CMV status; a mismatch here has greater implication for a lung recipient in the event of seroconversion or re-activation in the grafted tissue. However, blood group, lymphocyte cross-match and size are once again the important considerations.

Size can be assessed in a number of ways including comparison of measurements taken from donor and recipient chest radiographs. However, it is now generally recognised that donors should be matched to the predicted lung size of the recipient rather than the pathological size since thoracic capacity and chest wall mechanics will normalise after transplantation. Predicted total lung capacity is calculated by the formulae:

Male           $TLC = (7.99 \times height\ in\ m) - 7.08$
Female         $TLC = (6.60 \times height\ in\ m) - 5.79$

## Lung retrieval and preservation

As with heart retrieval, the median sternotomy is completed after initial mobilisation of the liver. Both pleurae are now opened widely and the lungs inspected. Any adhesions between visceral and parietal pleura are divided with electrocautery. The inferior pulmonary ligament on each side is divided up to the inferior pulmonary vein. The innominate vein is now ligated between ligatures and the pericardium is opened with the incision being continued up along the innominate artery which is similarly divided. For this reason central venous access must be via the right internal jugular vein and arterial monitoring from the left radial artery. The pericardium is now opened and the aorta, superior vena cava and inferior vena cava are mobilised as before. Once the superior vena cava has been mobilised the azygos vein can be identified, ligated and divided behind the SVC to facilitate the future removal of the bloc. It is now possible to mobilise the trachea above the aortic arch. It is important not to denude the trachea of its blood supply and a tape is simply passed around it. Perfusion cannulae are now inserted into the ascending aorta and into the main pulmonary artery.

When perfusion apparatus has been set up for perfusion of the abdominal organs, removal of the heart and lung bloc can proceed. The SVC is divided between ligatures and the IVC is clamped above the diaphragm. The aorta is now cross-clamped and the heart is cardio-pleged as described before with St Thomas' crystalloid cardioplegia. However, under these circumstances the cardioplegia is vented from the heart by incision of the tip of the left atrial appendage leaving the pulmonary veins intact. Once electromechanical arrest has been achieved, infusion of preservative into the lungs can proceed through the pulmonary artery catheter. Simultaneous topical cooling of heart and lungs proceeds throughout the procedure.

The anaesthetist is now asked to ventilate the lungs by hand with air to prevent alveolar collapse. Occasional cessation of ventilation will facilitate excision of the bloc which proceeds when cardioplegia and pulmonary preservative solution have both been given. The heart is elevated and the pericardium incised posteriorly below the inferior pulmonary veins joining right and left pleural spaces. It is now possible to elevate the heart, the back of the left atrium and both hila dividing the connective tissue between these structures and the descending aorta and oesophagus and vertebral column posteriorly. As the surgeon proceeds up the descending aorta the ligamentum arteriosum is encountered and divided. On the right hand side, the divided azygos vein is seen as dissection proceeds in a cephalad direction. At this point the heart–lung bloc is placed back in the chest and attention turned to the aorta which is divided below the cross-clamp. The anaesthetist is now asked to withdraw the endotracheal tube into the upper trachea whilst still ventilating.

A clamp can now be placed across the trachea below the endotracheal tube and the trachea divided above. All that remains is to divide the connective tissue behind the ascending aorta and trachea and remove the entire heart–lung bloc. The trachea is stapled to allow removal of the clamp whilst leaving the lungs inflated for transfer.

The heart–lung bloc is packed as described for heart transport if it is to be used as a complete bloc.

If the lungs are to be sent to a different destination from the heart, it is now necessary to split the bloc. This is performed by incising the left atrium anterior to the hilum on each side to separate pulmonary veins from the left atrium. It is important to leave a small cuff of left atrium on the pulmonary veins to facilitate implantation in the lung recipient. The pulmonary artery is divided at its bifurcation leaving a good length of pulmonary artery attached to each lung. All that remains now is to separate the ascending aorta and heart from the pulmonary arteries on each side and from loose connective tissue connecting it to the carina posteriorly. Lungs and heart can now be transported separately to different destinations as required.

Preservation is achieved by cooling with extracorporeal circulation in some centres but most units use a hypothermic cold flush perfusion technique. Cold Euro–Collins[18] is the most commonly used perfusate though suitably buffered autologous blood can also be used with good effect.[19] Prostaglandins may help prevent leucocyte sequestration and also optimise perfusion of the pulmonary capillary bed. Ischaemic times of 6–8 h can be safely achieved with these techniques.

### Single lung implantation

Anaesthesia is established with a double lumen endotracheal tube to permit ventilation of the native lung whilst implantation proceeds. A pulmonary artery flotation catheter is used to monitor pulmonary artery pressure during implantation and full arterial and venous monitoring is established. Facilities for cardiopulmonary bypass are made available but are used only if unacceptable desaturation during implantation occurs or if systemic hypotension or pulmonary hypertension develop.

A lateral thoracotomy is performed and the native lung is excised with ligation of inferior and superior pulmonary veins and pulmonary artery. The bronchus is divided flush with the mediastinum and the native organ removed. Care is taken not to spill endobronchial contents into the pleural space. Meticulous haemostasis at the hilum is established. The pericardium is now incised adjacent to the pulmonary veins and these are mobilised through this incision to free them with a small cuff of the left atrium. The pulmonary artery is mobilised in a similar fashion. The donor lung is now prepared by trimming the left atrial cuff appropriately, cutting the pulmonary artery to length and excising the stapled end of the bronchus to deflate the lung.

Implantation commences with the bronchial anastomosis. The membranous part of the bronchus is anastomosed with a continuous 3/0

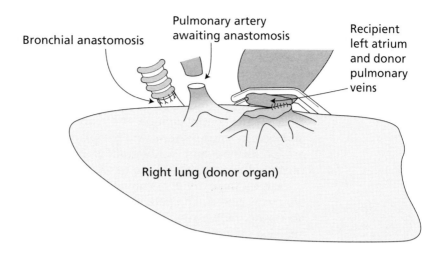

**Figure 11.8** *The left atrial anastomosis is performed after the bronchial connection.*

Prolene suture. A series of figure-of-eight interrupted sutures are now placed on the anterior cartilaginous part of the bronchus and left untied until all have been inserted. These are now tied to complete the anastomosis. A degree of telescoping of one bronchus within the other can be useful at this point. Loose connective tissue at the hilum of donor lung can now be used to wrap around the anastomosis and obliterate dead space adjacent to it. A long side-biting clamp is next placed across the native left atrial cuff and pulmonary veins and these are opened longitudinally. The left atrial anastomosis is now performed with a continuous 5/0 Prolene suture and the clamp is left applied (Fig. 11.8). The pulmonary artery anastomosis is performed in the same fashion and the donor organ is now de-aired by cautiously releasing the clamp from the pulmonary artery and de-airing through the left atrial anastomosis. The left atrial clamp can now be removed. Ventilation of the new lung commences.

Apical and basal chest drains are now inserted. The thoracotomy is closed and the patient is returned to the intensive care unit for further monitoring and care. It is usually possible to extubate the stable patient after the insertion of an epidural analgesic catheter. Typically the patient will return to the ward after approximately 24 h.

### Bilateral sequential lung implantation

Single lumen intubation for anaesthesia is all that is required. Cardio-pulmonary bypass is routinely used. Approach to the chest is through a submammary 'clam shell' incision. A median sternotomy is a less painful incision which can be used in some cases though access is not as good.

The patient is fully heparinised, the pericardium is opened and the patient is placed on cardiopulmonary bypass with an ascending aortic inflow cannula and venous drainage from a single two-stage venous cannula inserted through the right atrial appendage. Excision of each lung now proceeds with electrocautery division of adhesions. Care is taken to preserve the phrenic nerve while mobilising structures at each hilum especially in patients with septic lung disease where large lymph nodes and dense hilar adhesions make excision of the lung difficult. Excision of each lung proceeds in turn. Implantation of the donor lungs is performed in exactly the fashion described for single lung transplantation, the right side being anastomosed first. The patient is usually cooled to 32°C during implantation, the heart being allowed to continue to beat and eject in sinus rhythm. After implantation, de-airing and reperfusion are performed and ventilation is re-commenced. At normothermia cardiopulmonary bypass can be weaned.

Each thoracic cavity is drained with basal and apical drains and the wound is closed. The patient is then returned to the intensive care unit for further monitoring and can usually be extubated at 8–12 h. Epidural analgesia is essential following the 'clam shell' incision. Return to the ward is usually at about 24 h.

## Peri- and postoperative care for lung transplants

On notification of a possible donor the selected recipient is admitted and reassessed for deterioration or unexpected infection.

Antibiotic prophylaxis is largely directed by the known flora of the recipient but flucloxacillin is used for Gram-positive cover and metronidazole for Gram-negative cover in the absence of other positive cultures. Colomycin is administered by nebuliser in the immediate postoperative period. Antibiotic therapy is modified in the first few days after transplant as the results of peroperative donor and recipient bronchoalveolar lavages become available. In the absence of infection antibacterial agents are stopped after the first routine bronchoscopy and biopsy at one week, provided airway anastomoses appear healthy. Acyclovir, antifungal agents and pneumocystis prophylaxis are used routinely as in cardiac transplantation. It will be apparent from these comments that infection and colonisation of the airway and lung is a major feature of lung transplant and a leading cause of morbidity and mortality in the postoperative period.

Immunosuppression, as in heart transplantation, commences preoperatively with the administration of azathioprine and CsA. Methyl prednisolone is administered at reperfusion and continued for 24 h with commencement of oral steroids. However, since many pulmonary recipients have malabsorption and early CsA levels may be erratic, ATG is administered routinely for the first week with dosage and timing being regulated by daily flow cytometry count. With this exception, immunosuppression is managed in an identical fashion with the same dosage regimens as in cardiac transplantation.

If any lung injury is present in the immediate postoperative period, ventilation can present great difficulties. Lungs may be oedematous or infected with poor gas exchange. Meticulous control of fluid balance, optimisation of ventilation and microbiological control are needed in this situation. In the case of the single lung transplant for emphysema the

**Table 11.9**  *Grading of pulmonary allograft rejection*

| A acute rejection | 0 | none |
|---|---|---|
| | 1 | minimal – scattered mononuclear infiltrates |
| | 2 | mild – frequent infiltrates of activated lymphocytes 'endothelialitis' |
| | 3 | moderate – vascular cuffing, alveolar macrophages, extension of infiltrate into perivascular and air spaces |
| | 4 | severe – intra-alveolar necrosis, hyaline membrane, haemorrhage |

With or without

| B airway inflammation | 0–4 according to severity | |
|---|---|---|
| C chronic airway rejection | a | active |
| | b | inactive |
| D chronic vascular rejection | | |

residual lung can overinflate with air trapping and resultant mediastinal shift if the expiratory period of ventilation is insufficient. Modification of the ventilatory cycle can help but sometimes independent ventilation of each lung through a double lumen endotracheal tube is needed. When the time comes to wean the recipient from the ventilator an epidural catheter to administer analgesics is essential. Such an epidural infusion can be continued for some days after extubation to assist useful cough and expectoration of secretions.

Transbronchial biopsy and bronchoalveloar lavage with a flexible bronchoscope under sedation is performed at one week, one month and then every three months before reverting to annual biopsies to detect rejection and direct antimicrobial intervention. Additional biopsies are taken if rejection is suspected on the grounds of unexplained fever, symptomatic deterioration with arterial desaturation or a fall in pulmonary function tests including spirometry and transfer factor.

Rejection grading in lung transplants is summarised in Table 11.9.[20] Treatment is by augmentation of steroid therapy (three days of intravenous methyl prednisolone (500 mg) and subsequent augmentation of oral steroids). Treatment is required for Grades 3 and 4 and for Grade 2 if there is additional clinical concern.

## Outcomes and complications of lung transplantation

The actuarial survival of recipients of pulmonary transplants in the CsA era is shown in Fig. 11.9. Again these are aggregate world-wide data and survival in the Freeman Hospital series is also shown. Survival curves for BSLT are a little better than for SLT. A similar early shoulder to that seen in heart transplant survival reflects operative mortality, donor organ

**Figure 11.9** *The actuarial survival of recipients of lung transplants.* Freeman and ISHLT Registry data.

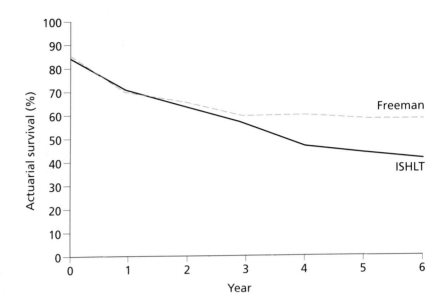

dysfunction, infection and rejection. Paediatric survival is similar to adult data though numbers are small.

Quality of life is significantly improved by transplantation for pulmonary failure.[21] Studies in populations of mixed pathology and transplant type and single pathology groups consistently show improvements in functional status and perception of symptoms.[22]

The causes of perioperative mortality are similar to those seen in cardiac transplantation with unsuspected donor lung injury (infection, oedema, embolic disease or poor preservation) and reperfusion injury. Specific technical difficulties include anastomotic stenoses with pulmonary oligaemia (arterial restriction) or pulmonary oedema (venous stenosis) and airway ischaemia and dehiscence with resultant mediastinitis.

The diagnosis and treatment of acute rejection has been discussed. Diagnosis is often made more difficult by concurrent infection and the decision to treat can also be complicated by fears of worsening such infection. As in cardiac grafts persistent or repeated episodes of rejection are managed with cytolytic therapy (ATG), monoclonal therapy or a change in immunosuppressive agent.

Fungal and viral infections are seen commonly in the early postoperative period (*Aspergillus* and CMV) and carry a significant morbidity. *Pseudomonas* colonisation is common in the cystic population. If preoperative data suggest that multiply-resistant pseudomonads are present antibacterial therapy is kept to a minimum to allow growth of sensitive organisms.

CMV infection can be a major clinical problem. Diagnosis is by immunofluorescence at lavage, by transbronchial biopsy, estimation of antigenaemia and culture on BAL samples. Infection is common in all except the donor-negative and recipient-negative transplants. Prophylactic ganciclovir can reduce the incidence of clinical CMV disease but is uneconomical (thus supporting matching CMV negative donors and recipients).[23] Pneumonitis is seen most commonly in donor-positive grafts irrespective of recipient status. Treatment is with intravenous ganciclovir or phoscarnate if neutropenia supervenes.

Lymphoproliferative disease and other malignancies are seen as in cardiac transplantation though lymphomas are more common (one series reports an incidence of 3.4% in heart recipients and 7.9% in lung recipients).[24] Mortality is significantly higher in lymphomas appearing after the first year after transplantation. Antiviral therapy (acyclovir or ganciclovir) with reduction in immunosuppression can be highly effective in early disease but later conventional chemotherapy may be required.

The vascular supply of bronchial and tracheal anastomoses is compromised and early dehiscence with ischaemia is a life-threatening complication with prolonged air leak and mediastinitis. Attention to detail when the anastomosis is performed with care not to denude the airway minimises this risk. It is no longer thought necessary to wrap the anastomosis in a vascularised pedicle or omentum.[25] Concurrent steroid therapy (once considered a contraindication to lung transplantation) may even reduce dehiscence as development of capillaries at the anastomosis is enhanced. Longer-term airway complications can also arise with overgrowth of granulation tissue at the anastomosis, especially in the presence of chronic infection, or fibrotic stricture formation (ischaemic in origin). Treatment is local with laser or electrocautery therapy. Use of expandable stents can also be helpful.[26]

Chronic rejection in lung transplantation manifests itself as obliterative bronchiolitis or vascular atherosclerosis the former being the greatest cause of long-term morbidity and mortality in recipients. Gradual deterioration in exercise tolerance and lung function arouse suspicion. Characteristic appearances are seen on the chest radiograph and CT scan and the diagnosis is confirmed by transbronchial biopsy. Predisposing factors may include multiple episodes of acute rejection in the postoperative period[27] and CMV infection may be an aetiological factor.[28] Treatment is directed towards decreased intensity of immunosuppression. Total lymphoid irradiation may also help.

## Recent advances and controversies in thoracic transplantation

Most recent changes in practice in cardiac transplantation are driven by a need to optimise the donor pool. To this end donation has been considered from both older and more marginal donors. As age limits for donation have crept upwards so the assessment of donor hearts has become more sophisticated. In the older donor, coronary and other structural disease is more common. The donor surgeon must be prepared to examine the heart closely for coronary artery disease and take and interpret accurate haemodynamic data. If coronary disease is seen it is possible to retrieve the heart and then perform 'bench angiography' to accurately define the anatomy and extent of the coronary lesions.

Whereas a donor heart with significant left main stem disease would obviously be unsuitable for use, less than 50% single vessel lesions can be accepted. Between these extremes significant single vessel disease can be managed with conventional coronary bypass surgery (with arterial or venous conduit) at the time of implantation. Recipients of hearts from donors over the age of 50 years where coronary disease has not been seen or palpated undergo routine coronary angiography six weeks after transplantation to ensure that no unsuspected prognostic narrowing or occlusion is present. The results of transplantation with older donor hearts do not differ significantly from those with younger donors in terms of long-term survival or the development of transplant-associated coronary disease. The need to perform simultaneous coronary surgery is, however, associated with reduced one year survival.[29]

Donors reported to have marginal haemodynamic performance, once rejected for use, are now often resuscitated by aggressive manipulation of inotropes and afterload assisted by data from a pulmonary artery flotation catheter and 'hormonal resuscitation'.[30] Reports of this approach suggest that up to 30% of such hearts could subsequently be used successfully for transplantation.[5]

There is increasing interest in conventional surgical techniques in patients who might otherwise be considered for transplantation. Improved myocardial preservation techniques in patients with ischaemic cardiomyopathies and failing ventricles make revascularisation feasible. Patients who might have viable (hibernating) myocardium are identified on clinical grounds (angina) and objectively with radionucleotide scanning, positron emission scanning and dobutamine stress echocardiography. Results in correctly selected patients are gratifying though in many ways this must be seen as a way of delaying rather than avoiding transplantation for many patients. Patients with preserved ventricular function but 'inoperable' coronary disease can be helped with new techniques such as transmyocardial laser revascularisation in which the heart is mobilised and precise channels are cut from the ventricular cavity into the myocardium to supply the myocardial capillary bed with a new supply of oxygenated blood.

Mechanical bridging of patients in heart failure until a donor organ becomes available has long been a contentious issue. The belief that transplants performed 'in extremis' with concurrent multiorgan failure and the real risk of on-going sepsis were likely to fare badly (a waste of a donor organ) and the philosophy that in an era of donor shortage, increasing the recipient pool was unhelpful has restricted this approach. However, the development and use of better assist devices has resurrected interest in mechanical bridging.[31] The awareness that left heart assist alone is sufficient to support the patient and the discovery that with scrupulous avoidance of sepsis patients can be supported for sufficient time for secondary organ failure (renal impairment for example) to correct[32] has led to reports showing that outcome for transplantation after bridging is as good as in the unbridged population.[33] Many patients supported on these devices are able to leave hospital with them in place whilst awaiting transplantation, some for over a year with a reasonably normal life style.

The next advance in the management of patients with end-stage cardiac failure will be the use of totally implantable devices to support the left ventricle. These will become an alternative to allotransplantation rather than a bridge.[34] The decision as to which surgical modality to use will be analogous to the choice between mechanical and biological prosthetic heart valves. Current devices rely on a power supply which must cross the skin from battery to pump with a consequent risk of device sepsis. The use of induction coils implanted beneath the skin to supply power will make pumps truly totally implantable. This advance together with improvements in quietness will make permanent left ventricular assist a realistic and clinically applicable technique.

In lung transplantation, also, developments have been directed by a shortage of donor organs. Living related donation of lungs by blood relatives of patients needing pulmonary transplantation is becoming popular. This technique is most applicable to paediatric transplantation for cystic fibrosis where lobar transplantation alone may provide sufficient lung tissue to fill the recipient chest. Early reports show good results but donor morbidity can also be significant.

A resurgence of interest in lung reduction surgery for symptomatic, non-prognostic emphysematous disease has diverted some patients who might otherwise have been transplanted on the grounds of symptomatic restriction away from transplant lists. Lung reduction surgery selectively excises the overexpanded underventilated and underperfused areas of emphysematous lung. The reduction in lung volume permits better aeration of remaining lung and improves the ventilatory performance of the thoracic cavity by normalising its previously overexpanded volume.

The next quantum leap in thoracic transplantation technology, however, will be the introduction of xenotransplantation. The thoracic organs and especially the heart are potentially well suited to replacement by xenogeneic alternatives since they have simple physiological functions (a pump and a gas exchange device) without complex metabolic and synthetic functions which may be species restricted at a biochemical level. The practical current limitation to xenotransplantation is the aggressive hyperacute rejection seen in discordant grafts (analogous in pace to a second set allograft rejection though probably mediated by the alternative pathway of complement in addition to heterophile antibody).[35] Other considerations are an ignorance of what processes will damage the graft if hyperacute rejection can be circumvented, a limited knowledge of comparative physiology and the potential for recipient infection by donor species pathogens. Donors will be discordant (distantly related species) for ethical reasons and pigs are most likely to be used but despite this selection there is likely to be considerable ethical debate of the propriety of using specially bred animals in this way. It seems that although this is a fruitful and challenging area for scientific research clinical application is still some way off.[36]

# References

1. Hosenpud JD, Novick MD, Bennett LE, Keck BM, Fiol B, Daily OP. The Registry of the International Society for Heart and Lung Transplantation: Thirteenth Official Report – 1996. J Heart Lung Transplant 1996; 15: 655–74.

2. Iberer F, Wasler A, Tscheliessnigg K et al. Prostaglandin $E_1$-induced moderation of elevated pulmonary vascular resistance. Survival on waiting list and results of orthotopic heart transplantation. J Heart Lung Transplant 1993; 12: 173–8.

3. Smith JA, Ribakove GH, Hunt SA et al. Heart retransplantation: the 25 year experience at a single institution. J Heart Lung Transplant 1995; 14: 832–9.

4. Yoshioka T, Sugimoto H, Uenishi M et al. Prolonged haemodynamic maintenance by the combined administration of vasopressin and epinephrine in brain death: a clinical study. Neurosurgery 1986; 18: 565–7.

5. Wheeldon DR, Potter CDO, Oduro A, Wallwork J, Large SR. Transforming the 'unacceptable' donor: outcomes from the adoption of a standardized donor management technique. J Heart Lung Transplant 1995; 14: 734–42.

6. Jeevanandam V, Furukawa S, Prendergast TW, Todd BA, Eisen HJ, McClurken JB. Standard criteria for an acceptable donor heart are restricting heart transplantation. Ann Thorac Surg 1996; 62: 1268–75.

7. Keogh A, Kaan A, Doran T, Macdonald T, Bryant D, Spratt P. HLA mismatching and outcome in heart, heart–lung and single lung transplantation. J Heart Lung Transplant 1995; 14: 444–51.

8. Drinkwater DC, Rudis E, Laks H et al. University of Wisconsin solution versus the Stanford cardioplegic solution and the development of cardiac allograft vasculopathy. J Heart Lung Transplant 1995; 14: 891–6.

9. El Gamel A, Yonan NA, Grant S et al. Orthotopic cardiac transplantation: a comparison of standard and bicaval Wythenshawe techniques. J Thorac Cardiovasc Surg 1995; 109: 721–30.

10. Billingham ME, Cary NRB, Hammond et al. A working formulation for the standardization of nomenclature in the diagnosis of heart and lung rejection. J Heart Transplant 1990; 9: 587–93.

11. Walker RC, Paya CV, Marshall WF et al. Pretransplantation seronegative Epstein–Barr virus status is the primary risk factor for post-transplant lymphoproliferative disorder in adult heart, lung and other solid organ transplantations. J Heart Lung Transplant 1995; 14: 214–21.

12. Kobashigawa JA, Miller L, Yeung A et al. Does acute rejection correlate with the development of transplant coronary artery disease? J Heart Lung Transplant 1995; 14: S221–6.

13. Fisher DC, Lake KD, Reutzel TJ, Emery RW. Changes in health-related quality of life and depression in heart transplant recipients. J Heart Lung Transplant 1995; 14: 373–81.

14. Grady KL, Jalowiec A, White-Williams C. Improvement in quality of life in patients with heart failure who undergo transplantation. J Heart Lung Transplant 1996; 15: 749–57.

15. Buxton MJ. Resource implications of heart transplantation. In: Wallwork J (ed.) Heart and heart–lung transplantation. Philadelphia: Saunders, 1989.

16. Yacoub MH, Banner NR, Khagani A et al. Heart–lung transplantation for cystic fibrosis and subsequent domino heart transplantation. J Heart Transplant 1990; 9: 459–67.

17. Waller DA, Thompson AM, Wrightson WN et al. Does the mode of donor death influence the outcome of lung transplantation? A review of lung transplantation from donors involved in major trauma. J Heart Lung Transplant 1995; 14: 318–21.

18. Locke TJ, Hooper TL, Flecknell PA et al. Preservation of the lung: comparison of topical cooling and cold crystalloid pulmonary perfusion. J Thorac Cardiovasc Surg 1988; 96: 789–95.

19. Wallwork J, Jones K, Cavarocchi A et al. Distant procurement of organs for clinical heart–lung transplantation using the single flush technique. Transplantation 1987; 44: 654–8.

20. Yousem SA, Berry GJ, Cagle PT et al. Revision of the 1990 working formulation for the classification of pulmonary allograft rejection: Lung Rejection Study Group. J Heart Lung Transplant 1996; 15: 1–15.

21. Ochoa L. Discussion of 'Quality of life evaluation after heart–lung transplantation: a retro-

spective study' by C. Dromer *et al*. In: Lung Transplantation. Current Topics in General Thoracic Surgery, Vol. 3, Amsterdam: Elsevier Science BV, 1995.

22. Ramsey SD, Patrick DL, Lewis S, Albert RK, Raghu G. Improvement in quality of life after lung transplantation: a preliminary study. J Heart Lung Transplant 1995; 14: 870–7.

23. Smyth RL, Scott JP, Borysiewcz LK *et al*. Cytomegalovirus infection in heart–lung transplant recipients: risk factors, clinical association and response to treatment. J. Infect Dis 1991; 164: 1045–50.

24. Armitage JM, Kormos RL, Stuart RS *et al*. Posttransplant lymphoproliferative disease in thoracic organ transplant patients: ten years of cyclosporine-based immunosuppression. J Heart Lung Transplant 1991; 10: 877–87.

25. Miller JD, de Hoyos A, Patterson GA. An evaluation of the role of omentopexy and early postoperative corticosteroids in clinical lung transplantation. J Thorac Cardiovasc Surg 1993; 105: 247–52.

26. Couraud J, Nashef SAM. Airway complications. In: Lung transplantation. Current Topics in General Thoracic Surgery, Vol. 3, Amsterdam, Elsevier Science BV, 1995.

27. Yousem SA, Dauber JA, Keenan R, Paradis IL, Zeevi A, Griffith BP. Does histologic acute rejection in lung allografts predict the development of bronchiolitis obliterans. Transplantation 1991; 52: 306–9.

28. Keenan RJ, Lega ME, Dummer JS *et al*. Cytomegalovirus serological status and post-operative infection correlated with risk of developing chronic rejection after pulmonary transplantation. Transplantation 1991; 51: 433–8.

29. Drinkwater DC, Laks H, Blitz A *et al*. Outcomes of patients undergoing transplantation with older donor hearts. J Heart Lung Transplant 1996; 15: 684–91.

30. El Oakley RM, Yonan NA, Simpson BM, Deiranita AK. Extended criteria for cardiac allograft donors: a consensus study. J Heart Lung Transplant 1996; 15: 255–9.

31. Portner PM, Oyer PE, Pennington DG. Implantable electrical left ventricular assist system: bridge to transplantation and the future. Ann Thorac Surg 1989; 41: 142–50.

32. Levin HR, Chen JM, Oz MC *et al*. Potential of left ventricular assist devices as outpatient therapy while awaiting transplantation. Ann Thorac Surg 1994; 58: 1515–20.

33. Mehta SM, Aufiero TX, Pae WE, Miller CA, Pierce WS. Combined Registry for the clinical use of mechanical ventricular assist pumps and the total artificial heart in conjunction with heart transplantation: Sixth Official Report – 1994. J Heart Lung Transplant 1995; 14: 585–93.

34. Loisance DY, Deleuze PH, Mazzucotelli P, Le Besnerais P, Dubois-Rande J. Clinical implantation of the wearable Baxter Novacor ventricular assist system. Ann Thorac Surg 1994; 58: 551–4.

35. Forty J, White DJG, Wallwork J. Activation of the alternative pathway of complement in hyperacute xenograft rejection of rabbit hearts by human blood. J Heart Lung Transplant 1993; 12: 283–6.

36. Lin SS, Platt JL. Immunologic barriers to xenotransplantation. J Heart Lung Transplant 1996; 15: 547–55.

# 12 The depressed immune system in the transplant patient (infection risk and increased malignancy)

*Gareth Morris-Stiff*
*Rozanne H. H. Lord*

## Infectious complications

### Introduction

Solid organ transplantation has now become widely accepted as the therapeutic option of choice for many chronic and some acute diseases which lead to organ failure of the kidneys, liver, heart or lungs. Despite numerous improvements in surgical technique, postoperative care and the benefits of modern immunosuppressive therapy, infectious complications together with rejection remain the major causes of morbidity and mortality to the transplant patient especially during the first year. These two factors are strongly interrelated with underimmunosuppression being associated with breakthrough rejection and high-dose therapy with an increased incidence of infective episodes. Thus successful immunotherapy involves striking the correct balance which is often clinically challenging.

Postoperative infections are very common among transplant patients. Ho *et al.*[1] reported an overall incidence of infection following solid organ transplantation of 70–80% whereas Dummer *et al.*[2] found infections to be associated with 85% of post-transplant deaths.

Patients undergoing transplantation require intense postoperative monitoring and usually have several intravenous cannulas and urinary catheters, and in addition many will require a period of prolonged mechanical ventilation. Therefore, common bacterial and nosocomial infections of the wound, respiratory and urinary tracts are common in the immunosuppressed patient. In addition to the threat posed by 'conventional' bacterial infections, there is also a greater risk of developing opportunistic infections.

Infections occurring in this first postoperative month are similar to those experienced by general surgical patients but in addition there are infections which may have been transmitted with the host organ. From the first to sixth months, opportunistic infection secondary to immuno-suppression predominate whereas after 6 months there is a return to more typical bacterial pathogens although fungal infections may also present in this period.[3]

This review will concentrate on the opportunistic infections which occur following organ transplantation.

## Viral infections

Viral infections are common following transplantation and may be due to primary infection or from reactivation of a latent virus following a previous infection. All viruses which affect the general population may infect the immunocompromised patient though it would appear that the DNA viruses are clinically more important.

### Cytomegalovirus (CMV)

Cytomegalovirus is the commonest cause of infection after the first postoperative month. Paya et al.[4] in a prospective study noted an overall prevalence of CMV infection following liver transplantation of 49%, with half of the patients being symptomatic. The group identified to be most vulnerable are seronegative patients who receive seropositive organs. Infections are rarely seen before 1 month and classically manifest at between 2 and 3 months though late presentation is not uncommon.

CMV is a herpes virus which may lead to primary infection (CMV-positive donor to a CMV-negative recipient), or secondary infection which may be either a superinfection (CMV-positive donor to CMV-positive recipient) or reactivation of dormant recipient CMV during immunosuppression (CMV-negative donor and CMV-positive recipient). Primary infection is the commonest mode of infection in the paediatric community but is rarely seen in adults where secondary infections predominate.

### Presentation

In its mildest forms CMV infection may be asymptomatic or present with a mild self-limiting febrile episode due to shedding of virus from infected cells. The classical presentation of CMV infection is of a high swinging pyrexia up to 39 or 40°C, with malaise and lethargy. There may be symptoms and signs specific to organ involvement such as hypoxia and dyspnoea with interstitial pneumonitis, deranged liver function in hepatitis or defective vision in CMV retinitis. Infection of the gastro-intestinal tract may manifest as abdominal pain, diarrhoea or rectal bleeding in the case of CMV colitis or with retrosternal pain and haematemesis with upper tract infection. Disseminated CMV may be life-threatening as patients may develop hypotension and respiratory failure and there is a significant mortality.[5] Patients with CMV are also at an increased risk of secondary infections including bacterial, *Pneumocystis carinii* and *Candida*, the diagnosis of which may be masked by the CMV.[6]

## Diagnosis

The diagnosis of CMV has in the past relied on the identification of CMV inclusion bodies in biopsy specimens or an increase in serum antibody titres following transplantation. The accuracy and speed of diagnosis has improved with the introduction of direct detection of CMV antigen in peripheral leucocytes (buffy coat), polymerase chain reaction techniques to detect CMV DNA or RNA and culture amplified virus antigen detection techniques.[7] In the case of organ specific involvement, samples should be obtained by means of bronchoalveolar lavage, liver biopsy or endoscopic biopsy in order to confirm the diagnosis.

## Prevention

Prophylactic measures to prevent CMV infection include the matching of CMV-seronegative donors to CMV-negative recipients whenever possible and the administration of seronegative blood products to CMV-negative patients.[6] The risk of transfusion may also be reduced by the use of in-line white cell filters which remove the leucocytes.[8] The risk of CMV infection is greater in the United States where antilymphocyte preparations are regularly used as part of the immunosuppressive regimen and pre-emptive therapy with ganciclovir is recommended for all patients under these circumstances.[9] Some centres also advocate the use of acyclovir or CMV immune globulin as part of prophylaxis.[10]

## Treatment

In the presence of an established infection ganciclovir should be prescribed at a dose of $5\,mg\,kg^{-1}$ twice daily for 14 or 21 days though doses need to be adjusted if there is renal impairment.[11] The main side effect of ganciclovir is bone marrow toxicity leading to a neutropenia. This is reversed on discontinuing therapy.

### Epstein–Barr virus (EBV)

The Epstein–Barr virus has been associated with several clinical scenarios following solid organ transplantation including asymptomatic viraemia, hepatitis and mononucleosis syndrome.[6] The most important link however is with the post-transplant lymphoproliferative disorder (PTLD) which develops as a result of the virus infecting the recipient's B lymphocytes and mutating their DNA.[12] The main risk factor for PTLD is the transplantation of a seropositive donor with an active infection into a seronegative recipient since recipient B-cells become infected and in the immunosuppressed state a lymphoma may develop.[13] PTLD is more commonly seen with primary infection[14] and is also associated with high-dose immunosuppression and the use of the monoclonal antibodies OKT3.[15]

*Presentation*
Patients with EBV viraemia usually present with non-specific symptoms such as lethargy and those developing PTLD will have a varied presentation depending on the site of the lymphoma since these tumours may develop in the donor organ or in the reticuloendothelial system of the host, usually in the tonsil or gastrointestinal tract.

*Diagnosis*
Diagnosis of viraemia may be made on estimation of plasma viral titres whereas histological examination of a biopsy specimen for immunoblasts, lymphocytes and plasma cells with EBV nuclear staining confirms the diagnosis of PTLD.

*Prevention*
There are no recognised effective prophylactic measures, however avoidance of mismatching seropositive donors with seronegative recipients is recommended.

*Treatment*
Most patients with PTLD respond to a reduction in immunosuppressive therapy together with the administration of high-dose acyclovir.[16] However, if there is no response the patient should be treated as for a lymphoma with systemic chemotherapy.[17]

### Herpes simplex (HSV)
There are two recognised herpes simplex viruses, type 1 (oral) and type 2 (genital) which usually remain dormant in the dorsal root ganglia of the nerves supplying the lips and perineum, respectively. The majority of HSV infections occurring in the transplant population are due to reactivation of the dormant virus and are generally seen between 1 week and 1 month after transplantation.

*Presentation*
Type 1 HSV typically presents with cold sores whereas type 2 HSV causes genital vesiculation or ulceration. In the immunocompromised host there may be marked local ulceration or widespread dissemination leading to oesophagitis, pneumonitis, hepatitis or encephalitis.[18] Ophthalmic infections are also seen following autoinfection caused by the patient rubbing their eyes.

*Diagnosis*
Localised HSV may be diagnosed on clinical features and confirmed with viral isolation. In the presence of disseminated disease electron microscopy is used to identify the HSV virus or alternatively monoclonal antibodies directed at the virus may be used.

*Prevention*

For patients who are seropositive, especially if there are high antibody titres, prophylactic acyclovir has been shown to significantly reduce the incidence of reactivation following transplantation.[19]

*Treatment*

Acyclovir is the treatment of choice for HSV infections and should be administered systemically either orally for localised infections or intravenously for disseminated disease. The recommended treatment dose is 800 mg five times per day though dose alteration is required in the presence of abnormal renal function. Eye infections may be treated by topical application of acyclovir cream.

### Varicella zoster (VZV)

Varicella zoster infections in the immunocompromised patient are usually the result of reactivation of dormant virus in the dorsal root ganglia following a previous chickenpox infection. Reactivation leads to shingles with dermatomal distribution, usually following the lower thoracic nerves or less commonly the cranial nerves. VZV presents later than many of the other post-transplant viral infections, usually after 2–3 months.

*Presentation*

The typical presentation is with unilateral dermatomal pain which develops over a period of days into an itchy vesicular rash. In contrast to the non-immunocompromised patient, transplant recipients develop extensive vesicles involving both the epidermis and dermis which are often haemorrhagic or necrotic. Individuals presenting with disseminated VZV disease require urgent diagnosis and treatment since the condition carries a considerable mortality. Children not previously exposed to the virus may develop an aggressive chickenpox which has a high mortality if not promptly treated.

*Diagnosis*

The diagnosis of localised infection may be made on clinical grounds and the presence of VZV confirmed by viral identification. In the case of disseminated VZV infection urgent electron microscopy, monoclonal antibodies and immunofluorescence may be used to rapidly establish the diagnosis.

*Prevention*

Children and seronegative patients may benefit from the administration of a live, attenuated vaccine[20] though this is not recommended for all patients since the incidence of VZV is relatively low and when it occurs it does so several months after transplantation.

*Treatment*
Treatment of established VZV infection, either chickenpox or shingles, is based on acyclovir which may be administered either orally or intra-venously in the case of disseminated disease.

### Papilloma virus (HPV)

There are many subtypes of HPV which infect the skin through breaches in the mucous membranes and then lay dormant in the basal layer. As skin cells naturally migrate towards the epidermis the virus is activated to produce an infection and stimulate proliferation of cells leading to the typical warty appearance. This process is regulated by T cell suppressor activity and thus HPV infections are common in the immunosuppressed patient and lesions may be large and numerous. It has been postulated that HPV may be important in the aetiology of cervical, anal and penile cancers[21] and therefore surveillance programmes for these tumours are recommended.

*Presentation*
The typical presentation is with warts which may be larger and more numerous than in the non-immunocompromised patient. Unfortunately, some patients present with carcinomas.

*Diagnosis*
Clinical and histological results usually suffice in the diagnosis of HPV.

*Prevention*
There is no effective prevention.

*Treatment*
Warty lesions may be locally excised whereas more extensive procedures will be required for carcinomas depending on their extent.

### Hepatitis B (HBV)

Infection with HBV is endemic in south-east Asia and parts of Africa. In these regions in addition to the horizontal transmission through body fluids, there is also a significant vertical transference from mother to child during pregnancy. Following an acute HBV infection there may be complete resolution of the virus, however there is often residual damage to the liver varying from a chronic persistent hepatitis, through chronic active hepatitis to cirrhosis. In these endemic regions there is also a high incidence of hepatocellular carcinoma. Patients with end-stage liver disease secondary to HBV have undergone liver transplantation; however, results are generally poor because of a high incidence of disease recurrence due to reactivation of infection.[22]

### Presentation

HBV infection of the immunosuppressed patient varies from being asymptomatic to fulminant hepatic failure. The classical presentation is one of fever, right upper quadrant pain and jaundice. Liver function is abnormal with elevated transaminase levels.

### Diagnosis

The diagnosis may be confirmed by the identification of HBcAg and HBeAg in the peripheral blood and recurrence confirmed by performing a liver biopsy.

### Prevention

Before transplantation, the donor must be screened for HBV and if HBsAg is positive the organs should not be transplanted. Similarly recipients who are HDV (Hepatitis delta virus) DNA or HBeAg positive should not be transplanted since both parameters indicate the presence of active HBV infection. Administration of prophylactic anti-HBs hyper-immune globulin on its own or in combination with interferon alpha to recipients with fulminant HBV infection or associated HDV infection has been shown to be successful in reducing disease recurrence and improving both patient and graft survival.[23,24]

### Treatment

Treatment is based on alpha interferon therapy, but there is significant graft loss to recurrent disease. Other antiviral preparations have also been tried with varying degrees of success.

## Hepatitis C (HCV)

The mode of transmission is identical to HBV although until recently the extent of world distribution of HCV was not appreciated. Half the HCV seropositive patients develop abnormal liver function and 20% progress to cirrhosis.[25]

### Presentation

Presentation of HCV is similar to that of HBV, but the symptoms are usually milder.

### Diagnosis

Diagnosis is established by the identification of antibodies to HCV in the peripheral blood and may be confirmed by liver biopsy.

### Prevention

Blood products are now routinely screened for HCV. The organs of potential donors that are found to be HCV positive should not be transplanted. Interferon alpha has been used with some success at prophylaxis in an attempt to prevent recurrence in seropositive patients prior to transplantation.

*Treatment*
Interferon alpha is effective in suppressing HCV infection. Clinical trials are also in progress evaluating other antiviral agents.

## Bacterial infections

Bacterial pathogens are responsible for the majority of infections seen following transplantation, especially during the early postoperative phase. The majority of these are caused by the same common Gram negative and Gram positive organisms that infect general surgical patients. There are, however, several opportunistic infections which are worthy of mention.

### Mycobacterium

Mycobacterial infections are not infrequently seen following solid organ transplantation, with an incidence of between 0.8% and 3% for renal transplant recipients which compares with 0.1% in the general population.[26,27] The majority are due to *M. tuberculosis* but up to 30% are due to atypical infections such as *M. kansasii, M. marinum* and *M. avium-intracellulare*.[27] The majority of cases are due to reactivation of latent organisms but transmission at the time of grafting and nosocomial infections have also been reported.

*Presentation*
The commonest presentation is with pulmonary disease and the classical symptoms of cough, pleuritic chest pain and dyspnoea. Extrapulmonary and disseminated disease have also been reported at presentation, however, many immunosuppressed patients will have few if any symptoms.

*Diagnosis*
Diagnosis is established on the basis of tissue culture and identification of acid-fast bacilli in sputum, urine and bronchopulmonary lavage specimens.

*Prevention*
Patients with a past history of tuberculosis or positive skin testing prior to transplantation should receive prophylactic isoniazid and should be closely monitored for reactivation.[28]

*Treatment*
The treatment of mycobacterial infections in transplant recipients should follow the same multidrug regimens as for the non-immunosuppressed patients including isoniazid, pyrazinamide and ethambutol, however rifampicin should be avoided due to the recognised interaction with cyclosporin.[29]

### Listeria

*Listeria monocytogenes* is an intracellular pathogen which is rarely seen in patients with a normally active immune system. Listerial infections appear to be seen more commonly in association with immunosuppressive regimens containing azathioprine.[6] Listerial infections may be primary or secondary.

### Presentation

Transplant patients infected with *Listeria* usually present with disease affecting the central nervous system including meningitis, brain abscess or encephalitis and thus neurological symptoms are common and varied, including headache, seizures or focal localising symptoms.[6] It may also present with respiratory symptoms secondary to a pneumonia.

### Diagnosis

Patients presenting with neurological symptoms should undergo a lumbar puncture to obtain a sample of cerebrospinal fluid together with a CT or MRI scan of the brain. The stools of these patients should also be cultured since *Listeria* is an enteric organism.

### Prevention

The use of sulphamethoxazole as prophylaxis for potential *Pneumocystis carinii* has had the additional benefit of drastically reducing the frequency of *Listeria monocytogenes*.

### Treatment

Listerial infections respond well to penicillin and this should be given early to reduce both morbidity and mortality which is otherwise significant.

### Nocardia

Nocardial infections are most commonly seen following thoracic organ transplantation but have been reported following renal grafting.[30] Disease may result from either pulmonary or secondary infection.

### Presentation

The organism usually causes a pneumonia but infection may become disseminated spreading to the skin and central nervous system.

### Diagnosis

Diagnosis is based on the histological identification of filamentous Gram-positive organisms in specimen cultures.

### Treatment

Nocardial infections respond well to either sulphamethoxazole or penicillin antibiotic therapy.

## Fungal infections

Fungal infections are common following solid organ transplantation with incidences varying between 5% for renal allograft recipients to 40% in liver transplant patients.[31] The majority of infections are seen within the first 2 months and more than 80% of infections are due to either *Candida* or *Aspergillus*. If left untreated fungal infections carry a high mortality.

### Candida

Candidal infections in transplant patients are usually due to *Candida albicans* and are often associated with prolonged use of broad-spectrum antibiotic therapy. Infection usually commences with colonisation of either the oral or genital tract mucosa but in contrast to the non-immunocompromised patient, oral infections in transplant patients rapidly spread distally leading to an oesophagitis or they may disseminate causing a candidaemia.

#### Presentation

The typical symptoms of mucocutaneous *Candida* are of a white, itchy rash which in the case of oral infections leads to odynophagia. If there is any oesophageal candidiasis there may be the additional symptoms of dysphagia and retrosternal pain.

#### Diagnosis

Diagnosis of oral and genital infections is made on clinical grounds and confirmed by culture of *Candida* from swabs. Invasive infection is diagnosed on the basis of detection of antigens in blood cultures whereas endoscopy and oesophageal biopsy are required for candidal oesophagitis.

#### Prevention

Standard prophylaxis against *Candida* consists of either nystatin or amphotericin B.

#### Treatment

Candidal infections in transplant patients require treatment with oral or intravenous or fluconazole or amphotericin B.

### Aspergillus

*Aspergillus* infections usually occur in the lung but may also disseminate to the central nervous system. The incidence of *Aspergillus* infection after renal transplantation was noted by Weiland *et al.*[32] to be 3%. The fungus is widespread in the soil and air and infection is believed to be from these sources though reactivation of dormant spores may also occur.

*Presentation*

The commonest manifestation is pulmonary disease whilst central nervous system infections and widely disseminated disease are less common.[32]

*Diagnosis*

The diagnosis of *Aspergillus* infection is often missed on sputum culture and lung biopsy or bronchoalveolar lavage is often required. Chest radiographs occasionally show the classic appearance of an aspergilloma but usually the appearance is of diffuse pulmonary infiltrates.

*Prevention*

The use of modern air filters has dramatically reduced the airborne spread of *Aspergillus*.

*Treatment*

Infections limited to the lung may be successfully treated however disseminated and cerebral disease responds poorly and carries a high mortality.[32] Surgical excision should be considered for aspergillomas.

## Parasitic infections

Several parasitic organisms may infect the immunosuppressed patient, the most important being *Pneumocystis carinii*.

### Pneumocystis carinii (PCP)

PCP infections usually occur within the first 6 months after transplantation and are often seen in association with CMV.[6] Pneumocystis infection is most common following thoracic organ transplantation[33] where it causes a pneumonia.

*Presentation*

Patients present with rapidly deteriorating respiratory function and untreated the mortality is high.

*Diagnosis*

Diagnosis is based on bronchoscopic biopsy or bronchoalveolar lavage.

*Prevention*

Prophylaxis with cotrimoxazole has dramatically reduced the incidence of PCP in the transplant community.

*Treatment*

The standard treatment of PCP is sulphatrimoxazole administered intravenously.

*Conclusion*

Transplant recipients are more prone to infections in general. The risk may be reduced by the following: avoidance of CMV +ve and EBV +ve donors in CMV −ve and EBV −ve recipients respectively, and antibacterial and antiviral prophylaxis at the time of transplantation. Regular surveillance for CMV is recommended with prompt initiation of ganciclovir in the advent of CMV infection or disease. Regular 'flu' and pneumovax vaccinations are recommended by many units. If travelling to 'tropical' climes vaccination should exclude 'live' vaccines due to the risk of a 'live' innoculum.

## Increased risk of malignancy post-transplantation

### Introduction

Improved immunosuppression has led to improved graft survival, but also an increased risk of developing post-transplant malignancy. Cancer registries have been in existence for many years and include Israel Penn's worldwide registry (CTTR, Cincinnati Transplant Tumour Registry), Ross Shiel's Australasian registry and many national registries.

Over 300 000 transplants have been performed worldwide. The prevalence of malignancy in renal graft recipients varies from 4 to 18%.[34] The overall risk ratio of developing a malignancy post-transplantation is increased threefold for all cancers apart from cancers of the breast and ovary (Table 12.1).[35] The risk ratio is highest when a viral aetiology has been implicated, as in lymphomas, cancers of the perineum, skin cancers and Kaposi's sarcoma. In the general population cancers tend to occur within 5–20 years of carcinogen exposure, whereas post-transplant

**Table 12.1** *Cancer other than skin which occurred in 420 (6%) of 6596 recipients of cadaveric donor renal allografts*

| Type of cancer | Observed CA | Expected CA | Risk ratio |
|---|---|---|---|
| Genitourinary | 156 (34%) | 35.9 | 4.3 |
| Digestive organs | 90 (20%) | 35.8 | 2.5 |
| Lymphoma | 48 (12%) | | |
|    Diffuse non-Hodgkin's | 38 | 5.1 | 7.4 |
|    CNS | 16 | 0 | >1000 |
| Respiratory system | 40 (9%) | 19.9 | 2.0 |
| Leukaemia | 22 (5%) | 3.9 | 5.6 |
| Breast | 26 (5%) | 20.6 | 1.3 |
| Kaposi's sarcoma | 14 (3%) | 0 | >1000 |
| Endocrine | 9 (2%) | 0 | 289 |
| Miscellaneous | 48 (10%) | 10.5 | 4.6 |
| Totals | 459 | 131.7 | 3.5 |

Reproduced from Sheil *et al.*[35]

**Table 12.2** *Times of presentation*

| Cancer | % of total | Time post-transplant | |
|---|---|---|---|
| | | Range (months) | Mean (years) |
| Lymphoma (central nervous system) | 4 | 4–106 | 2 |
| Kaposi's sarcoma | 3 | 4–218 | 5 |
| Endocrine glands | 2 | 8–117 | 5 |
| Lymphoma (diffuse) | 8 | 3–168 | 6 |
| Lung | 9 | 3–218 | 6.5 |
| Genitourinary | 34 | 4–249 | 7 |
| Breast | 5 | 4–197 | 8 |
| Leukaemia | 5 | 11–225 | 8 |
| Alimentary tract | 20 | 5–246 | 8.5 |

Reproduced from Sheil *et al.*[36]

malignancies may occur within months or a few years of transplantation (Table 12.2);[36] they also occur in a younger age group than the general population and behave more aggressively with earlier dissemination. The 1993 CTTR average age at the time of transplantation was 42 years (range 3 months–80 years) and the average age at the time of diagnosis of malignancy is 47 years.[34] The ratio of male:female in transplant patients developing cancer is 2:1 and reflects the ratio of transplant patients overall.[34]

The post-transplant cancer risk is linked to the dose of immuno-suppression and the use of polyclonal and monoclonal antibody therapy and recipient age. The aetiology of post-transplant malignancy is complex and varies for different tumours, but includes reduced immunosurveillance, repeated antigenic stimulation from the graft and blood transfusions, impaired deoxyribonucleic acid (DNA) repair, genetic influences, original cause of organ failure, viral factors and increased susceptibility to carcinogens. It has been suggested that cyclosporin A and antilymphocyte antibodies inhibit T cell function and allow unrestricted B cell activation and proliferation in response to primary viral infection or activation of latent virus. Viral infection of B cells may lead to DNA mutation. The following viruses are implicated: EBV virus in lymphoma, human papilloma virus (HPV) and herpes simplex virus in uterine cervical cancer, hepatitis B in hepatoma and herpes-like viruses in Kaposi's sarcoma (KS).

Treatment of post-transplant malignancies may include reduction or withdrawal of immunosuppression, antiviral agents and interferon treatment as supplements to conventional treatment of malignancies. However, reduction of immunosuppression is only an option in renal transplant recipients, where patients may be supported by a period of haemodialysis, but is not an option in liver, heart and lung transplant recipients, where graft failure leads to death. Cytotoxic therapy must be used with caution following immunosuppression, as cure may be followed by overwhelming infection and death. When prescribing cytotoxics prednisolone may be safely continued, but azathioprine should be stopped.

### Skin cancers

*Incidence*

The risk of skin cancer is increased 40-fold in transplant recipients living in high risk areas, but in areas of limited sun exposure there is only a 4–7-fold increase.[34] Skin cancer is rare in patients of non-Caucasian origin. About 50% of Australasian recipients have developed skin cancers 20 years post-transplantation.[37] Females have a marginally lower incidence than males.

In the general population, basal cell carcinomas (BCC) predominate over squamous cell carcinomas (SCC) (BCC:SCC = 5:1). This ratio is reversed in transplant recipients: SCC:BCC = 1.8:1.[34] Skin malignancy occurred in 1293 (20%) of Australasian patients, of these 71% had SCC, 52% BCC and 3% malignant melanoma.[35] Skin cancers tend to occur in a younger age group (i.e. 30–40 years) in this group of patients, compared to 60–70 years in the general population.[13] Of the transplant recipients with skin cancers 42% have multiple tumours.[34] Skin cancers tend to be more aggressive in transplant patients: 8% of Australasian transplant recipients with SCC developed metastases with a 4% mortality.[38] In patients with malignant melanoma the incidence of metastases rose to 28% and mortality to 20%.[38]

*Aetiology*

Aetiological factors in skin malignancy post-transplantation include skin type, exposure to ultraviolet light, impaired DNA repair from human papilloma virus and decreased number and decreased function of Langerhan cells.[38,39] Moreover, 6-mercaptopurine and methyl-nitro-thio-imidazole, two major azathioprine derivatives, may cause photo-sensitisation and photoallergy.[40] The active metabolite of azathioprine, thioguanine is thought to be a skin carcinogen.[41] Approximately 40% of transplant recipients develop warts, which may be associated with HPV infection (Fig. 12.1).

*Management*

Pre- and post-transplant counselling should include advice about protective clothing in the summer months (long sleeves, gloves to protect the dorsum of the hands, long trousers/long skirts and sun hats) and factor 20–30 sun block. Careful skin surveillance and early biopsy of suspicious lesions is mandatory. Treatment includes surgical excision, cryotherapy, topical application of 5-fluorouracil and retinoids.[41] In cases of multiple lesions or metastatic spread, reduction or even cessa-

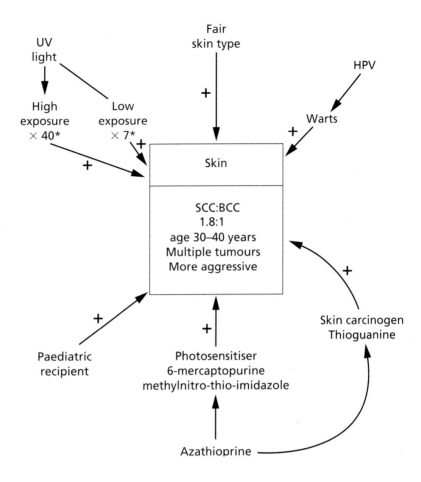

**Figure 12.1** *Factors influencing the development of skin cancer post-transplantation. *Risk compared to normal population.*

tion of immunosuppression, may be considered in renal transplant recipients.

## Lymphomas

### *Incidence*

In the general population lymphomas represent 5% of all cancers. The incidence is increased to 12–33%[34,36] in transplant recipients and represents a preponderance of non-Hodgkin's lymphoma (Table 12.3). These lymphomas tend to be termed post-transplant lymphoproliferative disorders (PTLD). About 80% are B cell in origin, 12.6% T cell in origin and 0.4% null cell.[38] Multiple organ involvement is seen in 52% of transplant recipients. The incidence of cerebral lymphoma is dramatically increased with up to a 1000-fold increased risk ratio.[35] Cerebral lymphomas only represent 1% of malignancies in the general population and occur in the presence of multiple metastases, whereas up to 56% of CNS lymphomas in transplanted recipients are limited to the brain.[34] Involvement of the graft is seen in 23% of patients and may be misdiagnosed as acute rejection.[42–44]

**Table 12.3** *Analysis of lymphomas from the Cincinnati Transplant Tumor Registry*

| Type of lymphoma | General population | Transplant population |
|---|---|---|
| Hodgkins | 12% | 2.7% |
| Myeloma | 21% | 3.8% |
| Non-Hodgkin's | 67% | 93.6% |

Adapted from Penn.[34]

Lymphomas occurred on average 32 months post-transplantation (range 1–254 months) in the Dec 93 CTTR.[34] However, the Australasian registry analysed diffuse and CNS lymphomas separately (Table 12.2). CNS lymphomas presented earlier at an average of 2 years compared to diffuse lymphomas at 6 years post-transplantation.[36]

## Aetiology

Epstein–Barr virus (EBV) infection is associated with benign polyclonal hyperplasia leading to frank B cell lymphoma. Viral infection of B cell may lead to DNA mutation. Cyclosporin and anti-T cell agents may play a more important role than other immunosuppressive agents. Maximal risk occurs in recipients with primary EBV infection at the time of transplantation. Lymphomas are more common in paediatric recipients; this may be due to the increased lymphoid mass, the need for increased immunosuppression and the increased incidence of primary EBV infection in this group of recipients. A similar aetiology is probably implicated in PTLD in small bowel transplant recipients. Furthermore, in these recipients the lymphoid mass is increased further by donor lymphoid tissue (Peyer's patches and mesenteric lymph nodes) (Fig. 12.2).

## Management

Investigations are performed in the standard manner and include tissue diagnosis. Histological examination of a biopsy specimen for immunoblasts, lymphocytes and plasma cells with EBV nuclear staining confirms the diagnosis of PTLD. The recipient's antibody status to EBV is compared in pre- and post-transplant sera. There are no recognised effective prophylactic measures; however, avoidance of mismatching seropositive donors with seronegative recipients is recommended.

Most patients with PTLD respond to a reduction in immunosuppressive therapy together with the administration of high dose acyclovir.[16] If there is no response the patient should be treated as for a lymphoma, with radiotherapy or systemic chemotherapy.[17] In a series of 729 patients with PTLD, 560 (77%) were treated and of these 227 (41%) had complete remissions. In 48 (21%) of the latter the only treatment was reduction or cessation of immunosuppressive therapy.[34]

**Figure 12.2** *Factors influencing the development of lymphomas post-transplantation. *Risk compared to normal population.*

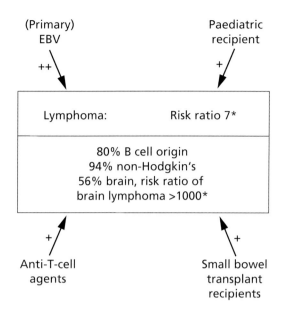

(Primary)
EBV

Paediatric
recipient

++

+

Lymphoma:                    Risk ratio 7*

80% B cell origin
94% non-Hodgkin's
56% brain, risk ratio of
brain lymphoma >1000*

+

+

Anti-T-cell
agents

Small bowel
transplant
recipients

## Kaposi's sarcoma

### Incidence

Kaposi's sarcoma (KS) occurs as frequently in transplant recipients, as in tropical Africa and represents 3–9% of all neoplasms in this group of patients.[42–45] The incidence in the USA before the advent of the AIDS epidemic was low: 0.02–0.07% malignancies. The risk ratio of KS in transplant recipients is >1000 when compared to the general population.[35,36]

Normally males predominate with a ratio 9:1 or 15:1. In transplant recipients this ratio is only 3:1.[42–45] As in the general population the incidence of KS in graft recipients was greatest in those of Arabic, Jewish, black or Mediterranean origins. Of transplant patients with KS 60% had non-visceral disease (skin, conjunctiva and otopharyngolaryngeal-mucosa) and 40% visceral disease. About 24% of patients with visceral disease had no skin involvement.[34]

### Aetiology

Kaposi's sarcoma is associated with HIV, but very few transplant patients with KS have tested positive for HIV. Oncogenic viruses of the herpes type have been implicated in the aetiology of KS.[42,44]

### Management

Clinical recognition of KS may be delayed in patients with visceral disease alone. Patients with visceral disease may present with abdominal pain, haematemesis or rectal bleeding. Diagnosis is confirmed by histology: the neoplasm has a multicentric origin and is characterised by tumours with vascular and fibroblastic elements. The 1993 CTTR of 7316 transplant recipients identified 311 with KS.[34] Of the patients with non-visceral disease 47% had complete remission and 33% of these remissions occurred when the only form of treatment was a dramatic reduction in immunosuppression. Only 20% of patients with visceral disease had complete remissions. Interestingly, 54% of the remissions in visceral KS followed reduction or cessation of immunosuppression. Of the patients with visceral KS 66% died and of these 73% died of the malignancy itself.[34]

## Carcinomas of the vulva and perineum

### Incidence

Neoplasms of the vulva, perineum, scrotum, penis, perianal skin and anus are increased 100-fold in transplant recipients and represent 3.6% of post-transplant cancers, compared to 0.6% of cancers in the general population.[34] The risk ratio for carcinomas of the vulva and vagina was increased to 35.5 in the 1992 Australasian registry.[38] One-third of the patients presented with *in situ* lesions. They are more common in females than males = 2.5:1,[34,38] unlike most other post-transplant malignancies (M:F = 2:1). In women the condition is often multicentric with lesions involving the vulva, vagina and anus.[42–44,46] The average age at diagnosis was only 42 years compared to 60–70 years in the general population. Patients presented on average 112 months (range 1.5–285.5 months) post-transplantation.[34]

### Aetiology

One-third of patients have a history of condylomata acuminata (genital warts) associated with the HPV.

### Management

Many patients with neoplasms of the vulva and perineum respond well to local excision and reduction of immunosuppression; some succumb despite extensive excision and abdoperineal resections. Analysis of 18 Australasian transplant recipients, with vulva/perineal cancer, revealed inguinal node involvement in three patients, but no deaths from malignancy to date.[36]

## Carcinoma of the uterus

### Incidence

The incidence of *in situ* carcinoma of the cervix is increased fourfold in transplant recipients. The risk ratio was measured at 3.6 for *in situ* carcinoma and 4.5 for invasive carcinoma when Australasian transplant recipients were compared to the general population.[38] The risk ratio for carcinoma of the uterus was lower (2.2).[38] In the CTTR, carcinoma of the cervix represented 11% of post-transplant cancers in women. At least 72% presented with *in situ* lesions. The CTTR data failed to show an increased incidence of carcinoma of the cervix. This is surprising as two studies have shown a 14–16-fold increase in transplant recipients.[47,48]

## Aetiology

There is a known association between carcinoma of the cervix and human papilloma virus, and thus an increased risk of immunocompromised patients who are more susceptible to viral infections and their sequelae.

## Management

The main emphasis should be preventative with yearly screening in female postadolescent transplant recipients. Ideally screening should include colposcopy, but most units offer yearly smears and reserve colposcopy for those patients with abnormal smears. Established disease is treated in the standard manner by cryotherapy, cone biopsy or hysterectomy, but may include reduction of immunosuppressive agents.[44]

## Renal carcinomas

### Incidence

Renal cancers constitute 4.8% of cancers in transplant recipients in the 1993 CTTR compared to 2% of cancers in the general population.[34] The increase is seen mainly in renal graft recipients. In 265 patients with renal neoplasms identified in the 1993 CTTR, 74% had renal cell cancers, 12% transitional cell cancers and 13% miscellaneous cancers. Up to 25% of the neoplasms were discovered incidentally at the time of nephrectomy for other reasons (i.e. infection, hypertension, polycystic kidneys) or at autopsy.[34] The risk ratios for renal, bladder and uteric cancers were increased to 9.2, 4.9 and 198, respectively in the Australian 1992 registry. Approximately one-third of renal, bladder and uteric cancers proved fatal.[38]

### Aetiology

Renal cell cancers are known to be more common in patients with polycystic kidney disease and in end-stage polycystic kidneys. In addition, the immune system plays an important role in the progression of renal cell cancer, as modulation with immunotherapy, in the form of interleukin-2, interferons and LAK (lymphokine activated killer) cells may induce remission of this tumour.[49,50] The increased incidence of transitional cell cancers is linked with a history of analgesic abuse as the initial cause of renal failure and abnormalities of the urinary tract.

### Treatment

Standard surgical management is combined with a reduction of immunosuppression where possible.

## Hepatobiliary tumours

### Incidence
A 20–38-fold increase is seen in transplant recipients. The increase is seen in particular in liver graft recipients and in patients with a history of hepatitis B.

### Aetiology
Hepatitis B is known to be an important factor in the aetiology of hepatomas. In some liver graft recipients, the tumour represents recurrence of pretransplant disease. In the Australian combined liver transplant registry (577 patients) the five-year survival for patients transplanted for primary liver cancer or with a finding of incidental liver cancer was 20% compared to 70% for patients who received a liver transplant for benign disease.[51]

## Effect of immunosuppression in pre-existing cancers

Cadaveric organ retrieval includes a thorough laparotomy to exclude pre-existing donor malignancy. If donor malignancy is missed, and micrometastases are transplanted with the organs, disseminated carcinomatosis may occur within months.

The timing of transplantation in recipients with pre-existing malignancy is a vexed issue and recommendations vary according to the institution and the tumour. Analysis of 855 recipients with treated pretransplant malignancy or an incidental finding of malignancy at the time of transplantation revealed a 22% (191/855) recurrence rate.[52] Some of the recurrences were *de novo* cancers of similar aetiology, particularly in tumours arising from paired organs. A total of 53% (101/191 of 855) recurrences occurred in recipients grafted within 2 years of treatment of the cancer. The percentage of recurrences fell to 34% if transplantation was delayed to 2–5 years post-malignancy and to 13% if the delay was extended to 5 or more years. A wait of five years may be unacceptable in older patients or in non-renal patients and therefore a compromise of 2 years is recommended by many units.[52,53] In early cases of renal call cancer a wait of only one year is considered acceptable, if the potential recipient is free of tumour.[53] Tumours with recurrence rates greater than 26% in this series[52] included bladder cancers, sarcomas, malignant melanomas, symptomatic renal cell cancers, non-melanotic skin cancers and multiple myeloma.

Liver transplantation is often performed for primary liver carcinomas and the high recurrence rate is well documented: by six years 15% have recurrent or *de novo* liver malignancy.[51]

### *De novo* cancer in paediatric transplant recipients

The pattern of post-transplant malignancy differs in paediatric recipients. In children, 50% of post-transplant tumours are lymphomas[22,26] compared to 12–23% in adult recipients.[34–6] Of the children with lymphoma 60% were recipients of non-renal organs.[22,26] The second most common malignancy in paediatric recipients were skin cancers (20%), but occurred less frequently than in adult recipients in whom skin cancers represent 38% of neoplasms.[54] Malignant melanomas were more common in paediatric than adult recipients, as were lip cancers. Spread to lymph nodes was also more common in paediatric recipients (13% v 6%). The third most common tumour in paediatric transplant patients was carcinoma of the vulva, perineum/anus which occurred after puberty in females at an average of 140 months (range 43–262 months) post-transplantation.[54]

### Long-term survival after renal transplantation

It is interesting to note that 26% of patients with transplants functioning for 10 years died from cancer, whereas only 1% of patients died from cancer after 10 years on dialysis and only 3% after a failed graft and 10 years on dialysis.[55] In Australia 17.4% (38/219) of cadaveric renal transplant recipients survived for 20–26 years post-transplant with a functioning graft. The average age at the time of transplantation was 33 years (range 17–55 years). Carcinoma occurred in 79% (30/38) of survivors. Of the 74% who developed skin cancers, the majority had more than three lesions. Three deaths occurred from metastatic disease (one skin, two colon primaries).[37]

### Conclusion

The transplant cancer registries represent a disparate group of patients receiving different forms of transplants, with differing follow-up periods and range from neonates to 80 year olds. Data accuracy depends on cooperation from units around the world. Once collated the data must be compared with age-matched epidemiological data from the general population. The long-term results of modern aggressive immunosuppression will not be seen for many years. A trend upwards has already been noticed in carcinoma of the breast, where the risk ratio in the Australasian series has increased from 1 to 1.3.[35] It is possible that a similar increase will also be seen in carcinomas of the bowel and lung. Extrapolation of Shiel's data suggests that between 30 and 40 years post-transplantation virtually all patients will have some form of cancer (Fig. 12.3).[36]

**Figure 12.3** *The proportions of patients surviving following cadaveric donor renal transplantation in Australia and New Zealand who develop skin, non-skin or any malignancy. Reproduced from Sheil.*[38]

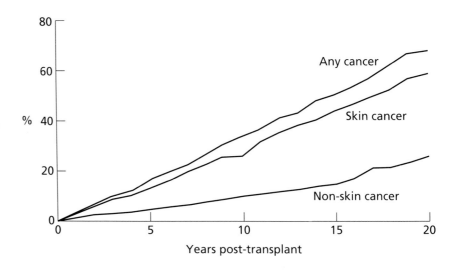

## References

1. Ho M, Wajszezuk CP, Har *et al.* Infections in kidney, heart and liver transplant recipients on cyclosporine. Transplant Proc 1983; 15 (Suppl 1): 2768–72.
2. Dummer JS, Hardy A, Poorsatter A *et al.* Early infections in kidney, heart and liver transplants. Transplantation 36: 259–67.
3. Rubin RH. Pre-emptive therapy in immunocompromised hosts. N Engl J Med 1991; 324: 1057–9.
4. Paya CV, Wiesner RH, Hermans PE *et al.* Risk factors for cytomegalovirus and severe bacterial infections following organ transplantation: a prospective multivariate time-dependent analysis. J Hepatol 1993; 18: 185–95.
5. Peterson PK, Balfour HH, Marker SC *et al.* Cytomegalovirus disease in renal allograft recipients: a prospective study of the clinical features, risk factors and impact on survival. Medicine 1980; 59: 283–300.
6. Nicholson V, Johnson PC. Infectious complications in solid organ recipients. Surg Clin North Am 1994; 75: 1223–45.
7. Patel R, Snydman DR, Rubin RH *et al.* Cytomegalovirus prophylaxis in solid organ transplantation. Transplantation 1996; 61: 1279–89.
8. Gilbert GL, Hayes K, Hudson IL, James J. Prevention of transfusion-acquired cytomegalovirus infection in neonates by blood filtration to remove leucocytes. Neonatal cytomegalo-

virus infection study group. Lancet 1989; i: 1228–31.
9. Merigan TC, Renlund DG, Kaey S *et al.* A controlled trial of ganciclovir to prevent cytomegalovirus disease after heart transplantation. N Engl J Med 1992; 1182–91.
10. Snydman DR, Werner BG, Heinze-Lacey B *et al.* Use of cytomegalovirus immune globulin to prevent cytomegalovirus disease in renal-transplant recipients. N Engl J Med 1987; 317: 1049–54.
11. Dunn DL, Mayoral JL, Gillingham KJ *et al.* Treatment of invasive CMV disease in solid organ transplants with ganciclovir. Transplantation 1991; 51: 98–106.
12. Griffiths PD. Viral complications after transplantation. J Antimicrob Chemother 1995; 36 (Suppl B): 91–106.
13. Cen H, Breinig MC, Atchison RW, Ho M, McKnight JL. Epstein–Barr virus transmission via the donor organs in solid organ transplantation: polymerase chain reaction and restriction fragment length polymorphism analysis of IR2, IR3 and IR4. J Virol 1991; 65: 976–80.
14. Cockfield SM, Preiksaitis JK, Jewell LD *et al.* Post-transplant lymphoproliferative disorder in renal allograft recipients. Transplantation 1993; 56: 88–96.
15. Swinnen LJ, Costanzo-Nordin MR, Fisher SG *et al.* Increased incidence of lymphoproliferative

disorder after immunosuppression with the monoclonal antibody OKT3 in cardiac-transplant recipients. N Engl J Med 1990; 323: 1723–8.

16. Hanto DW, Frizzera G, Gajl-Peczalska KJ et al. Epstein–Barr virus-induced B-cell lymphoma after renal transplantation: acyclovir therapy and transition from polyclonal to monoclonal B-cell proliferation. N Engl J Med 1982; 306: 913–18.

17. Benkerrou M, Durandy A, Fischer A. Therapy for transplant-related lymphoproliferative diseases. Hematol-Oncol Clin N Am 1993; 7: 467–75.

18. Kusne S, Schwartz M, Breinig MK et al. Herpes simplex virus hepatitis after solid organ transplantation in adults. J Infect Dis 1991; 163: 1001–7.

19. Berry NJ, Grundy JE, Griffiths PD. Radioimmunoassay for the detection of IgG antibodies to herpes simplex virus and its use as a prognostic indicator for HSV excretion in transplant recipients. J Med Virol 1987; 21: 147–54.

20. Kitai IC, King S, Gafni A. An economic evaluation of varicella vaccine for pediatric liver and kidney transplant recipients. Clin Infect Dis 1993; 17: 441–7.

21. Bavin PJ, Giles PJ, Hudson E et al. Comparison of cervical cytology and the polymerase chain reaction to identify women with cervical disease in a general practice population. J Med Virol 1992; 37: 8–12.

22. O'Grady JG, Smith HM, Davies SE et al. Hepatitis B reinfection after orthotopic liver transplantation. Serological and clinical implication. J Hepatol 1992; 14: 104–11.

23. Didier S, Muller R, Alexander G et al. Liver transplantation in European patients with the hepatitis B surface antigen. N Engl J Med 1993; 329: 1842–7.

24. Neuhaus P, Steffen R, Blumhardt G et al. Experience with immunoprophylaxis and interferon therapy after liver transplantation in HBsAg positive patients. Transplant Proc 1991; 23: 1522–4.

25. Valeri M, Pisani F, De Paolis P et al. Hepatitis C infection in kidney transplant recipients. Transplant Proc 1993; 25: 2284–5.

26. Delaney V, Sumrani N, Hong JH et al. Mycobacterial infections in renal allograft recipients. Transplant Proc 1993; 25: 2288–9.

27. Quinbi WY, Al-Sibai B, Taher S et al. Mycobacterial infection after renal transplantation. Q J Med 1990; 77: 1039–60.

28. Kusne S, Ryers J et al. Mycobacterium tuberculosis after liver transplantation: management and guidelines for prevention. Clin Transplant 1992; 6: 81–90.

29. Van Buren D, Wideman CA, Reid M et al. The antagonistic effect of rifampin upon cyclosporine bioavailability. Transplant Proc 1984; 16: 1642–5.

30. Arduino RC, Johnson PC, Miranda AG. Nocardiosis in renal transplant recipients undergoing immunosuppression with cyclosporine. Clin Infect Dis 1993; 16: 505–12.

31. Paya CF. Fungal infection in solid-organ transplantation. Clin Infect Dis 1993; 16: 677–88.

32. Weiland D, Ferguson RM, Peterson PK et al. Aspergillosis in 25 renal transplant recipients. Ann Surg 1983; 198: 622–9.

33. Dummer SJ, Montero CG, Griffith BP et al. Infections in heart–lung transplant recipients. Transplantation 1986; 41: 725–9.

34. Penn I. Malignancy. Surg Clin North Am 1994; 74.

35. Sheil AGR, Disney APS, Mathew TH, Amiss N. De novo malignancy emerges as a major cause of morbidity and late failure in renal transplantation. Transplant Proc 1993; 25: 1383–4.

36. Sheil AGR, Disney APS, Mathew TG, Amiss N, Excell L. Malignancy following renal transplantation. Transplant Proc 1992; 24: 1946–7.

37. Mahoney, Caterson RJ, Coulshed S, Stewart JH, Sheil AGR. Twenty and 25 years survival after cadaveric renal transplantation. Transplant Proc 1995; 27: 2154–5.

38. Sheil AGR. Development of malignancy following renal transplantation in Australia and New Zealand. Transplant Proc 1992; 24: 1275–9.

39. Sontheimer RD, Bergstresser PR, Gailiunas JR et al. Perturbation of epidermal Langerhans cells in immunosuppressed human renal allograft recipients. Transplantation 1984; 37: 168–74.

40. Trush MA, Mimnaugh EG, Glamm TE. Laboratory of Medicinal Chemistry and Biology, developmental therapeutics program, division of cancer treatments,

National Cancer Institute, National Institutes of Health, Bethesda, MD. Biochem Pharmacol 1982; 31: 3335–46.

41. Lennard L, Thomas SE, Harrington CI *et al*. Skin cancer in renal transplant recipients is associated with increased concentrations of 6-thioguanine nucleotide in red blood cells. Br J Dermatol 1985; 113: 723–9.

42. Penn I. Immunosuppression and opportunistic tumours: Do viruses play a role? In: Dammaco F (ed.) Advances in tumor immunology and allergic disorders. Immuno Incontri 1992; 6: 139.

43. Penn I. Tumors after renal and cardiac transplantation. Hematol Oncol Clin North Am 1993; 7: 431.

44. Penn I. Why do immunosuppressed patients develop cancer? CRC Crit Rev Oncogenesis 1989; 1: 27.

45. Penn I. Posttransplant kidney cancers and skin cancers (including Kaposi's sarcoma). In: Schmoahl D, Penn I (eds) Cancer in organ transplant recipients. Berlin: Springer-Verlag, 1991, p. 46.

46. Penn I. Cancers of the anogenital region in renal transplant patients: Analysis of 65 cases. Cancer 1986; 58: 611.

47. Porreco R, Penn I, Droegemueller W *et al*. Gynecologic malignancies in immunosuppressed organ homograft recipients. Obstet Gynecol 1975; 45: 359.

48. Sillman F, Stanek A, Sedlis A *et al*. The relationship between human papillomavirus and lower genital intraepithelial neoplasia in immunosuppressed woman. Am J Obstet Gynecol 1984; 150: 300.

49. Rosenberg SA, Mule JJ, Spiess PJ, Reichert CM, Schwarz SL. Regression of established pulmonary metastases and subcutaneous tumour mediated by the systemic administration of high-dose recombinant interleukin-2. J Exp Med 1985; 161: 1169–88.

50. Rosenberg SA, Mule JJ. Immunotherapy of cancer with lymphokine-activated killer cells and recombinant interleukin-2. Surgery 1985; 93: 437–44.

51. Sheil AGR. Malignancy following liver transplantation: a report from the Australian combined liver transplant registry. Transplant Proc 1995; 27: 1247.

52. Penn I. Effect of immunosuppression on pre-existing cancers. Transplant Proc 1993; 25: 1380–2.

53. Penn I. Kidney transplantation in patients previously treated for renal carcinomas. Transplant Int 1993; 6: 350.

54. Penn I. De novo malignancy in pediatric organ transplant recipients. J Pediatr Surg 1994; 29: 221–6; discussion 227–8.

55. Penn I. Occurrence of cancers in immunosuppressed organ transplant recipients. Clin Transplant 1994; 99–109.

# 13 The economics of transplantation

*Keith M. Rigg*

**Introduction**

Health economics is an area where the medical profession as a whole is becoming increasingly aware and involved. An epidemic of health care reforms is taking place in the United Kingdom (UK), North America, Europe and Australasia. Spending on health care has increased, but this has not kept pace with demand and there is still relative underfunding. Many reforms are aimed towards maximising efficiency and cost effectiveness, and basing health care interventions on good scientific evidence. It is likely, however, that funding will remain a problem.

Nowhere is this more apparent than in the field of transplantation where expensive treatments are given to a small proportion of the population. Solid organ transplantation of kidneys, liver, heart, lung and pancreas is now well established. However, with increased public expectation and an ageing population there is an increasing demand for the latest technologies and treatments. Older and higher risk patients are now receiving organ transplants. New drugs such as cyclosporin, tacrolimus and mycophenolate mofetil, albeit effective, are expensive. Funding for transplantation has to come from the same pot as hip replacements, vaccination programmes, coronary artery bypass grafts and cancer treatment. Clearly resources are finite and are likely to remain so. Extra funding will increasingly come from internal savings, efficiency gains and shifting costs from another person's budget. It therefore behoves the transplant clinician, (a) to provide a service that makes maximum use of these finite resources, and (b) to understand the principles of health economics and how they can be used to benefit transplantation.

The following facets of the economics of transplantation will be considered:

1. Models of funding
2. Cost effectiveness
3. Clinical issues
4. Pharmacoeconomics
5. Future direction

**Models of funding**

There are three basic models of funding in operation:

1. Funding from central government via taxation, e.g. UK, Australia, Italy and Sweden
2. Public/private health insurance schemes, e.g. Belgium, France, Germany and the Netherlands
3. Individual resources

The last may be practised by the rich in countries where there is no established transplant programme with access to all; as such it will be considered no further.

With an older population and technological and pharmacological advances, expenditure on health care in the 1970s and early 1980s increased more than the growth in the economy in most countries of Western Europe, North America and Australasia.[1] Since then the growth rate of the gross national product (GDP) has slowed and in Sweden, Denmark and Germany expenditure on health care expressed as a percentage of the GDP has fallen. However, despite the high cost of transplantation in relation to other treatments, there is still little reliable and accurate information about the costs involved.[2] Most of the published data on the economics of transplantation are from North America. In the UK, costs for renal transplantation in 1995/96 varied between units from £13 000 to £25 000 (first year costs), liver transplantation approximately £30 000–40 000 (first year costs), cardiopulmonary transplantation £25 000 (first three months cost) and small bowel transplantation £40 000 (first year costs). Similar variations are reported from North America in kidney, liver and heart transplantation.[2,3] This disparity does not necessarily mean that some units are more expensive than others, although they may be; but rather that case mix varies and costs are calculated in different ways.

In broad terms purchasers (e.g. health authorities, insurance companies) 'buy' health care from providers (e.g. hospitals). Providers may (1) negotiate a contract with the purchaser and be allocated a budget or (2) be reimbursed according to a system such as diagnosis related groups (DRG) or managed care. Within either system it is important to distinguish between elements and components of cost. The main elements of cost to the hospital are direct and indirect costs. Direct costs include pay, non-pay (diagnostic services, consumables and disposables) and drugs whereas indirect costs cover support services and other hospital overheads.

To take account of the case mix these costs need to be averaged. For example a young, otherwise healthy patient receiving a kidney transplant that functions immediately with no rejection or other complication and requiring minimal immunosuppression will incur lower costs than an elderly diabetic recipient who has delayed graft function, develops steroid-resistant rejection and cytomegalovirus disease, and requires prolonged hospitalisation. It is not difficult to see why costs vary between centres and why there are few accurate data available.

At present the major obstacle to increasing the transplantation rate is the limited availability of suitable cadaveric organs. Since kidney transplantation is cost effective compared to dialysis most purchasing authorities are willing to fund extra kidney transplants beyond contract numbers. At present this is also the case for other solid organ transplants even though the cost-effectiveness of these procedures cannot be so clearly demonstrated. However, it is unclear, in the USA and other countries, whether adequate funding for liver transplantation will continue.[3] Larger proportions of finite health care resources are going towards disease prevention rather than expensive, high technology treatments that only benefit a few. In the UK and other countries where there is a national health service extra transplants performed above a certain agreed number are usually paid/reimbursed at marginal rather than full cost. Typically for a renal transplant marginal costs are 30–40% of the full first year costs. In countries that operate the model of public/ private health insurance full costs, including pay, are recouped for each transplant performed. However, this is changing in some countries with the introduction of managed care. This was initiated in the US in response to the health care crisis where an increasing number of patients were uninsured. Managed care is an umbrella term whereby 'for-profit' organisations contract with their provider hospitals and physicians to provide a defined package of care for a fixed fee. These contracts are based on price, volume and quality. Although managed care is not without its problems, it is one way forward in providing healthcare for all without increasing costs.[4] When funding comes via central government a certain degree of external control exists. In the UK, liver, heart and lung transplantation are currently funded supraregionally via the Department of Health, although this situation is likely to change in the next year. In Australia, lung and pancreas transplantation are still funded nationally. This allows the number of centres to be restricted with better identification and control of costs and probably improved results. This contrasts with the USA and other European countries where there is no such restriction and there are many centres performing relatively few transplants. This centre/volume effect will be discussed later.

## Cost effectiveness

Technological and immunological advances in transplantation have resulted in improved graft and patient survival. One year first cadaver transplant graft survival of at least 85% (kidney), 70% (liver), 80% (heart) and 65% (lung) is now expected. However, transplantation is expensive and when there are finite health care resources, concern has been expressed about the cost effectiveness of these procedures. In the industrialised countries governments are wanting to see measures of quality, efficiency and effectiveness in health care provision, although at the same time providers are increasingly having to give an account of the resources used. This can only be done by measuring the outcome of their interventions and how these meet specified objectives.[5] Detsky and

Naglie[6] listed five principles involved in evaluating new or existing health care interventions. These principles are equally applicable in the field of transplantation; whether it be with established (renal, heart and lung, liver and pancreas) or innovative organ transplant programmes (small bowel, cluster and islet cell). The five principles are as follows.

1. Demonstrate efficacy: can the intervention achieve its stated goal when used in optimal circumstances?
2. Assessment of effectiveness: does the intervention do more good than harm when used in the normal clinical situation?
3. Assessment of efficiency or cost effectiveness: how effective is the intervention and what resources are needed to provide it? Efficiency can be defined as the maximum improvement in health obtained for a fixed amount of resources.
4. Availability: will the intervention be accessible to the person requiring it?
5. Distribution: who are the winners and losers if resources are allocated to one health care programme at the expense of another?

There is no doubt that kidney transplantation, in general, is cost effective. First year transplantation costs in the UK are on average £15 000–20 000 compared to dialysis costs of £12 000–18 000 for peritoneal dialysis and £20 000–25 000 for haemodialysis. However from year 2 transplants cost £1500–3000 clearly demonstrating their cost effectiveness. The arguments are not so compelling for heart and liver transplantation. Costs of transplantation have to be compared with that of no treatment at all, which is the cost of dying with end-stage disease. Evans[7] reviewed the literature; the treatment of end-stage renal, cardiac and hepatic failure without a transplant is expensive and may be more so than a transplant. Furthermore, caring for the dying patient was also shown to be a costly business. Allowing a patient with end-stage cardiac or hepatic failure to die without treatment is not an alternative, unless there is little or no chance for recovery. Supportive treatment of these patients in intensive care facilities is undoubtedly expensive, but with the availability of successful transplantation, and a resultant improvement in quality and duration of life, it is easier to argue for the cost effectiveness of the transplant. There are ethical, as well as economic, considerations to bear in mind and whereas the clinician wants to give the best available treatment for the patient, the health economist may take a more global view in determining where the scarce health care resources should go. The issues become less clear when retransplantation and transplantation of marginal recipients are considered where the likelihood of success is less and the financial price to pay may be greater.

## Definitions

Cost effectiveness so far has been used as a generic term to determine how the cost of an intervention correlates with the effectiveness of it in terms of outcome. Four main types of economic evaluation of health care are commonly used – cost minimisation, cost effectiveness, cost utility and cost–benefit analysis.[8,9]

1. Cost minimisation analysis where the outcomes of the health care interventions under analysis are similar.
2. Cost effectiveness analysis where effectiveness is measured in terms of clinical outcome, such as graft or patient survival in years.
3. Cost utility analysis where outcomes are measured in 'utility based' units that relate to a persons quality of life, e.g. quality adjusted life year (QALY).
4. Cost–benefit analysis where benefit is measured in terms of 'willingness to pay', translating clinical outcomes into a monetary value. What would the individual be willing to pay to receive a defined health care benefit?

It is important to define clearly what the two health care interventions are, e.g. haemodialysis and renal transplantation or the use of cyclosporin as opposed to tacrolimus-based immunosuppression; and what the costs and clinical outcomes of both interventions are. Improved outcomes may be achieved with fewer resources, but often improved outcome is associated with increased costs. In analysing the effectiveness, utility and benefit of any intervention over another it is possible to derive a ratio for each.

These approaches can be used, theoretically at least, to help in the distribution of health care resources. Cost–benefit analysis 'requires several value judgements that are based on controversial issues' and therefore economists prefer the use of utility over benefit as an outcome measure.[6] However, these approaches can cause confusion and have not, as yet, gained widespread acceptance and use. Caution is advised as it is essential that the costs of an intervention and measurement of the outcome, be it clinical or quality of life, be recorded in a standard, reproducible fashion that is applicable to each centre performing that intervention. Clearly this standard has not yet been reached.

## Outcomes

Up until the last ten years the effectiveness of a procedure or treatment in transplantation has generally been measured in terms of clinical outcomes, which look at outcomes from primarily the clinician's viewpoint. The simple, but relatively crude, measure of patient and graft survival has been used more or less exclusively. Although this is important, it does not distinguish between the graft that functions well with minimal complications and immunosuppression, and the graft that has poor function with a large number of complications. Therefore more sensitive means of measuring clinical outcomes need to be developed. Over the last ten years there has been a burgeoning interest in looking at outcomes from the patient's point of view and an increasing number of tools have been developed for measuring patient quality of life. Furthermore, it is recognised that clinical outcomes may correlate with quality of life and in particular health-related quality of life.[10]

### Clinical outcomes

Clinical outcomes are one way of determining the quality and effectiveness of a healthcare intervention, but it is a complex issue. Recently in the UK the government has discussed producing 'league tables' of mortality following different procedures. Not surprisingly this has generated widespread opposition. There are other factors, such as accuracy of data collection and casemix, that need to be considered before coming to a conclusion that one hospital has better results than another.

In the transplant setting other measurable outcomes apart from graft and patient survival should be considered. If I were to need a transplant, what would constitute a good outcome?

- Short wait for a transplant
- Immediate function
- No rejection
- Minimal immunosuppression
- Excellent graft function
- Few hospital admissions
- Early return to work
- Long-term health

It is important that clinicians take the lead in measuring and recording these types of clinical outcomes; hospital statistics are generally too crude and the accuracy can be open to question. Two large international databases; the Collaborative Transplant Study (CTS) and the UNOS registry record many of these outcomes from participating centres. Great emphasis is placed on accuracy of data collection although submission of data is entirely voluntary. In addition many transplant centres do record these types of outcome measures on databases generated internally and regularly submit these data to clinical audit. Over the next few years it is increasingly likely that purchasers of health care will wish to see these data to demonstrate clinical effectiveness and allocate resources and funding upon that.

Comparative studies of similar health care interventions performed in different centres often reveal differences in outcome, the so called 'centre effect'. Assuming that data collection is accurate and complete, there are two major reasons for this – case mix and the volume effect.

Case mix is a complex issue that includes patient and diagnostic variables. Attempts have been made to measure case mix using Diagnosis Related Groups (DRGs) and in the UK, Healthcare Resource Groups (HRGs). DRG is a case mix measure developed in the USA which groups hospital inpatients who are expected to consume similar amounts of health care resource. HRG is a similar measure that is applicable to the UK. Both require an inpatient minimum dataset of information which includes primary diagnosis, secondary diagnosis (complication or comorbidity), principal and secondary procedures (if any), age, specialty and discharge status. Cases can then be assigned using computer software called groupers into a particular DRG of HRG by using a decision pathway. Analysis of groups is then based on comparing length of stay, which is a surrogate marker for resource consumption. The aim of DRGs and HRGs is primarily to act as a resource management tool for managers. Much of this approach is still conceptual and is difficult to apply to transplantation[11] although DRGs are used in Sweden as a basis for reimbursement of costs. Further work to refine patient groupings will include need-based groupings and prognosis-based groupings which will be essential for accurate case mix-adjusted outcome data.[5]

It is generally accepted that the quality of patient care improves with the experience of those providing it. Therefore surgical mortality rates will be lower in those hospitals that perform a higher volume of a given procedure and this volume effect is more marked for complex procedures.[12] This type of data does, however, have to be adjusted for case mix. Evans[13] showed that patient, donor and transplant centre variables could all adversely affect kidney graft and patient survival. After adjusting for patient and donor variables, transplant centre volume was associated with improved results. Transplant physician experience was positively related with improved graft and patient survival whereas the experience of the transplant surgeon only affected patient survival. Similar findings could be expected in non-renal solid organ transplantation and have been reported in heart transplantation.[14] From the outcome point of view there is a strong argument for 'regionalising' transplant centres to ensure an adequate number of transplant procedures are performed, thereby maintaining the developed experience. The numbers of cardiopulmonary and liver transplant centres in the UK have been restricted by central government with a resultant large surgical volume. These restraints are not seen in other countries, notably USA and France, where there are many transplant centres performing a relatively small number of transplants each, often with inferior clinical outcomes. There is also a strong economic argument for having larger, rather than small units. Staff and hospital resources can be used in a more cost-effective manner. If graft survival is improved, there will also be cost savings in terms of retransplantation and treatment associated with failing or failed grafts.

## Patient outcomes – 'quality of life'

'The quality of life is more important that life itself' Alexis Carrel. It is naive to assume that clinical outcomes are the only result that matters after a health care intervention. It is also important to know how the patient perceives the result of that intervention and how their quality of life is affected. Usually the two are positively related, but it may not always be the case. A poorly functioning graft, drug side effects or employment difficulties will affect quality of life, but may not be identified in measurement of clinical outcomes. Quality of life (QOL) is difficult to define but encompasses how the individual functions and interacts in the physical, psychological, emotional and social domains. Numerous questionnaires have been designed to measure QOL and these can be classified as generic, disease specific or dimension specific. The design of these questionnaires needs to take into account the validity, reliability and responsiveness; ease of administration and cultural setting.[15,16] Scores controlled for age, sex and social class have been determined for the general population.

Generic questionnaires, such as the Sickness Impact Profile (SIP), Nottingham Health Profile (NHP) and the Short Form-36 (SF-36) Health Survey, measure perceived health in the physical, psychological, emotional and social domains. The Sickness Impact Profile was developed in the USA and has 136 questions covering 12 dimensions. Scores are expressed on a scale of 1–100, with higher scores denoting a worse state. The Nottingham Health Profile was developed in the UK, although it has been adapted for use in other countries. The questionnaire is in two parts. Part I comprises 38 questions encompassing the dimensions of sleep, physical mobility, energy, pain, emotional reactions and social isolation. Each question is answered yes or no and the answers weighted to give a maximum of 100. Part II of the profile relates to seven areas of daily living most often affected by health. The NHP has been criticised because of its inability to detect low levels of disability. Although the SF-36 was first developed in the USA an anglicised version has been produced in the UK. It has 36 questions covering eight dimensions; physical and social functioning, role limitations due to physical and emotional problems, mental health, energy and vitality, pain and general perception of health. Again the scores are weighted and transformed on a scale of 0–100, where 100 is the best possible.

There are a number of disease-specific questionnaires that have been designed for patients with renal disease, although many of these are specifically for people on dialysis.[17] These look at the effect of renal specific symptoms and the effect of renal replacement therapy on the individual. Dimension-specific questionnaires concentrate on individual areas and a number of measures may be required for assessment. These include measures of physical well-being, social well-being, emotional and psychological well-being.[17,18]

In assessing QOL a composite questionnaire may often be constructed which includes generic, disease and dimension specific components. These are all subjective observations made by the patient themselves either through self-completion of the questionnaire or by interview. An objective view from the patient can also be gained by including indicators such as ability to work, the self-assessed Karnofsky performance index and functional impairment.[19] A number of studies measuring QOL following kidney, liver, pancreas, heart and lung transplantation have been performed. Renal transplant recipients score consistently higher than haemodialysis or peritoneal dialysis patients, but are still slightly less than the general population in most domains.[18,20,21] Similar findings are found in recipients of liver,[22,23] pancreas[24] and heart transplants.[25]

## Correlating clinical and patient outcomes

Clinical and patient outcomes are inextricably linked. There are two approaches to linking clinical to patient outcomes; the approach of the clinician and that of the health economist.

### Clinician's approach

The clinician is primarily interested in seeing the effect a health care intervention, e.g. transplantation, immunosuppressive regimen or the effect of any complication has on a patient's QOL. Health-related QOL is being increasingly used as a valid outcome measure in clinical trials. Another approach is the time trade-off method (TTO) which has been used to measure QOL longitudinally following renal transplantation.[26]

Correlating clinical and patient outcomes is a complex issue and Wilson[10] has proposed a model to classify different measures of health outcome. There are five levels: biological and physiological factors, symptoms, functional status, general health perceptions and overall quality of life. These relate to each other, but the higher the level the more difficult it is to measure the outcome. In addition there are external influences such as patient personality, environmental factors and non-medical factors that cannot be controlled by the clinician. However, this approach is deserving of further work.

### Health economist approach

The main approach of the health economist in correlating clinical outcomes with patient outcomes, i.e. quality of life, has been cost–utility analysis. The most commonly used measure of utility is the quality adjusted life year (QALY). The QALY is a number representing a unit of benefit that combines a measure of life expectancy with a measure of quality of life. One QALY is equivalent to one year of life in perfect health. QALYs are then calculated by measuring life years gained by a particular health care intervention and weighting each year to reflect the QOL. It is then theoretically possible to compare different health care interventions on the basis of cost per QALY gained.

The generic QOL measures do not generate a single score, but rather scores for different domains. The 'quality' part of QALYs is therefore measured using the Rosser Index where health status is measured using the two dimensions of disability and distress. There are eight categories of disability ranging from no disability to being unconscious; and four categories of distress (none, mild, moderate and severe). A matrix can then be constructed giving 32 different states of health, each of which has been scored on a scale ranging from $-1$ = worse than death through 0 = dead to 1 = perfect health. On the basis of this any state of health can be assigned a quality of life score.

Multiplying this quality of life score by the likely number of life years gained by the health care intervention gives the number of QALYs gained.

By introducing the cost of the intervention it is then possible to derive a cost per QALY although with the information available this has to be viewed as a 'guesstimate'. Not surprisingly clinicians have viewed the QALY approach with scepticism and criticism, but even health economists recognise that QALYs need further development and at present should be used cautiously. Other measures have been described but these have yet to be validated.

## Clinical issues

The importance of case mix in determining transplantation costs have already been highlighted above. A number of variables affecting the delivery and outcome of care need to be considered in this equation:

1. Donor-related variables
2. Selection criteria (which patients are suitable for transplantation?)
3. Allocation criteria (which patient gets any individual organ?)
4. Immunosuppression (benefits and adverse effects)
5. Failed grafts and retransplantation

### Donor-related variables

There are two main sources for organs at present – cadaveric heart beating donors and live (related or unrelated) donors – and for kidneys cadaveric non-heart beating donors are also an option. The shortage of organs for transplantation means that more cadaveric organs are being removed from marginal donors who may be elderly and have coexisting disease. Donor age of >55 years for kidneys and >40 years for hearts is associated with a significant increase in graft failure[27,28] and therefore cost effectiveness has to be looked at very carefully in this context. Similarly an increasing number of kidney transplant centres are using non-heart-beating kidneys. Although there is a higher incidence of delayed graft function, the long-term results are encouraging.[29] The early increase in costs will be offset by the effect of graft function.[30]

The shortage of organs is in part related to fewer deaths from head injuries and intracerebral haemorrhage, but also to lack of intensive care facilities. This is particularly acute in the UK. It is of interest that donor hospitals are reimbursed £1000 per donor in the UK which contrasts with Spain where reimbursements of up to £40 000 may be made. Proper reimbursements to the donor unit that truly reflect the costs associated with organ donation may improve the supply of organs. For kidney transplantation this cost would be offset by the successful transplantation of two organs and the resultant cost savings on dialysis.

Live donor renal transplantation is well established and graft survival is superior to when cadaveric organs are used. Recently this approach has been applied to liver, lung and small bowel transplantation.

Although there are increased costs associated with donor assessment, these are abrogated by the reduced waiting time for the transplant and improved results. In developing countries live donor renal transplantation is the preferred method of renal replacement therapy because of the limited dialysis facilities available and restricted health care resources.

### Selection criteria

Not all patients with end-stage organ failure are suitable for transplantation. Some patients are clearly not suitable because of coexistent medical conditions, but there is a grey area where acceptance or rejection for transplantation depends on the transplant centre. In general the larger centres, who have more experience and human resources, have more liberal selection policies than smaller units whose selection criteria are more stringent. Consequently costs for transplantation from the larger centres may be higher. This can be explained by the increased resources required by the 'marginal' recipient and a higher retransplantation rate.

There is an increasing number of patients >65 years old who are developing end-stage organ failure and are considered for transplantation. There is clearly increased cardiovascular and other morbidity in this age group and patients need to be carefully screened. The cost of a failed transplant can be measured not only in financial terms, but also in increased morbidity and mortality. Other coexistent disease also needs to be considered. Diabetic patients undergoing renal transplantation have similar graft survival, but inferior patient survival compared to non-diabetic patients.[31] Evans *et al.*[3] summarises a number of studies demonstrating that increasing severity of liver disease pretransplant is associated with increased length of stay and more than double the one year costs.

### Allocation criteria

The prime allocation criteria used for kidney transplantation are blood group compatibility, HLA matching and a negative cytotoxic cross-match; although for non-renal organs blood group compatibility and clinical criteria are important. The underlying principle is to transplant the organ into the recipient who will gain maximum benefit from it.

In renal transplantation the main dilemma from a clinical and economic point of view is balancing the advantages of HLA matching with the disadvantages of prolonged cold ischaemia times. For cadaveric organs the ideal match is a 'favourable' match, i.e. 0 or 1 mismatch at the A and/or B locus, but good results are achieved with a 0 DR mismatch alone. If matching does result in superior graft survival this will reduce the costs of transplantation by delaying the return of the patient to dialysis and the need for retransplantation. The pool of potential recipients in any one centre is not large enough to provide a 'favourable' or 0 DR mismatch for any kidney to be retrieved locally. Consequently organ sharing networks have been set up, e.g. UKTSSA (UK) and

Eurotransplant (Europe) which facilitate the distribution of organs to well-matched recipients. This theoretically improves graft survival, but the effect can be annulled by the travelling times required. Once cold ischaemic storage times extend beyond 24 h there is an increased incidence of delayed graft function (DGF). DGF results in increased initial hospitalisation times, increased dialysis requirements, intensive graft monitoring and inferior graft survival – all of which increase the costs. The use of University of Wisconsin (UW) preservation solution has been shown to be cost effective in this situation.[32]

Centres are adopting three different approaches to this dilemma:

1. Some are dispensing with matching and stressing the importance of minimising the cold ischaemic time:
2. Some are encouraging geographical 'zoning' of centres with a common waiting list which increases the recipient pool and reduces travelling time;
3. Others are adopting the status quo.

### Immunosuppression

This will be considered below under 'Pharmacoeconomics'

### Failed grafts and retransplantation

Loss of a graft is a catastrophic event for the patient. There may be associated morbidity and compromised quality of life. It is clear that the financial consequences of graft loss are also high. Manninen et al.[33] showed in renal transplants that failed in the initial admission the average transplant procedure costs were $80 000, compared with $30 522 for the functioning grafts. Follow-up charges were also significantly higher in those grafts that failed later. Indirect costs associated with transplant failure included inability to work, greater functional impairment, poorer health status and a decreased quality of life score. At least in kidney transplantation there is dialysis to fall back on, whereas in liver and heart transplantation there is death or retransplantation. Graft survival of retransplants is inferior to primary grafts for all organs. In addition retransplants are more expensive than primary transplants. Evans et al.[34] calculated that transplant procedure charges (excluding outpatient follow-up) for kidney, heart and liver retransplants were greater than primary grafts by 9%, 26% and 156%, respectively. There is clear doubt raised as to the cost effectiveness of liver and possibly heart retransplants.

## Pharmaco-economics

Apart from azathioprine and steroids, immunosuppressive agents for the prevention and treatment of rejection are expensive. Health care resources are limited and in introducing new pharmaceutical agents it is essential that they can be shown to make maximum use of health care currency. This has been illustrated with the recent availability of the new and effective, but expensive, immunosuppressive agents – mycophenolate mofetil and tacrolimus. It is therefore important to have an understanding of pharmacoeconomics – economic analysis that compares the costs and therapeutic consequences of different pharmaceutical agents in treating a particular medical condition.[35]

### Principles of pharmacoeconomics

The principal methods of pharmacoeconomic analysis are those that have already been defined above:

- Cost-minimisation analysis
- Cost-effectiveness analysis
- Cost–utility analysis
- Cost–benefit analysis

Freund and Dittur[35] emphasise the need to select the relevant perspective before deciding which economic analysis to perform. Society, the individual, the direct provider of health care, e.g. the transplant unit, the hospital, purchasers of health care and makers of health policy all wish to see the economic analysis from a slightly different perspective. Society may wish to see the cheapest drug used as this appears to be the best use of the limited resources (cost-minimisation analysis). However, if the use of this drug results in more side effects affecting quality of life the patient will not think it was the best drug to use, even though it was cheaper (cost–utility and cost–benefit analysis). If this drug related morbidity then results in an increased use of hospital resources, the providers and purchasers of health care will then have increased costs to contend with (cost-effectiveness analysis). Furthermore, not every type of analysis will be relevant to a particular situation.

Jolicoeur et al.[36] described ten basic steps for performing a pharmacoeconomic analysis. Although this is not a simple procedure to perform it does increase the likelihood of producing accurate, relevant and useful results.

Pharmacoeconomic analysis should also be an important consideration in the designing and undertaking of clinical trials. In the past it has been sufficient to demonstrate that a new drug is more effective and has a better side effect profile than the established drug without regard to the cost differences. In the current economic climate it is difficult to introduce a new and expensive drug into routine clinical practice unless a valid cost effectiveness ratio can be presented. Traditionally clinicians and statisticians have been involved in determining sample sizes for clinical trials. Torgerson et al.[37] argue the case for involvement of health economists in design of clinical trials. From the economic perspective the likely relative costs of the two treatments need to be considered. If there is a large cost difference, only a small sample size is required as the expensive treatment must have major advantages to justify its use. Conversely if there is a small cost difference a large sample size is required to show any small improvements that would justify the smaller extra costs.

## Pharmacoeconomics of immunosuppressive agents

The first breakthrough in immunosuppression was in the early 1960s with the introduction of azathioprine. In combination with steroids this formed the mainstay of maintenance immunosuppression until the early/mid 1980s when cyclosporin came into routine clinical practice. The last few years have seen the introduction of tacrolimus and mycophenolate mofetil as new immunosuppressive agents, as well as Neoral[R] the new oral formulation of cyclosporin. A number of other promising agents including sirolimus (rapamycin), deoxyspergualin and a range of monoclonal antibodies are currently in clinical trial; these too may be available for clinical use in the next 5–10 years. With this expanding armamentarium of effective and expensive drugs, decisions as to which drugs to use will need to be based on sound clinical and economic evidence.

In the pharmacoeconomic analysis of immunosuppressive agents the approaches of cost-effectiveness[38–40] and cost–utility[18] are well recognised. Cost–benefit analysis is a theoretically attractive approach since it attributes a monetary value to both the input (cost) and output (benefits), but it does rely on some subjective judgements in measuring benefit. Cost minimisation is probably an inappropriate method since it is difficult to show that the outcome of two immunosuppressive regimes is the same. Most analyses are directed towards showing that one regimen is better than another.

In order to measure cost effectiveness of immunosuppression outcomes need to be considered which relate both to the benefits and to the adverse effects of the immunosuppressive agent. Benefits include prevention of rejection and short- and long-term graft survival. Adverse effects include side effects of immunosuppression (infection and malignancy), non-immune toxicity and death. If rejection is prevented costs will be reduced since there will be fewer hospitalisations, fewer biopsies and other diagnostic procedures, less use of drugs to treat rejection (intravenous steroids, polyclonal and monoclonal antibodies), improved graft survival and less dialysis costs. On the other hand, if there is an increased drug-associated morbidity, costs may rise due to an increased use of diagnostic services, more inpatient and outpatient hospital attendances and treatment of infections and malignancy. By calculating the average cost savings per patient for benefits accrued and average cost gains per patient for adverse events occurring it is possible to determine if the extra cost of the immunosuppressive is offset by net cost savings. In practice these data can be very time consuming to collect, retrieve and analyse. Canafax et al.[38] compared the effects of three immunosuppressive drug protocols (ALG/azathioprine/prednisone (ALG/AZA/P); cyclosporin/prednisone (CyA/P); sequential quadruple therapy) on cadaveric renal transplantation costs after four years of therapy. Total hospital costs for the three groups after four years were \$60 821 (ALG/AZA/P), \$57 670 (CyA/P) and \$45 337 (ALG/AZA/CyA/P). The cost improvements for the CyA group were explained by fewer rejection episodes, less infection and reduced steroid requirement. There was a reduced initial hospitalisation in the quadruple therapy group because of a shorter duration of delayed graft function. A pilot economic analysis of 30 stable renal transplant patients (>6 months post-transplant) receiving Sandimmun[R] ($n$ = 6) or Neoral[R] ($n$ = 24) was reported by Keown et al.[39] Total direct medical costs per patient were \$2228 for the Neoral[R] group and \$3000 for the Sandimmun[R] group. Other studies have shown that Neoral[R], because of its improved bioavailability, will result in an average 10% dose reduction in patients transferred from Sandimmun[R].[41] Lake et al.[40] reported total one-year inpatient charges (excluding professional fees and outpatient charges) of 322 patients participating in the US trial comparing tacrolimus to cyclosporin in liver transplantation. Six centres participated and, although there was a wide range, charges in the tacrolimus group were \$122 279 compared to \$141 569 in the CyA group. The lower costs in the tacrolimus arm were attributed to different rejection profiles. The European and US multicentre studies of mycophenolate have recently been published and these too show a significant reduction in the incidence of biopsy proven rejection in the first six months.[42,43] It is likely that economic analysis of these studies will also show significant cost savings that will partly offset the cost of the drug. In the current climate of cost effectiveness it is clear that future clinical trials of immunosuppressive agents will need to include an economic analysis. On the negative side immunosuppression also results in adverse events and increased costs. McCarthy et al.[44] analysed the impact of cytomegalovirus disease on one-year post-renal transplant costs where mean total institutional costs were 2.5 times higher for patients with CMV disease compared to controls.

Owing to the expense of current immunosuppressive agents, a number of therapeutic manoeuvres have been described to minimise immunosuppressive usage while maintaining the efficacy. Diltiazem has been used to decrease the requirements of cyclosporin in cardiac transplantation, and ketoconazole has been used in a similar fashion in both cardiac and renal transplantation. Although this decreased cyclosporin requirement does result in significant cost savings the practice has not gained widespread acceptance. Clark et al.[45] described flow cytometric monitoring of CD3 counts during ATG administration. This led to decreased ATG requirements resulting in less infection and an average cost saving of £1440 per patient course, but with no reduction in efficacy.

Pharmacoeconomic analysis in the first year of transplantation is relatively straightforward, when the main variables to measure are the diagnosis and treatment of rejection, periods of hospitalisation, drug costs and graft failure. Long-term effects of immunosuppression are more difficult to quantitate. The withdrawal of steroid therapy may improve immediate quality of life, lead to fewer bone problems with fewer fractures and reduce overall morbidity, but this may be at the expense of decreased graft survival in some individuals. There needs to be better measurement of the total costs associated with transplantation in order to determine which transplants and which treatments are most cost effective.

## Future direction

Clinical transplantation has developed much in the last 30 years and it is likely that it will continue to do so for the foreseeable future. Graft survival rates for kidney, liver, heart, lung and pancreas transplantation have reached very acceptable levels; small bowel and islet cell transplantation are in their infancy with the prospect of clinical xenotransplantation on the horizon. The recent introduction of tacrolimus and mycophenolate mofetil and the development of sirolimus and new humanised monoclonal antibodies will expand the immunosuppressive repertoire; significantly reducing the incidence and severity of acute rejection and making possible inroads into chronic rejection. This is all occurring at a time when resources for health care are scarce and there is increasing competition for the limited available funding. In exploring the economics of transplantation over the next decade, three areas need careful consideration.

### Introducing new therapeutic options

There will undoubtedly be new therapeutic options available in all areas of clinical transplantation in the years to come. It is also clear that many of these will be costly. In the UK the assessment of new technologies is coming under the aegis of the Department of Health. It is unlikely that purchasers of health care will sanction the introduction of such technologies unless there is proven cost effectiveness. The provider will need to be able to provide accurate and inclusive costings for the first year and subsequent years. The effectiveness of the intervention must be based on scientifically based research evidence using the principles of evidence-based medicine. As new development moneys are unlikely to be forthcoming, the cost of the intervention should be met, where possible, from the resultant cost savings. Purchasers and providers of health care need to enter an evaluative culture where both sides are seeking to provide a high quality, cost effective service.[46] The latest initiative in the UK national health service is 'Clinical Effectiveness' that encompasses these principles. Transplant clinicians need to be at the forefront of this new culture.

### Priority setting

Priority setting is a less emotive term than rationing. Surgeons have operated a system of 'rationing' for years in putting non-urgent cases at the bottom of the waiting list. Priority setting is recognising that there are infinite demands and finite resources for health care and targeting resources on those activities which are most cost effective. Traditionally, clinicians want maximum resources for their patients and transplant clinicians are no exception. Economists and purchasers of health care have to view the situation from a broader perspective and make choices regarding the allocation of the limited resources. Someone is always going to be disappointed! Priority setting, in practice, is still in its infancy although initial experience has been gained in Oregon, the Netherlands and New Zealand.[47] Purchasers and health policy makers in the US and the UK have already indicated that liver and heart transplantation are not high priorities.[3] Over the next decade it is important that transplant clinicians operate sensible selection and allocation criteria and endeavour to provide the necessary high quality and cost-effective transplant programmes.

### Accurate costing and measurement of outcomes

Most of the published data on costs associated with transplantation derive from North America where the structure of the health care system encourages this. Accurate data for renal transplantation exist through Medicare although not for non-renal transplants as yet. In the future, accurate costings for all components of transplantation need to be available in a form that is standard between centres. In addition, transplants need to be compared with the cost of treating end-stage organ failure without a transplant.[2]

The measurement of outcomes of transplantation, both clinical and patient centred, will become increasingly important if clinicians take the initiative in demonstrating the provision of a cost-effective and clinically effective service. It is relatively easy to measure the clinical outcomes following transplantation, but further work is required to develop measures of patient-centred outcomes. Transplantation has faced head on the challenges of surgical technique, immunology, immunosuppression and donor organ supply since its early days; it will do the same with the economic challenge that it is currently facing.

## References

1. Smith T. European health care systems. In: Richards T (ed) Medicine in Europe. London: BMJ, 1992, pp. 23–9.
2. Eggers PW, Kucken LE. Cost issues in transplantation. Surg Clin North Am 1994; 74: 1259–67.
3. Evans RW, Manninen DL, Dong FB. An economic analysis of liver transplantation. Gastroenterol Clin North Am 1993; 22: 451–73.
4. Friedman EA. View from across the Atlantic. America struggles with health care reform. Nephrol Dial Transplant 1996; 11: 203–7.
5. Orchard C. Comparing healthcare outcomes. BMJ 1994; 308: 1493–6.
6. Detsky AS, Naglie IG. A clinicians guide to cost-effectiveness analysis. Ann Intern Med 1990; 114: 147–54.

7. Evans RW. Cost-effectiveness analysis of transplantation. Surg Clin North Am 1986; 66: 603–16.

8. Robinson R. Economic evaluation and health care – what does it mean? BMJ 1993; 307: 670–3.

9. Coyle D, Davies L. How to assess cost-effectiveness: elements of a sound economic evaluation: In: Drummond MF, Maynard A (eds) Purchasing and providing cost-effective health care. Edinburgh: Churchill Livingstone, 1993; pp. 66–79.

10. Wilson IB, Cleary PD. Linking clinical variables with health-related quality of life. JAMA 1995; 273: 59–65.

11. Gould FK, Dark JH. The economics of transplantation. J Antimicrob Chemother 1995; 36 Suppl B: 135–40.

12. Luft HS, Bunker JP, Enthoven AC. Should operations be regionalised? N Engl J Med 1979; 301: 1364–9.

13. Evans RW, Manninen DL, Dong F. The center effect in kidney transplantation. Transplant Proc 1991; 23: 1315–17.

14. Laffel GL, Barnett AI, Finkelstein S et al. The relation between experience and outcome in heart transplantation. N Engl J Med 1992; 327: 1220–5.

15. Fitzpatrick R, Fletcher A, Gore S et al. Quality of life measures. I: Applications and issues in assessment. BMJ 1992; 305: 1074–7.

16. Fletcher A, Gore S, Jones D et al. Quality of life measures in healthcare. II: Design, analysis, and interpretation. BMJ 1992; 305: 1145–8.

17. Welch G. Assessment of quality of life following renal failure. In: McGee H, Bradley C (eds) Quality of life following renal failure. Chur: Harwood Academic Publishers, 1994, pp. 55–97.

18. Simmons RG, Abbess L, Anderson CR. Quality of life after kidney transplantation. Transplantation 1988; 45: 415–21.

19. Gokal R. Quality of life in patients undergoing renal replacement therapy. Kidney Int 1993; 43, Suppl 40: S23–7.

20. Evans RW, Manninen DL, Garrison LP et al. The quality of life of patients with end-stage renal failure. N Engl J Med 1985; 312: 553–9.

21. Khan IH, Garratt AM, Kumar A et al. Patients perception of health on renal replacement therapy: evaluation using a new instrument. Nephrol Dial Transplant 1995; 10: 684–9.

22. Lowe D, O'Grady JG, McEwan J et al. Quality of life following liver transplantation: a preliminary report. J R Coll Physicians Lond 1990; 24: 43–6.

23. Tarter RE, Switala J, Arria A et al. Quality of life before and after orthotopic hepatic transplantation. Arch Intern Med 1991; 151: 1521–6.

24. Nathan DM, Fogel H, Norman D et al. Long-term metabolic and quality of life results with pancreatic/renal transplantation in insulin-dependent diabetes mellitus. Transplantation 1991; 52: 85–91.

25. Buxton M, Acheson RM, Caine N et al. Costs and benefits of the heart transplant programmes at Harefield and Papworth hospitals: final report. London: HMSO, 1985.

26. Russell JD, Beecroft ML, Ludwin D et al. The quality of life in renal transplantation – a prospective study. Transplantation 1992; 54: 656–60.

27. Renal Transplant Audit 1984–1993. Bristol: UKTSSA, 1995.

28. Thoracic Organ Transplant Audit 1985–1992. Bristol: UKTSSA, 1994.

29. Wijnen RMH, Booster MH, Stubenitsky BM et al. Outcome of transplantation on non-heart-beating donor kidneys. Lancet 1995; 345: 1067–70.

30. Bibo JC, Engel GL, Kootstra G et al. Cost analysis of transplantation with ischemically damaged kidneys: preliminary results. Transplant Proc 1995; 27: 2959–61.

31. Catalano C, Goodship THJ, Tapson JS et al. Renal replacement treatment for diabetic patients in Newcastle upon Tyne and the Northern region, 1964–88. BMJ 1990; 301: 535–40.

32. Rutten FFH, Ploeg RJ, McDonnell J et al. The cost-effectiveness of preservation with UW and EC solution for use in cadaveric kidney transplantation in the case of single kidney donors. Transplantation 1993; 56: 854–8.

33. Manninen DL, Evans RW, Dugan MK et al. The costs and outcome of kidney transplant graft failure. Transplant Proc 1991; 23: 1312–14.

34. Evans RW, Manninen DL, Dong FB et al. Is retransplantation cost effective? Transplant Proc 1993; 25: 1694–6.

35. Freund DA, Dittus RS. Principles of pharmacoeconomic analysis of drug therapy. PharmacoEcon 1992; 1: 20–32.

36. Jolicoeur LM, Jones-Grizzle AJ, Boyer JG. Guidelines for performing a pharmacoeconomic analysis. Am J Hosp Pharm 1992; 49: 1741–7.

37. Torgerson DJ, Ryan M, Ratcliffe J. Economics in sample size determination for clinical trials. Q J Med 1995; 88: 517–21.

38. Canafax DM, Carleton BC, Matas AJ *et al.* Effects of three immunosuppressive drug protocols on cadaver renal transplantation costs after 4 years of therapy. Transplant Proc 1993; 25: 1692–3.

39. Keown P, Lawen JG, Landsberg D *et al.* Economic analysis of Sandimmune Neoral in Canada in stable renal transplant patients. Transplant Proc 1995; 27: 1845–8.

40. Lake JR, Gorman KJ, Esquivel CO *et al.* The impact of immunosuppressive regimes on the cost of liver transplantation – results from the US FK506 multicenter trial. Transplantation 1995; 60: 1089–95.

41. Neumayer HH, Farber L, Haller P *et al.* Substitution of conventional cyclosporin with a new microemulsion formulation in renal transplant patients: results after 1 year. Nephrol Dial Transplant 1996; 11: 165–72.

42. European mycophenolate mofetil cooperative study group. Placebo-controlled study of mycophenolate mofetil combined with cyclosporin and corticosteroids for prevention of acute rejection. Lancet 1995; 345: 1321–5.

43. Sollinger HW. Mycophenolate mofetil for the prevention of acute rejection in primary cadaveric renal allograft recipients. Transplantation 1995; 60: 225–32.

44. McCarthy JM, Karim MA, Krueger H *et al.* The cost impact of cytomegalovirus disease in renal transplant recipients. Transplantation 1993; 55: 1277–82.

45. Clark KR, Forsythe JLR, Shenton BK *et al.* Administration of ATG according to the absolute T lymphocyte count during therapy for steroid resistant rejection. Transpl Int 1993; 6: 18–21.

46. Hutton J. How providers should respond to purchasers' needs. In: Drummond MF, Maynard A (eds) Purchasing and providing cost-effective health care. Edinburgh: Churchill Livingstone, 1993, pp. 145–56.

47. Maynard A. Future directions for health-care reform. In: Drummond MF, Maynard A (eds) Purchasing and providing cost-effective health care. Edinburgh: Churchill Livingstone, 1993, pp. 242–54.

# Index

Page numbers in *italic* refer to illustrations and tables; **bold** page numbers indicate a main discussion

A77 1726 102
ABO blood grouping 50
  matching 177
Acute fulminant hepatic failure (AFHF) 159, 165
  as indication for liver transplantation 148–9
Acute rejection
  definition **64–5**
Adhesion molecules 76–8, *76*
Age matching **45–8**
Age, donor 27
  hormonal resuscitation of hearts 278
Age, recipient
  heart transplantation 47, 252–3, 257
  kidney transplantation 46, 126–7, 143
  liver transplantation 47–8, 155–6, 165
  pancreas transplantation 170, 175, 184
  *see also* Age matching
Alcohol abuse
  morality of liver transplantation in 9
  organ donation and 28, 29
Alcoholic liver disease (ALD)
  liver transplantation and 148
Allocation of organs 38, 58–9
  cadaveric **7–9**
  criteria **317–18**
  ethics 7–9
Allogeneic transplants 63
Allopurinol 31, 90
Altruism 11, 12
Amphotericin 36
Antigen presenting cells (APC) 66, *66*, 74
Antithymocyte globulin (ATG) 99, 140
alpha1-Antitrypsin deficiency 151, 152
Aprotinin (Trasyslol) 154
Aspergillosis following small bowel transplantation 248
*Aspergillus*
  in lung transplantation 276
  post-transplant **292–3**
Azathioprine 54, 89–91

B cell lymphoma following small bowel transplantation 249
Balloon dilatation 162
Benzylpenicillin 32
beta2 integrins 76
beta2-microglobulin 69
Biliary atresia 149, 157
Bovine spongiform encephalopathy 84
Brain stem death 3, **19–20**
  clinical criteria *20*
Brain stem function tests 19
Brenner's hyperfiltration hypothesis 48–9
Brequinar sodium **100–1**
Budd–Chiari syndrome as cause of acute fulminant liver failure 148

Cadaver donors
  allocation 7–9
  ethics **3–7**
Cancer
  kidney transplantation and 128–9
  *see also* Carcinoma
*Candida albicans*
  following small bowel transplantation 248
  post-operative infection 292
Candida infection 285
  in pancreas transplantation 181
*Candida tropicalis*
  following small bowel transplantation 248
Carcinoma
  of the cervix 300–1
  hepatobiliary 302
  renal 301
  of the uterus 300–1
  of vulva and perineum 300
  *see also under types*
Cardiovascular disease following kidney transplantation 141–2
Case mix measurement 312–13
Cataract formation 195
Catecholamines 25

CD45 77
CD45RA 77
CD45RO 77
Cefuroxime 32
Chickenpox, post-operative infection 287
Children
    biliary atresia in 149
    chronic liver disease as indication for liver
        transplantation 148
    heart transplantation 252–3, *264*
    as liver donors 48
    liver transplant surgical technique 155–6, *156*
    liver transplantation survival in 165
    living related donors 156–7
    post-transplantation malignancy in 303
Cholangiocarcinoma 148
    hilar 150, 152
Cholangiocellular carcinoma 150
Chronic active hepatitis (CAH)
    as indication for liver transplantation 148
Chronic ambulatory peritoneal dialysis (CAPD)
        124–5
Chronic rejection 65
    antibodies and 81
    15-deoxyspergualin (DSG)  and 112
    FK506 and 109
    of heart 265
    of kidney 142, 143
    leflunomide and 102–3
    of liver 160, 163
    of lung *275*
    MMF in reversal of 96, 100
    of pancreas 188
    rapamycin and 104–5
    of small bowel 243
Cigarette smoking, allocation and 9
Cirrhosis, alcohol-related
    allocation and 9
    HLA matching and 54
    liver transplantation and 148
Cirrhosis, primary biliary
    HLA matching and 54
    as indication for liver transplantation 147
    size matching in 49
Clonal expansion 66
Cold ischaemic times (CIT) 59
Colistin 36
Commercialisation of donation 12–13
Complement 69
Computerised tomography (CT) 187
    in assessment for lung transplantation 266–8
Consent for organ donation 3–4

Corneal transplants, HLA matching 54
Coronary angiography 174
Coronary artery disease, allocation and 9
Corticosteroids 90
Cost–benefit analysis 311, 319, 320
Cost effectiveness 309–10
Cost effectiveness analysis 311, 319, 320
Cost minimisation analysis 311, 319, 320
Cost utility analysis 311, 319
Costimulation 74–6
Crigler–Najjar syndrome 150, 11
Cross-matching **71–2**
CTLA-4-Ig 82
Cyclophosphamide 56
Cyclosporin A 19, 90, **91–4**, 100, 131, 139, 160, 193
    effect on HLA matching 54
    in kidney immunosuppression 142
    liver transplant survival and 47
    side effects *93*
    toxicity 139
Cystic fibrosis 152
    allocation and 8
Cytokines 78–80
Cytomegalovirus (CMV) 100, 161, **284–5**
    diagnosis 285
    following small bowel transplantation 246, 247
    in lung transplantation 270, 276–7
    presentation 284–5
    prevention 285
    treatment 285
Cytotoxic T lymphocytes (CTL) 80

Death, definition of 3
Decay accelerating factor (DAF) 83
Delayed hypersensitivity (DTH) 79
Dendritic cells 74
15-Deoxyspergualin (DSG) 110–12
Desmopressin 26
Diabetes insipidus 26
Diabetes mellitus
    age of onset 195
    donation and age 46
    effect of pancreas transplantation on 193–5
    liver donation and 48
    recurrence after pancreas transplantation 188
    Type I (insulin dependent diabetes mellitus;
        IDDM) 167–8, **169–70**, **203–5**
    Type II (non-insulin dependent diabetes
        mellitus; NIDDM) 168, **169–70**, **203–4**
        as contraindication for pancreas
            transplantation 28
        as contraindication for liver transplantation 28

Diabetes mellitus (*cont.*)
  *see also* Pancreas islet cell transplantation; Pancreas transplantation
Diagnosis Related Groups (DRGs) 312–13
Dialysis, allocation and 8–9
Dihydro-orotic acid dehydrogenase (DHODH) 100, 102
Discordant transplantation 83
Distributive justice, theory of 7
Dithiothreitol 55
DNA typing **52–3**
Dobutamine 26
Donor assessment **26–8**
  contraindications 27–8
  exclusion criteria 27
Donor cards 21–2
Donor co-ordinator network (Spain) 21–2
Donor medical management **25–6**
  medical problems 25
Donor retrieval team 30
Donor transplant co-ordinator 22–3
Dopamine 25
Doppler ultrasound 162
Drug abusers, intravenous as donors 27
Duffy blood groups 50
Duplex ultrasound 187

e-selectin 78
Economics of transplantation
  clinical issues **316–18**
    allocation criteria 317–18
    donor-related variables 316–17
    failed grafts and retransplantation 318
    selection criteria 317
  clinical outcomes **312–13**
  correlating clinical and patient outcomes **315–16**
    clinician's approach 315
    health economist approach 315–16
  cost–benefit analysis 311, 319, 320
  cost effectiveness 309–10
  cost effectiveness analysis 311, 319, 320
  cost minimisation analysis 311, 319, 320
  cost utility analysis 311, 319
  costs 308–9
  definitions 310–11
  future direction **322–3**
    accurate costing and measurement of outcomes 323
    new therapeutic options 322
    priority setting 322–3
  models of funding 308–9

outcomes 311–12
pharmacoeconomics **318–22**
  of immunosuppressive agents 320–2
  principles 319–20
quality of life **313–15**
Effector limb of rejection 80–1
Eisenmenger's syndrome 253
Elective ventilation 21
ELISA 55, 80
Emphysema
  allocation and 8
  single lung transplantation (SLT) and 266, 274–5
Endoscopic retrograde cholangiography (ERCP) 161, 162, 163
Endothelium, role in immune responses 78
Enzyme linked immunoabsorbent assay (ELISA) method 55, 80
Epithelioid haemangioendothelioma 150
Epstein–Barr virus (EBV) 264–5, **285–6**
  association with lymphoma 298
  following small bowel transplantation 247
  post-transplant cancer and 295
Ethics, medical
  autonomy 2, 5
  beneficence 2, 5, 10
  duty-based ethics (deontology) 1, 3–4, 5
  justice 2, 5, 7
  primum non nocere 2, 5, 10
  principles **1–3**
  utilitarianism 2, 4, 5, 10
*Eupenicillium brefeldianum* 94
EuroCollins solution 31
Eurotransplants 22
Extravesical ureteroneocystostomy 136

Fas ligand 80
Fatty liver of pregnancy
  as cause of acute fulminant liver failure 149
Femoral artery disease 195
Fine needle aspiration cytology 139
Flow cytometric analysis 71
  cross-matching 56–8, *57*
Frusemide 26
Fungal infection 283, **292–3**
  following small bowel transplantation 247–8
  following liver transplantation 161
  *see also under names*

Gancyclovir 161
Gene sequencing 83–4
Gene transfer techniques 83–4
Gentamycin 32

Glomerular filtration rate 174
Glomerular sclerosis 127
Graft delayed function (GDF) 59
Graft vascular disease (GVD) 100
Graft-versus-host disease 160, 243–4, 247, 249

H-Y antigen 72
Haemochromatosis 151
Haemorrhage
    of liver, post-transplantation 158–9
    variceal, in cirrhosis 151
Healthcare Resource Groups (HRGs) 312–13
Heart transplantation **251–65**
    age matching 47
    chronic rejection 265
    conventional surgical techniques as alternative
        to 278
    contraindications *255*
    effects of long-term immunosuppression 264–5
    grading of cardiac allograft rejection 263, *263*
    heart donor criteria and selection 28, 256–7,
        *256*
    heart implantation 258–60, *259*
    heart–lung implantation 260–1, *261*
    heart recipient assessment and selection 253–6,
        *254*
    heart recipient–donor matching 257
    heart retrieval and preservation 257–8
    hyperacute rejection 263–4
    immunosuppression 262–3
    indications 251–3, *252*
    mechanical bridging prior to 278–9
    mortality 263, *264*
    outcomes and complications 263–5
    paediatric 252–3
    paediatric survival rates *264*
    peri- and postoperative care 261–3
    prognostic indicators in heart failure 253, *254*
    pulmonary vascular resistance measurement
        255
    quality of life 265
    renal function 255–6
    retransplantation 256
    retrieval surgical technique 36
    size matching 49
    xenotransplantation 279
Heart-beating cadaveric retrieval 32–5, *33*, *34*
Heart–lung transplantation
    indications 266
    operative technique **260–1**, *261*
    survival rates 265
Heat shock protein 69

Heparin 37
Hepatic arterial thrombosis (HAT) 162
Hepatitis A as cause of acute fulminant liver failure
        148
Hepatitis B (HBV) 148
    association with hepatomas 302
    as cause of acute fulminant liver failure 148
    kidney transplantation and 128
    post-transplant **288–9**
    post-transplant cancer and 295
Hepatitis C virus 148–9, 151
    kidney transplantation and 128
    post-transplant **289–90**
Hepatitis non-A non-B as cause of acute fulminant
        liver failure 148
Hepatitis, viral
    chronic active 148
    chronic post-transplant 163–4
    as contraindication for organ donation 29
Hepatocellular carcinoma (HCC) 149, 150
    survival rates are liver transplantation 165
Hepatopulmonary syndrome 152
Hepatorenal syndrome 153, 159
Herpes simplex virus **286–7**
    post-transplant cancer and 295
Heterotopic transplantation 63
HIV 72, 73, 84
    as contraindication to kidney transplantation
        128
Human leucocyte antigen (HLA) 50, *51*, 67, 177
    HLA-A, -B and DR antigens 59
    HLA-A2 structure 69–70, *69*
    HLA-B27 structure 69–70
    HLA matching 8, 71
        benefit of 53–4
Human Organ Transplant Act (UK) (1989) 10, 144
Human papilloma virus (HPV) 288
    post-transplant cancer and **295**
Hydroxy-ethyl starch 31
Hyperacute rejection 64
Hyperamylasaemia 191
Hyperfiltration hypothesis **48–9**
Hyperglycaemia 169, 193
    in brain dead patients 26
Hyperlipidaemia following kidney transplantation
        141
Hypertension
    following kidney transplantation 141
    liver donation and 48
Hypoamylasuria 187
Hypoglycaemia 169, 193
Hypotension in brain dead patients 25

ICAM-1 77, 78
IFN-gamma 75, 77, 78, 79
Ig superfamily 76
Immunosuppressive agents
    anti-T cell agents **103–10**
    antipyrimidine agents **100–3**
    conventional, side-effects of *90*
    effect on late graft 91, *91*
    future **113–14**
    influencing purine biosynthesis **94–100**
    inhibiting antigen presentation **110–12**
    mechanism of action *93*
    monoclonal antibodies **112–13**
    pharmacoeconomics of **320–2**
    structures *106*
    *see also under names*
Infection, postoperative, incidence of 283
    bacterial **290–2**
    fungal **292–3**
    parasitic **293–4**
    viral **284–90**
    *see also under names*
Informed consent 11
Inosine monophosphate dehydrogenase (IMPDH)
    94, 96
Integrins 76
Intensive care unit (ICU), donor numbers and 21
Interferons 79
Interleukins
    IL-1 77
    IL-2 66, 78–9, 80
    IL-4 78, 79
    IL-5 79, 81
    IL-6 78, 79 81
    IL-10 78–79
    IL-13 79
Interventional ventilation **4–6**, 16
Intraoperative management **31–2**
Ischaemic heart disease, liver donation and 48
Isoprenaline 26

Kaposi's sarcoma (KS)
    aetiology 299
    incidence 299
    management 299–300
    post-transplant cancer and 295
Kasai operation 149
Kidney transplantation
    age matching 46
        donor 46
        recipient 46
    allocation, HLA matching as criterion for 8

assessment for **126–9**
    age 126–7
    blood transfusion 129
    cancer 128–9
    cause of renal failure 127
    co-morbidity 127
    infection 128
    peripheral vascular disease 128
    polycystic kidney disease 127
    recurring disease 127
    urological 128
    urological abnormalities 127
call-up for **129–31**
    antibiotic prophylaxis 130–1
    deep venous thrombosis prophylaxis (DVT)
        130
    examination 129–30
    history 129
    investigation 130
    prophylaxis against rejection 131
        delayed graft function 131
        procedure 131
        match 131
        rejection 131
cancer following 303
choice of immunosuppression 142–3
cost effectiveness 310
donation by living donors 10
donor selection 29–30
early postoperative phase **137–41**
    delayed graft function 138–41
        drug toxicity 139
        lymphocoele 140–1
        rejection 140
        ureteric leak 139–40
        ureteric obstruction 140
    primary function 137
future 143–4
graft survival 123
living-related donation 40
    donor surgery 40–1
longer-term problems **141–2**
    cardiovascular disease 141–2
    chronic rejection 142
    hyperlipidaemia 141
    hypertension 141
    renal artery stenosis 142
from non-heart beating donor 6–7
removal technique from non-heart-beating
    cadaver 23–5, *24*
retrieval, surgical technique 32–5, *33, 34*
size matching **48–9**

Kidney transplantation (*cont.*)
  surgical preparation of renal failure patient
    **123–6**
    creation of arteriovenous fistula 125–6
    insertion of peritoneal catheter 124–5
    jugular venous catheter 126
  transplant operation **132–7**
    incision 132–3
    preparation of donor kidney 132
    use of ureteric stent 137
    vascular abnormalities 135–7
    vascular anastomosis 134–5
  use of shipped organs 59
Kupfer cells 74

Leadbetter/Politano technique 136
Leflunomide (HWA 486) 100, 101–3
*Leishmania major* 79
Leucocyte adhesion deficiency syndrome (LAD)
    76–77
Leucocyte common antigen 77
*Listeria monocytogenes*, post-transplantation
    infection 291
Live-donor nephrectomy, mortality risk 10–11
Liver eaters 164
Liver failure, chronic, as indication for liver
    transplantation 147–8
Liver transplantation
  advances in operative technique 155–7
  age limit for 47–8
  basic operation **153–5**, *154*
  biliary anastomosis 157
  complications **158–64**
    haemorrhage 159
    immediate 158–9
    renal failure 159
  donation, complications 39
  donor selection 29–30, 153
  early complications after surgery **159–62**
    acute rejection 160
    biliary complications 161–2
    chronic rejection 160
    graft ischaemia 162
    infection 161
  future 165
  immunosuppression **157–8**
  indications **147–50**, *148*
  late complications **163–4**
    biliary 163
    chronic post-transplant hepatitis 163–4
    chronic rejection 163
    malignancy 164

lateral segment grafts 48
living-related donation 39, 40
marginal 48
patient assessment **151–3**
rates 147
recurrence of carcinoma 302
reduced size adult grafts 48, 49, 50
retransplantation 164–5
  indications *164*
retrieval surgical technique 32–5, *33*, *34*, 41
segment donation by living donors 10
size matching 49–50
split-liver grafts 48, 49
survival and quality of life 165
timing of referral 150–1
use of shipped organs 59
Living donor transplantation
  commercialisation and 12–13
  ethics **9–13**
  kidney, rate of 143–4
  non-related 12
Living-related organ donations **39–41**, 42
  complications 39
  donor selection and assessment 39–40
  donor surgery 40–1
    kidney 40–1
    liver 41
  long-term risks 39
  lung 279
  mortality 39
  risks 39
Lung transplantation **265–77**
  bilateral (sequential) lung transplantation
    (BSLT) 265, 273–4
  chronic rejection 277
  contraindications *269*
  immunosuppression 274
  indications 265–6, *267*
  infections 276
  by living donors 10, 11
  living related donation 279
  lung assessment tests *268*
  lung donor criteria and selection 29, 269–70, *270*
  lung recipient assessment and selection 266–9
  lung recipient–donor matching 270–1
  lung reduction surgery as alternative to 279
  lung retrieval and preservation 36, 271–2
  outcomes and complications 275–7
  peri- and postoperative care 274–5
  quality of life 276
  recent advances and controversies 277–9
  rejection grading 275, *275*

Lung transplantation (*cont.*)
  single lung transplantation (SLT) 265–6, 272–3
  size assessment 270
  survival 275–6, *276*
  xenotransplantation 279
Lymphocyte activated killer (LAK) cells 67, 80
Lymphocyte function associated antigen (LFA-1)
      76, 77
Lymphocytotoxic cross-matching **54–5**, 56, 71, 177
  kidney transplant and 130
Lymphoma 113, 297–8
  aetiology 298
  analysis of types *298*
  B cell lymphoma following small bowel trans-
      plantation 249
  following lung transplantation 277
  incidence 297–8
  management 298
Lymphoproliferative disorder, association of EBV
      with 285

Mac-1 76
Macrophages 80
Magnetic resonance imaging 187
Major histocompatibility antigens **67–9**, *68*
  molecular structure 69–71
Malignancy, post-transplant **294–303**
  incidence 303, *304*
  paediatric 303
  pre-existing, effect of immunosuppression on
      302
  prevalence 294
  times of presentation *295*
  treatment 295–6
  types *294*
  viral implication 295
  *see also* Cancer; Carcinoma; Lymphoma
Mannitol 26
Marshall's solution 31
Matching, graft
  age **45–8**
  DNA typing **52–3**
  flow cytometric cross-matching **56–8**
  HLA matching, benefit of 53–4
  local versus imported organ usage 58–9
  lymphocytotoxic cross-matching 54–5, 56
  panel reactivity 55–6
  size 48–50
  tissue typing **50–9**
Medawar, Sir Peter 64–5
Melanoma, malignant 164
  in children 303

Meningitis, meningococcal, organ donation and 28
6-Mercaptopurine (6-MP) 89
Methylprednisolone 131
  in renal transplantation 142
Microchimerism 245
Minor histocompatibility antigens 72
Mizoribine (Bredinin) 94–5
Monoclonal antibodies 51, 71, **112–13**
  OKT3 112, 140, 160, 285
Mononucleosis syndrome 285
Motives, donor 12
MRI cholangiography 162
*Mycobacterium avium-intracellulare* 290
Mycobacterium infection, post-operative **290**
*Mycobacterium kansasii* 290
*Mycobacterium marinum* 290
*Mycobacterium tuberculosis* 290
Mycophenolate mofetil (MMF) (Cellcept) 94,
      **95–100**, 104, 140
  animal studies
  human studies 96–100
  in kidney rejection 140, 143
  mechanism of action 95–6
  rejection *98*, 100
  in renal transplantation 143
  side effects *99*, 100
Mycophenolic acid 96

Natural killer (NK) cells 67, 80
Neomycin 36
Neoral 93, **109–10**
  in renal transplantation 142
  toxic effects 111, *111*
Nocardial infections, post-transplantation **291**
Non-compliance with medication,
      morality of second transplants following 9
Non-heart beating donation **23–5**
  ethics 4, 6–7, 16
  organ removal techniques 23–5
Non-Hodgkin's lymphoma 297
Nottingham Health Profile (NHP) 314
NSAIDs 139

Obesity, pancreas transplantation and 175, 177
Odynophagia 292
Oncostatin M 73
Opt in organ donation policies 22, 41
Opt out organ donation policies 22, 41
Organ donation **20–2**
Organ preservation 31
Organ shortages 1
Organisation of organ retrieval **30–1**

Orthotopic transplantation 63
Oxalosis, primary 150
Oxygen levels 26

p-selectin 78
p150.95 76
Pancreas islet cell transplantation 196
   clinical experience **215–20**
      islet after kidney (IAK) transplants 216–20
      simultaneous islet kidney (SIK) transplants
         216–20
   criteria for donors *205*
   donor operation **205–6**
   future **220–3**
      islet transplants alone (ITA) 221–3
      islet xenotransplantation 223
      pancreas whole organ graft or islet graft
         221
   preparation and quality control **206–11**
      islet isolation and purification 206
      islet number and volume 206–8
      islet purity 208
      islet sterility 210–11
      islet viability and endocrine function 209–10
   rejection of islet cells **211–15**
      gene therapy 214–15
      immunoalteration 212
      immunoisolation (micro- and macroencapsu-
         lation) 212–13
      induction of immunotolerance 211
      prevention of diabetes recurrence 213–14
Pancreas transplantation
   criteria for patient selection 174–5, *174*
   diabetes and 167–70
   diagnosis of rejection **185–91**, *186*
      acute rejection 188
      chronic rejection 188
      complications 188, *189*
      enteric conversion 191
      haematuria and dysuria 190–1
      mortality 189
      pancreatitis 190
      thrombosis 189–90
      urine leak 191
   donor age 176
   donor selection 29, **175–8**
   effect on secondary complications of diabetes
      **193–5**
      macroangiopathy 195
      nephropathy 193
      neuropathy 194–5
      retinopathy 195

future prospects 196
   glucose homestasis 192–3
   histological grading of rejection 188
   immunosuppression 185
   living donors 10
   living related pancreas transplantation 195–6
   pancreas preservation 177–8
   postoperative management **183–5**
      delayed dysfunction 183
      transplant venous thrombosis 184
   recurrence of autoimmune diabetes 188
   recipient categories **170–1**
      kidney transplantation alone (KTA) 170
      pancreas transplantation alone (PTA) 170,
         172
      pancreas transplantation after previous suc-
         cessful kidney transplantation 170, 173–4
      simultaneous pancreas kidney transplantation
         (SPK) 170, 171, 172–3
   recipient surgery **178–83**
      bench to preparation 179–81
      recipient procedure 181–3
      technique 36, 176–7
Panel reactivity 55–6
Paracetamol poisoning
   as cause of acute fulminant liver failure 150
Passenger leucocytes 74
PBC 151
Percutaneous transhepatic cholangiography (PTC)
   162, 163
Perforins 80
Persantin thallium scanning 174
Persistent vegetative state (PVS) 5
Pig, transplantation from 14–15
*Pneumocystis carinii* (PCP) 285
   following small bowel transplantation 248
   post-operative **293**
Polyclonal antibodies 160
Polycystic kidney disease 127
Polycystic nephrectomy 127
Polymerase chain reaction (PCR) 71, 78
Polymerase chain reaction-sequence specific oligo-
   nucleotides (PCR-SSO) 53
Post-reperfusion syndrome 158
Post-transplant lymphoproliferative disease
   (PTLD) 108, 113, 297
   following small bowel transplantation 247
Prednisolone 54, **89–91**, 193
Pregnancy
   fatty liver of, as cause of acute fulminant liver
      failure 148
   HLA antibodies in 55

Preservation injury 159
Primary non-function of liver, post-transplantation
        158–9
Primary sclerosing cholangitis (PSC) 151, 157
    as indication for liver transplantation 148
Pro-fibrotic cytokines 96
Procurement agency 22, 23
Prostitutes as donors 27
*Pseudomonas* in lung transplantation 276
Purine biosynthesis 96, *97*

Quality adjusted life years (QALY) 315–16

Rapamycin (RAPA) **103–5**
Rapid retrieval methods 37–8
Rates of organ donation 201
Rejection mechanism, origin of **65–7**
Restriction fragment length polymorphism (RFLP)
        analysis 53
Retransplantation
    economics 318
    heart 256
    liver 164–5
Rhesus blood groups 50
Rosser Index 315
Roux-en-Y jejunal loop 162, 163

Sarcomata 150
Selectins 76, 77
Self-induced disease, allocation and 9
Serine esterases 80
Shingles, postoperative 287–8
Short Form-36 (SF-36) Health Survey 314
Short gut syndrome 232, 248
Sickness Impact Profile (SIP) 314
Skin cancer 164, **296–7**
    aetiology 296
    factors influencing development *297*
    incidence 296
    management 296–7
Small bowel transplantation
    combined liver/small bowel transplantation
        **238–41**
        donor procedure 238–9, *239*
        recipient procedure 239–41, *240*
    future 249–50
    indications 229, *230*
    investigative techniques **230–2**
        donor selection 231–2
        recipient assessment 230–1
    isolated bowel transplantation **235–7**
        cadaveric donor procedure 235–6

live related donor procedure 236
        recipient procedure 236–7, *237*, *238*
    by living donors 10, 11
    management **232–4**
        non-transplant options 232–4
        transplant options 234
    pathophysiology 241–2
    postoperative complications **246–8**
        immunological 247
        infection 247–8
        motility disorders 247
        technical problems 246–7
    postoperative management **244–8**
        clinical observation 245
        feeding 244
        functional tests 245–6
        graft monitoring 245–6
        immunological assessment 245
        immunosuppression 244–5
        microbiology 246
        radiological imaging 246
    rejection, incidence of 245
    results and recommendations 248–9
    retrieval, surgical technique 36–7
    sequelae 242–4
        effect of denervation 242
        effect of lymphatic interruption 242
        effect on mucosal barrier mechanisms 242
        graft rejection 243
        graft-versus-host disease 243–4
Spanish donor co-ordinator network 21–2
Steroid therapy 131
    organ donation and 28
Success rates 1
Super-urgent exchange scheme 59
Surgical equipment for organ donation 303
Syngeneic transplants 63

T-cell receptor (TCR) 72–3
T helper cells 72
T lymphocytes 72–3, *73*
T-tubes, use in biliary anastomosis 161–2
Tacrolimus (FK506) 100, **105–9**, 131, 139, 140, 160,
        193
    in kidney rejection 140, 143
    in renal transplantation 143
    toxicity 139
TAP1 and TAP2 69
Temperature, brain stem death and 26
6-Thioinosinic acid 89
Thromboelectrogram (TEG) 154
Time trade-off method (TTO) 315

Tissue typing **71–2**
TNF-alpha 69, 77, 78, 113
TNF-beta 69
Tobramycin 36
Tolerance 81–2
Total parenteral nutrition 229–30
    adaptation to 233–4
    failure 232–3
    long-term effects 232
    operative procedures to improve effectiveness of
        233–4
    problems with 233
Transaminase, serum, organ donation and 29
Transjugular intrahepatic portosystemic shunts
        (TIPSS) 151
Transplant Support Service (UK) 22, 23
Tri-iodothyronine (T3) levels after brain death 26
Triple therapy 142–3, 157, 185
Tubulitis 80

Ultrasound 161, 162
University of Wisconsin (UW) solution 31, 36, 37
Urine output 26
Ursodeoxycholic acid 147

Vanishing bile duct syndrome (VBDS) 65, 160,
        163
Varicella zoster virus (VZV) 287–8
Vascular cell adhesion molecule 1 (VCAM-1) 77,
        78
Viral infections, postoperative 284–90
VLA-4 76

Wegener's granulomatosis 127
Welfare maximisation 8
Wilson's disease 151
    as cause of acute fulminant liver failure 148
Xanthine oxidase 90

Xenogeneic transplants *see* Xenotransplantation
Xenotransplantation 42
    concordant 63
    discordant 63
    ethics **13–15**
    heart 279
    immunology 82–4
    kidney 143
    lung 279
    pancreas islet 223